C0-DXE-271

A WORD BOOK IN PATHOLOGY AND LABORATORY MEDICINE

SHEILA B. SLOANE, C.M.T.
Formerly President, Medi-Phone, Inc.
Author, The Medical Word Book

JOHN L. DUSSEAU, M.A.
Vice President and Editor-in-Chief, Retired
W. B. Saunders Company

1984
W. B. SAUNDERS COMPANY
PHILADELPHIA □ LONDON □ TORONTO
MEXICO CITY □ RIO DE JANEIRO □ SYDNEY □ TOKYO

W. B. Saunders Company: West Washington Square
Philadelphia, PA 19105

1 St. Anne's Road
Eastbourne, East Sussex BN21 3UN, England

1 Goldthorne Avenue
Toronto, Ontario M8Z 5T9, Canada

Apartado 26370–Cedro 512
Mexico 4, D.F., Mexico

Rua Coronel Cabrita, 8
Sao Cristovao Caixa Postal 21176
Rio de Janeiro, Brazil

9 Waltham Street
Artarmon, N.S.W. 2064, Australia

Ichibancho, Central Bldg., 22-I Ichibancho
Chiyoda-Ku, Tokyo 102, Japan

Library of Congress Cataloging in Publication Data
Sloane, Sheila B. *N, Paulk*
  A word book in pathology and laboratory medicine.

  1. Pathology–Terminology.   2. Medical technology–Terminology.
I. Dusseau, John L.   II. Title. [DNLM: 1. Pathology–Terminology.
2. Diagnosis, Laboratory–Terminology.   QZ 15 S634w]
RB115.S56   1984   616.07'014   83-20261
ISBN 0-7216-1099-4

A Word Book in Pathology
  and Laboratory Medicine   ISBN   0-7216-1099-4

© 1984 by W. B. Saunders Company. Copyright under the Uniform Copyright Convention. Simultaneously published in Canada. All rights reserved. This book is protected by copyright. No part of it may be reproduced, stored in a retrieval system, or transmitted in any form or by any means, electronic, mechanical, photocopying, recording, or otherwise, without written permission from the publisher. Made in the United States of America. Press of W. B. Saunders Company. Library of Congress catalog card number 83-20261.

Last digit is the print number: 9   8   7   6   5   4   3   2   1

Dedicated
to
our children
Cheryl, Steve, and Donnie
whose achievements and happiness
are our greatest joy

PREFACE

Among the early entries of this book is ABC (absolute basophil count; aspiration-biopsy cytology; axiobuccocervical), and this is an appropriate beginning, for this is essentially an abecedarian work — a primer of vocabulary in pathology and laboratory medicine going progressively through the alphabet in what is inevitably an orderly and hopefully a useful progression.

The preface to any book should answer the question: Why was it written? We believe that the complex and difficult vocabulary of pathology and laboratory medicine needs an accurate and comprehensive listing for use by transcriptionists, medical secretaries, record librarians and laboratory technologists, who often need to find a word and its proper spelling in the context of its relation to other or similar technical terms or to whole phrases. This is why there are, on the pages to follow, many general headings under which are listed appropriate subentries, so that the user, familiar with only part of a complex phrase, will find entry points to its complete form. Logophilia is not a syndrome listed in this book; but it is a common condition in medicine — the love of words, especially new and polysyllabic ones. Hence perhaps even the working pathologist may find useful this workaday vocabulary of the discipline, for medical terms (and their ingenious abbreviations) are in number almost beyond computation and in their Greek and Latin roots often beyond comprehension. For the latter we have added plurals to those entries whose plural is often more singular than its singular form.

Therefore, this listing must be both accurate and current. To this purpose we have used many reference sources; but seven of them stand out as splendid in their scholarship and authority. They are

> Bennington: Saunders Dictionary and Encyclopedia of Laboratory Medicine and Technology. Saunders, 1984.
>
> Dorland's Illustrated Medical Dictionary, 26th Edition. Saunders, 1981.
>
> Robbins & Cotran: Pathologic Basis of Disease, 2nd Edition. Saunders, 1979.
>
> Stedman's Medical Dictionary, 24th Edition. Williams & Wilkins, 1982.
>
> Systematized Nomenclature of Pathology. The American College of Pathology, 1969.
>
> Tietz: Clinical Guide to Laboratory Tests. Saunders, 1983.
>
> Williams: Textbook of Endocrinology, 6th Edition. Saunders, 1981.

It is not to gainsay the accuracy of these works to observe that in details of terminology they sometimes differ from one another. Therefore this book had to become something more than compilation. Its putting-together frequently called for judgment and knowledge beyond the capacity of its authors, so that the Saunders editorial staff was often called upon for help, and this was always readily forthcoming, especially from Wynette Kommer and Baxter Venable. If errors remain, they are those of our own commission. Whatever their number, it would have been significantly greater without the help we herewith gratefully acknowledge. We also appreciate the role of the American Association for Medical Transcription, whose seminars and publications have been valuable to us and whose leaders and members have done so much to insure high standards of proficiency in a demanding and difficult profession.

We may also say of this book that it could easily enough have been twice its size and might, with some labor, have been reduced to half its size. We hope that we have followed the ancient advice of Pythagoras — moderation in all things is excellent — and have

PREFACE vii

achieved that happy course midway between superfluity and insufficiency.

Nowhere was the question of proper detail more troublesome than in the issue of how anatomy was to be treated. From Morgagni on, pathology has had its foundation in knowledge of human structure, so we make no apology for an abundance of anatomical terms. Further, we have not hesitated to include relatively simple terms whose spelling poses no problem to anyone, because such words round out the dimensions and define the scope of our subject. Similarly, the pages to follow are generously seasoned with abbreviations and eponyms, because the former are an international language of medicine and the latter are a puzzle in orthography.

We conclude by saying that one of the authors of this book has already fashioned for Saunders a Medical Word Book that has proved useful to its audience. It is our simple wish that this companion volume too will serve its purpose and its users well. Its last entry is Z.Z.'Z". (increasing degrees of contraction). This has a suspiciously soporific look; so we shall hope that we have succeeded in judicious contraction, vigilant selection of terms, and wakeful reading of proof.

SHEILA B. SLOANE
JOHN L. DUSSEAU

CONTENTS

PART I
THE VOCABULARY 1

PART II
APPENDICES

Appendix 1
NORMAL LABORATORY VALUES 546

Appendix 2
EPONYMIC DISEASES AND SYNDROMES.............. 569

Appendix 3
CULTURE MEDIA................................ 584

Appendix 4
TABLE OF ELEMENTS........................... 587

Appendix 5
TABLES OF WEIGHTS AND MEASURES 589

x CONTENTS

Appendix 6
COMBINING FORMS IN MEDICAL TERMINOLOGY 597

Appendix 7
RULES FOR FORMING PLURALS. 606

Appendix 8
SYMBOLS AND PREFIXES 608

PART I
THE VOCABULARY

A

A — absolute temperature
　　absorbance
　　acetum
　　ampere
　　Angström unit
　　anode
　　anterior
　　artery
　　atropine
　　axial
　　mass number
　　total acidity
A. — *Actinomyces*
　　Anopheles
A_2 — aortic second sound
a or A — ampere
　　anode
AA — acetic acid
　　alveolar-arterial
　　aminoacetone
　　arachidonic acid
　　ascending aorta
　　atomic absorption
$\overline{AA}$ or $\overline{aa}$ — of each (ana)
aa — arteries
AAA — abdominal aortic
　　aneurysm
　　amalgam

AAA *(continued)*
　　androgenic anabolic
　　agent
AAAS — American Association
　　for the Advancement of Science
AAC — antibiotic-associated
　　pseudomembranous
　　colitis
AACC — American Association
　　for Clinical
　　Chemistry
AACIA — American Association for Clinical
　　Immunology and
　　Allergy
AAI — American Association
　　of Immunologists
AAM — American Academy of
　　Microbiology
AAMI — Association for the
　　Advancement of
　　Medical Instrumentation
AAN — American Association
　　of Neuropathologists
AAP — American Association
　　of Pathologists

4 AAPA – ABERRATION

AAPA – American Association of Pathologist Assistants
AAPB – American Association of Pathologists and Bacteriologists
AAR – antigen-antiglobulin reaction
AAS – aortic arch syndrome
    atomic absorption spectrophotometry
AAT – alpha-antitrypsin
AAV – adeno-associated virus
AB – abnormal
    abortion
    alcian blue
    asbestos body
    asthmatic bronchitis
    axiobuccal
A/B – acid-base ratio
Ab – antibody
ABA – antibacterial activity
abacterial
A band
abasia
    a. astasia
    a. atactica
    choreic a.
    paralytic a.
    paroxysmal trepidant a.
    spastic a.
    a. trepidans
abatement
Abbe's condenser
ABC – absolute basophil count
    American Blood Commission
    aspiration-biopsy cytology
    axiobuccocervical
ABD, Abd or abd – abdomen
    abdominal
ABDOM, Abdom or abdom – abdomen
    abdominal
abdomen
abdominal
    a. aorta
    a. esophagus
    a. inguinal ring
    a. lymph node
    a. reflex
    a. viscera
    a. wall
abducens
    a. nerve
    a. nucleus
abducent
    a. nerve
abductor
    a. digiti minimi muscle
    a. longi and extensor brevis pollicis muscle
    a. pollicis muscle
ABE – acute bacterial endocarditis
aberrant
    a. ductule
    a. pancreas
    a. renal vessels
    a. tissue
aberration
    chromatic a.
    chromosome a.
    dioptric a.
    distantial a.
    heterosomal a.
    homosomal a.
    meridional a.
    newtonian a.
    penta-X chromosomal a.
    spherical a.
    tetra-X chromosomal a.
    triple-X chromosomal a.

abetalipoproteinemia
ABG — axiobuccogingival
abiotrophy
ABL — abetalipoproteinemia
    axiobuccolingual
ablastin
ablatio
    a. placentae
    a. retinae
ABLB — alternate binaural
    loudness balance
ablepharon
ABN, Abn or abn — abnormal
abnormal
    a. chorion
    a. chorionic villi
    a. endochondral ossification
abnormality
    bone marrow a.
    cytologic a.
    fetal a.
    morphologic a.
    traumatic a.
ABO
    antibodies
    antigens
    blood groups
    compatibility
    incompatibility
    typing
ABO-Rh typing
aborted
    a. ectopic pregnancy
abortion
    afebrile a.
    ampullar a.
    artificial a.
    cervical a.
    complete a.
    contagious a.
    criminal a.
    habitual a.

abortion *(continued)*
    imminent a.
    incomplete a.
    induced a.
    inevitable a.
    infected a.
    justifiable a.
    missed a.
    septic a.
    spontaneous a.
    therapeutic a.
    threatened a.
    tubal a.
abortive
    a. infection
abortus
    a. fever
ABP — arterial blood pressure
Abrams' test
abrasion
abrin
abruptio placentae
ABS — alkylbenzene sulfonate
abscess
    acute a.
    alveolar a.
    amebic a.
    apical a.
    Bartholin's a.
    Brodie's a.
    cerebral a.
    chronic a.
    epidural a.
    Kogoj's a.
    Monro's a.
    perinephric a.
    subdiaphragmatic a.
    subhepatic a.
    tubo-ovarian a.
abscissa
absence
    acquired a.

absence *(continued)*
   congenital a.
Absidia
   A. corymbifera
   A. ramosa
absolute
   a. alcohol
   a. eosinophil count
   a. temperature
   a. valve
   a. zero
absorb
absorbefacient
absorbency
   a. index
absorbent
absorption
   a. cavities
   a. cell
   a. coefficient
   a. constant
   a. of erythrocyte antibodies
   fat a.
   iron a.
   a. peak
   a. spectrum
abstinence
   alimentary a.
AC — acromioclavicular
   adrenal cortex
   air conduction
   anodal closure
   anterior chamber
   anticoagulant
   anticomplementary
   anti-inflammatory
     corticoid
   aortic closure
   atriocarotid
   auriculocarotid
   axiocervical
Ac — actinium

ac — acute
ACA — adenocarcinoma
acacia
acanthamebiasis
Acanthamoeba
   A. castellani
   A. hartmannella
acanthion
Acanthobdella
Acanthocephala
Acanthocheilonema
   A. perstans
   A. streptocerca
acanthocyte
acanthocytosis
acanthoid cell
acantholysis
acanthoma
   a. adenoides cysticum
   basal cell a.
   a. verrucosa seborrheica
acanthorrhexis
acanthosis
   a. nigricans
acapnia
acardiacus
acardius
acariasis
acaricide
Acaridae
Acarus
   A. folliculorum
   A. gallinae
   A. hordei
   A. rhyzoglypticus hyacinthi
   A. scabiei
   A. siro
acaryote
acatalasia
Acaulium
ACC — adenoid cystic
     carcinoma

ACC *(continued)*
    anodal closure contraction
accelerant
accelerated idioventricular rhythm
acceleration
    growth a.
    negative a.
accelerator
    a. globulin
    serum prothrombin conversion a.
    serum thrombotic a.
    a. urinae
accelerin
acceptor
    hydrogen a.
    oxygen a.
accessory
    a. adrenal cortex
    a. atrium
    a. breast
    a. cells
    a. nasal sinus
    a. nerve
    a. nucleus cuneatus
    a. obturator nerve
    a. pancreas
    a. pancreatic duct
    a. paraflocculus
    a. parotid gland
    a. saphenous vein
    a. sinus
    a. spleen
    a. structure
access time
accident
    cerebrovascular a.
ACCL — anodal closure clonus
acclimation
accommodation

accumulation(s)
    a. of carbohydrates
    a. of complex lipids
    a. of glycogen
    intracellular a.
    a. of pigments
    a. of protein
ACD — absolute cardiac dullness
    acid-citrate-dextrose
    anterior chest diameter
ACE — adrenocortical extract
A cell
acellular
acenocoumarin
acentric
acephalous
acephalus
    a. dibrachius
    a. dipus
    a. monobrachius
    a. monopus
    a. paracephalus
    a. sympus
acervulus (acervuli)
acetabulum (acetabula)
acetal
acetaldehydase
acetaldehyde
acetamide
acetaminophen
    a. hepatic toxicity
acetanilid
acetarsone
acetate
acetazolamide
Acetest
acetic
    a. acid
    a. anhydride
    a. naphthalene
    a. orcein

acetohydroxamic acid (urease inhibitor) [handwritten annotation]

8 ACETOACETIC ACID – ACHARD-THIERS SYNDROME

acetoacetic acid
acetoacetyl-coenzyme A
    a.-CoA reductase
    a.-CoA thiolase
acetoacetylglutathione hydrolase
acetoacetylhydrolipoate hydrolase
acetoarsenite
Acetobacter
    A. aceti
    A. melanogenus
    A. oxydans
    A. rancens
    A. roseus
    A. suboxydans
    A. xylinum
aceto-carmine
acetohexamide
acetoin
    a. dehydrogenase
acetol kinase
acetolysis
acetone
acetonemia
acetonitrile
acetonuria
acetophenazine
acetophenetidin
acetrizoate
acetyl
    a. chloride
    a. peroxide
    a. sulfisoxazole
acetylaminodeoxyglucosephosphate isomerase
acetylaminodeoxyglucose phosphomutase
beta-acetylaminodeoxyglucosidase
acetylaspartic acid

acetylation
acetylcarbromal
acetylcholine
acetylcholinesterase
acetyl-coenzyme A
    a.-CoA acetyltransferase
    a.-CoA acyltransferase
    a.-CoA carboxylase
    a.-CoA hydrolase
    a.-CoA synthetase
acetylcysteine
acetyldigitoxin
acetylene
    a. dichloride
    a. tetrachloride
    a. trichloride
acetylesterase
acetylgalactosamine
acetylgalactosaminidase
acetylglucosamine
N-acetyl-β-D-glucosaminidase
acetylmannosamine
acetylmethadol
acetylmethylcarbinol
acetylmuramic acid
N-acetylneuraminate lyase
N-acetylprocainamide
acetylsalicylic acid
acetylserotonin methyltransferase
ACG – apexcardiogram
AcG – accelerator globulin
ACH – adrenocortical hormone
ACh – acetylcholine
achalasia
    biliary a.
    esophageal a.
    pelvirectal a.
    sphincteral a.
Achard-Thiers syndrome

AChE — acetylcholinesterase
Achilles
    reflex
    tendon
achlorhydria
Acholeplasma laidlawii
Acholeplasmataceae
acholic
acholuria
achondroplasia
achondroplastic
    a. dwarf
Achorion
    A. schoenleini
    A. violaceum
achroacyte
achromasia
achromate
achromatic
    a. lens
    a. spindle
achromatophil
achromia
    congenital a.
    cortical a.
    a. parasitica
    a. unguium
Achromobacter
Achromobacteraceae
achromocyte
achromophil
Achucárro's stain
achylia
acid
    acetoacetic a.
    acetylsalicylic a.
    amino a.
    aminobenzoic a.
    aminocaproic a.
    aminoglutaric a.
    aminoisobutyric a.

acid *(continued)*
    aminolevulinic a.
    aminosuccinic a.
    a. anhydride
    argininosuccinic a.
    ascorbic a.
    Brönsted-Lowry a.
    chloranilic a.
    chlorophenoxyacetic a.
    a.-citrate-dextrose
    deoxyribonucleic a.
    diacetic a.
    ethacrynic a.
    folic a.
    a. formaldehyde hematin
    formiminoglutamic a.
    glucuronic a.
    glutamic a.
    a. glycoprotein
    a. halide
    a. hematin
    hippuric a.
    homogentisic a.
    homovanillic a.
    hydrochloric a.
    a. hydrolases
    5-hydroxyindoleacetic a.
    lactic a.
    nalidixic a.
    a. orcein
    phenylpyruvic a.
    a. phosphatase
    pyruvic a.
    ribonucleic a.
    teichoic a.
    tricarboxylic a.
    trichloroacetic a.
    uric a.
    valproic a.
    vanillylmandelic a.
    xanthurenic a.

Acidaminococcus
   A. fermentans
acid-base
   a.-b. balance
   a.-b. indicator
   a.-b. nomogram
acidemia
acid-fast
   a.-f. bacilli
   a.-f. stain
acidifiable
acidified serum test
acidifier
acidify
acidimetry
acidity
acidocyte
acidocytopenia
acidocytosis
acidogenic
acidophil
   alpha a.
   a. cell
   epsilon a.
acidophilic
   a. normoblast
acidosis
   metabolic a.
   respiratory a.
acid phosphatase
acid-Schiff stain
acid-secretion rate
aciduria
   acetoacetic a.
   beta-aminoisobutyric a.
   argininosuccinic a.
   methylmalonic a.
   orotic a.
   pyroglutamic a.
aciduric
acinar
   a. cell carcinoma

acinar *(continued)*
   a. cell tumor
   a. development
Acinetobacter
   A. anitratus
   A. calcoaceticus
   A. parapertussis
   A. lwoffi
acini
acinic
   a. cell adenocarcinoma
   a. cell tumor
aciniform
acinotubular
acinus (acini)
   liver a.
ACl — aspiryl chloride
ACLA — American Clinical Laboratory Association
Acladium
aclasis
   diaphyseal a.
   tarsoepiphyseal a.
ACLPS — Academy of Clinical Laboratory Physicians and Scientists
ACM — albumin-calcium-magnesium
acne
   a. atrophica
   a. conglobata
   a. rosacea
   a. vulgaris
acneiform
aconitase
aconitate hydratase
aconitine
aconitrate dehydrogenase
acoustic
   a. nerve
   a. neuroma

ACP — acid phosphatase
    acyl-carrier protein
    American College of
      Pathologists
    anodal-closing picture
    aspirin, caffeine, phena-
      cetin
acquired
    a. character
    a. hemolytic anemia
    a. immune deficiency syn-
      drome
acrania
Acremonium
acridine
acriflavine
acroanesthesia
acrocentric
acrocephalosyndactyly
acrocephaly
acrochordon
acrocyanosis
acrodermatitis
    a. chronica atrophicans
    a. continua
    a. perstans
acrodynia
acrokeratosis
    a. verruciformis
acrolein
    a. phenylhydrazine
acromegaly
acromioclavicular
acromion
acropachy
acropachyderma
acroparesthesia
acroscleroderma
acrosclerosis
acrosomal
    a. granule
    a. vesicle

acrosome
    a. reaction
acrospiroma
Acrotheca pedrosoi
Acrothesium floccosum
acrylamide
acrylonitrile
ACS — American Cancer
      Society
    American Chemical
      Society
    American Society of
      Cytology
    anodal-closing sound
    antireticular cytotoxic
      serum
    Association of Clinical
      Scientists
ACSV — aortocoronary
      saphenous vein
ACT — activated coagulation
      time
    anticoagulant therapy
ACTe — anodal-closure tetanus
ACTH — adrenocorticotropic
      hormone
ACTH test
actin
actinic
    a. keratosis
actinide
actinium
Actinobacillus
    A. actinomycetemcomitans
    A. lignieresii
    A. mallei
    A. pseudomallei
actinochemistry
Actinomadura
    A. madurae
    A. pelletierii
Actinomyces

Actinomyces (continued)
   A. bovis
   A. congolensis
   A. eriksonii
   A. israelii
   A. muris
   A. muris-ratti
   A. naeslundii
   A. necrophorus
   A. odontolyticus
   A. rhusiopathiae
   A. vinaceus
   A. viscosus
actinomyces
Actinomycetaceae
Actinomycetales
actinomycete
actinomycetes
actinomycetic
actinomycetoma
actinomycin
actinomycosis
actinomycotic
   a. mycetoma
actinophage
Actinoplanaceae
Actinoplanes
Actinopoda
action
   ball-valve a.
   buffer a.
   calorigenic a.
   capillary a.
   cumulative a.
   diastasic a.
   diastatic a.
   opsonic a.
   reflex a.
   specific dynamic a.
   tampon a.
   thermogenic a.
   trigger a.

action *(continued)*
   vitaminoid a.
action potential
   biphasic a. p.
   cardiac a. p.
   compound muscle a. p.
   compound nerve a. p.
   monophasic a. p.
   muscle a. p.
   polyphasic a. p.
   serrated a. p.
activated
   a. coagulation time
   a. partial thromboplastin time
activation
   lymphocyte a.
   ovum a.
   photometrazol a.
   plasma a.
actomyosin
Actonia
ACTP – adrenocorticotropic polypeptide
acute
   a. cardiovascular disease
   a. inflammation
   a. interstitial nephritides
   a. lymphocytic leukemia
   a. mastitis
   a. monocytic (monoblastic) leukemia
   a. myelocytic leukemia
   a. myelomonocytic leukemia
   a. promyelocytic leukemia
   a. pyelonephritis
   a. renal failure
   a. splenitis
   a. tubular necrosis
   a. undifferentiated leukemia

ACVD — acute cardiovascular
    disease
acycloguanosine
acyclovir
acyesis
acyl
    a. halide
    a. peroxide
acylation
acylcarnitine
acylcholine acylhydrolase
acyl-coenzyme A
    a. CoA dehydrogenase
    a. CoA synthetase
acylphosphatase
acylsphingosine
    a. deacylase
acyltransferase
AD — Aleutian disease
    anodal duration
    average deviation
    axiodistal
    axis deviation
A & D — ascending and
    descending
ADA — adenosine deaminase
    anterior descending
    artery
adactyly
adamantanamine
adamantinoma
adamantoblast
Adamkiewicz's test
adamsite
Adams-Stokes disease
adaptation
    cellular a.
    color a.
    dark a.
    enzymatic a.
    genetic a.
    light a.
    phenotypic a.

adaptation *(continued)*
    photopic a.
    retinal a.
    scotopic a.
adaptive
    a. enzyme
ADC — anodal-duration
    contraction
    average daily census
    axiodistocervical
ADCC — antibody-dependent
    cell-mediated
    cytotoxicity
addict
addiction
    alcohol a.
    drug a.
Addis count
addissonian crisis
addisonism
Addison's
    anemia
    disease
    keloid
additive
adductor
    a. brevis muscle
    a. canal
    a. hallucis muscle
    a. longus muscle
    a. magnus muscle
    a. pollicis muscle
Adelomycetes
ADEM — acute disseminated
    encephalomyelitis
adenasthenia
adendritic
adenine
    a. arabinoside
    a. deaminase
    a. hypoxanthine
    a. phosphoribosyltrans-
    ferase

adenitis
- acute epidemic infectious a.
- acute salivary a.
- cervical a.
- mesenteric a.
- phlegmonous a.
- a. tropicalis

adenoameloblastoma
adenocanthoma
adenocarcinoma
- acinic cell a.
- alveolar a.
- anaplastic a.
- bronchiolar a.
- clear cell a.
- colloid a.
- follicular a.
- gelatinous a.
- Hürthle cell a.
- infiltrating duct a.
- inflammatory a.
- a. in-situ
- lobular a.
- medullary a.
- mesonephric a.
- mucinous a.
- papillary a.
- sebaceous a.
- signet ring a.
- sweat gland a.
- trabecular a.
- undifferentiated a.

adenocystic carcinoma
adenofibroma
adenofibrosis
adenohypophysis
adenoid
- a. cystic carcinoma
- a. facies

adenoiditis
adenolymphoma

adenoma
- acidophilic a.
- adnexal a.
- adrenal cortical a.
- adrenocortical a.
- apocrine a.
- basophilic a.
- bile duct a.
- bronchial a.
- ceruminous a.
- chief cell a.
- chromophobe a.
- clear cell a.
- colloid a.
- embryonal a.
- eosinophil a.
- fetal a.
- follicular a.
- Hürthle cell a.
- islet cell a.
- liver cell a.
- macrofollicular a.
- malignant a.
- microfollicular a.
- oncocytic a.
- oxyphil a.
- papillary a.
- Pick's tubular a.
- polypoid a.
- sebaceous a.
- sweat gland a.
- trabecular a.
- tubular a.
- villous a.

adenomatoid
adenomatosis
- fibrosing a.
- pulmonary a.

adenomatous
- a. goiter
- a. hyperplasia

adenomatous *(continued)*
   a. polyp
adenomyoma
adenomyosarcoma
adenomyosis
adenopathy
adenosarcoma
adenosine
   a. 3', 5'-cyclic phosphate
   a. deaminase
   a. diphosphate
   a. kinase
   a. monophosphate
   a. phosphorylase
   a. triphosphatase, calcium-activated
   a. triphosphatase, magnesium-activated
   a. triphosphate pyrophosphohydrolase
adenosinediphosphate deaminase
adenosinetriphosphatase
adenosis
   blunt duct a.
   fibrosing a.
   sclerosing a.
   vaginal a.
adenosquamous carcinoma
adenosylhomocysteinase
adenovirus
adenyl
   a. cyclase
adenylate
   a. cyclase
   a. kinase
adenylic acid
adenylosuccinase
adenylosuccinate
   a. lyase
adenylpyrophosphatase
adenylyl
adenylylation
adenylylsulfate kinase
ADG — atrial diastolic gallop
        axiodistogingival
ADH — alcohol dehydrogenase
        antidiuretic hormone
ADH deficiency
adherence
   immune a.
adherent
   a. pericarditis
adhesion
   amniotic a.
   fibrinous a.
   fibrous a.
   sublabial a.
adhesive
   a. chronic pachymeningitis
   a. pericarditis
ADI — axiodistoincisal
adiadochokinesia
adiaspiromycosis
Adie's
   pupil
   syndrome
adiphenine hydrochloride
adipic
adipocere
adipocyte
adipokinesis
adipolysis
adiponecrosis
adipose tissue
adiposis
   a. cerebralis
   a. dolorosa
   a. hepatica
   a. tuberosa simplex
   a. universalis
adiposity
adiposogenital dystrophy
aditus (aditi)

adjuvant
    Freund's a.
    mycobacterial a.
Adler's test
adnexa
    a. oculi
    a. uteri
adnexal
    a. adenoma
    a. carcinoma
ADO — axiodisto-occlusal
adonidine
adoral
ADP — adenosine diphosphate
adrenal
    a. artery
    a. capsule
    a. cortex
    a. cortical adenoma
    a. cortical carcinoma
    a. cortical hyperplasia
    a. crisis
    a. feminizing syndrome
    a. function test
    a. gland
    a. gland virilizing syndrome
    a. insufficiency
    a. medulla
    a. rests
    a. scan
    a. vein
Adrenalin
adrenaline
adrenarche
    delayed a.
    precocious a.
adrenergic
adrenochrome
adrenocortical
    a. insufficiency
    a. rest
adrenocorticosteroid
adrenocorticotropic
    a. cell
    a. hormone
    a. hormone stimulation test
adrenocorticotropin
adrenodoxin
adrenogenital syndrome
adrenoreceptor
ADS — antibody deficiency syndrome
    antidiuretic substance
adsorb
adsorbate
adsorption
    agglutinin a.
ADT — adenosine triphosphate
adult
    a. cystic teratoma
    a. hemoglobin
adulteration
adulthood
adventitia tunica
adventitious
adynamia
    hereditary a.
adynamic ileus
AE — antitoxineinheit (antitoxin unit)
Aedes
    A. aegypti
    A. albopictus
    A. cinereus
    A. flavescens
    A. leucocelaenus
    A. scutellaris pseudoscutellaris
    A. sollicitans
    A. spencerii
    A. taeniorhynchus
AEG — air encephalogram
AEM — analytical electron microscope

AEP — average evoked potential
AEq — age equivalent
AER — aldosterone excretion rate
    auditory evoked response
    average evoked response
aerated
aeration
Aerobacter
    A. aerogenes
    A. cloacae
    A. lipolyticus
    A. liquefaciens
    A. subgroup A, B, C
aerobe
aerobia
aerobian
aerobic
    a. diphtheroids
aerobiosis
aerobiotic
Aerococcus
    A. viridans
aeroembolism
aerogenic
aerogenous
Aeromonas
    A. hydrophila
    A. liquefaciens
    A. punctata
    A. salmonicida
    A. shigelloides
aeropathy
aerophagia
aerophilic
aerosol
aerotaxis
aerotitis media
aerotolerant
aerotropism
AET — absorption-equivalent thickness
AF — acid-fast
    aldehyde fuchsin
    amniotic fluid
    antibody-forming
    aortic flow
    atrial fibrillation
    atrial flutter
AFB — acid-fast bacilli
AFC — antibody-forming cells
afebrile
affective
afferent
    a. arteriole
    a. lymph node
affinity
AFIB — atrial fibrillation
afibrinogenemia
AFIP — Armed Forces Institute of Pathology
AFL — atrial flutter
aflatoxin
AFP — alphafetoprotein
    anterior faucial pillar
African
    A. sleeping sickness
    A. tick borne fever
aftergilding
AG — antiglobulin
    atrial gallop
    axiogingival
A/G — albumin-globulin ratio
Ag — silver
AGA — appropriate for gestational age
agammaglobulinemia
    Bruton's a.
    Swiss-type a.
Agamodistomum
    A. ophthalmobium

AGAMONEMA – AGGLUTINATION

Agamonema
Agamonematodum migrans
aganglionosis
agar
  bile-esculin a.
  bird seed a.
  bismuth sulfite a.
  blood a.
  Bordet-Gengou a.
  brain-heart infusion a.
  brilliant green a.
  chocolate a.
  Christensen's urea a.
  citrate a.
  Columbia blood a.
  corn meal a.
  cystine trypticase a.
  Czapek-Dox a.
  deoxyribonuclease a.
  DNase a.
  egg-yolk a.
  EMB a.
  eosin-methylene blue a.
  Hektoen a.
  inhibitory mold a.
  lysine iron a.
  MacConkey a.
  Martin-Lester a.
  Middlebrook's a.
  Mueller-Hinton a.
  mycobiotic a.
  nitrate a.
  nutrient a.
  phenylalanine a.
  phenylethyl alcohol a.
  potato dextrose a.
  rabbit blood a.
  Sabhi a.
  Sabouraud's dextrose a.
  Salmonella-Shigella a.
  Schaedler blood a.
  sheep-blood a.

agar *(continued)*
  Simmons' citrate a.
  Thayer-Martin a.
  thistle seed a.
  Trichophyton a.
  triple sugar iron a.
  tryptic soy a.
  urea a.
  Wilkins-Chilgren a.
  xylose-lysine-deoxycholate a.
Agarbacterium
agarose
agenesis
agent
  activating a.
  adrenergic blocking a.
  adrenergic neuron blocking a.
  alkylating a.
  caudalizing a.
  chelating a.
  cholinergic blocking a.
  Eaton a.
  ganglionic blocking a.
  Gordon's a.
  levigating a.
  Marburg a.
  Marcy a.
  Norwalk a.
  A. Orange
  progestational a's
  reducing a.
  transforming a.
  vacuolating a.
  virus inactivating a.
  wetting a's
AGG – agammaglobulinemia
agglutination
  acid a.
  bacteriogenic a.
  cold a.

AGGLUTINATION – AGYRIA

agglutination *(continued)*
  H a.
  intravascular a.
  latex a.
  macroscopic a.
  mediate a.
  microscopic a.
  O a.
  platelet a.
  salt a.
  spontaneous a.
  T-a.
  Vi a.
agglutinator
agglutinin
  alpha a.
  anti-Rh a.
  beta a.
  chief a.
  cold a.
  febrile a.
  flagellar a.
  group a.
  H a.
  haupt-a.
  immune a.
  latex a.
  leukocyte a.
  Mg a.
  O a.
  platelet a.
  Rh a.
  somatic a.
  warm a.
agglutinogen
aggregate
  cytoplasmic a.
  nuclear a.
aggregation
aging
agitation

AGL – acute granulocytic leukemia
       aminoglutethimide
aglobulia
aglobuliosis
aglobulism
aglutition
aglycemia
aglycogenosis
aglycone
AGN – acute glomerulonephritis
agnathus
agnocobalamin
agnogenic
  a. myeloid metaplasia
agnosia
agonadal
agonadism
agonal
agonist
agoraphobia
agranular endoplasmic reticulum
agranulocyte
agranulocytic angina
agranulocytosis
agranuloplasia
agranuloplastic
agraphia
A/G ratio test – albumin-globulin ratio test
Agrobacterium
AGS – adrenogenital syndrome
AGT – antiglobulin test
AGTT – abnormal glucose tolerance test
ague
AGV – aniline gentian violet
agyria

AH – AKARYOCYTE

AH – acetohexamide
   amenorrhea and hirsutism
   aminohippurate
   antihyaluronidase
   arterial hypertension
   hypermetropic astigmatism
AHA – acquired hemolytic anemia
   autoimmune hemolytic anemia
ahaptoglobinemia
AHD – arteriosclerotic heart disease
   atherosclerotic heart disease
A hemoglobin
AHF – antihemophilic factor
AHG – antihemophilic globulin
   antihuman globulin
AHH – arylhydrocarbon hydroxylase
   alpha-hydrazine analog of histidine
AHLE – acute hemorrhagic leukoencephalitis
AHLS – antihuman lymphocyte serum
AHP – air at high pressure
AHT – antihyaluronidase titer
   augmented histamine test
AI – angiotensin I
   aortic incompetence
   aortic insufficiency
   apical impulse
   axioincisal
AIBA – aminoisobutyric acid
AIC – aminoimidazole carboxamide
AID – acute infectious disease
AIDS – acquired immune deficiency syndrome
AIEP – amount of insulin extractable from the pancreas
AIH – artificial insemination, homologous
AIHA – autoimmune hemolytic anemia
AIN – acute interstitial nephritides
ainhum
AIO – amyloid of immunoglobulin origin
AIP – acute intermittent porphyria
   automated immunoprecipitation
   average intravascular pressure
air
   alveolar a.
   a. embolus
   a. foil
   liquid a.
   a. monitor
   residual a.
   venous alveolar a.
airway
   oropharyngeal a.
   a. resistance
AITT – arginine insulin tolerance test
AIU – absolute iodine uptake
AIVR – accelerated idioventricular rhythm
AJCCS – American Joint Committee on Cancer Staging
Ajellomyces
   A. dermatitidis
akaryocyte

akathisia
Akeridae
akinesia
akinetic
AL — albumin
    axiolingual
Al — aluminum
ALA — aminolevulinic acid
    axiolabial
ala (alae)
    a. auris
    a. nasi
ALAD — abnormal left axis deviation
    aminolevulinic acid dehydrase
ALAG — axiolabiogingival
ALAL — axiolabiolingual
alamecin
alangine
alanine
    a. aminotransferase
    a. dehydrogenase
    a.-glutamate transaminase
    a.-ketoacid aminotransferase
    a.-ketoglutarate transaminase
    a.-oxoglutarate aminotransferase
    a. transaminase
alaninemia
alaninuria
alanyl-RNA synthetase
alastrim
alb — albumin
Albers-Schönberg disease
albinism
albino
Albright's
    disease
    syndrome

albumin
    a. A
    acetosoluble a.
    acid a.
    aggregated a.
    alkali a.
    Bence Jones a.
    caseiniform a.
    chromated serum a.
    coagulated a.
    derived a.
    a./globulin (A/G) ratio
    hematin a.
    iodinated serum a.
    macroaggregated a.
    a. microspheres
    normal human serum a.
    Patein's a.
    radio-iodinated serum a.
    serum a.
    a. suspension test
    a. tannate
    triphenyl a.
albuminocytological
albuminoid
albuminous
albuminuria
    march a.
    orthostatic a.
albumosuria
    Bence Jones a.
    Bradshaw's a.
    enterogenic a.
    pyogenic a.
ALC — approximate lethal concentration
    axiolinguocervical
Alcaligenes
    A. bookeri
    A. bronchosepticus
    A. denitrificans
    A. faecalis

Alcaligenes (continued)
   A. marshallii
   A. metalcaligenes
   A. odorans
   A. recti
   A. viscolactis
alcaptonuria
alcohol
   alkyl a.
   amyl a.
   benzyl a.
   butyl a.
   caprylic a.
   a. dehydrogenase
   diacetone a.
   ethyl a.
   grain a.
   isoamyl a.
   isobutyl a.
   isopropyl a.
   methyl a.
   octyl a.
   phenylethyl a.
   propyl a.
   wood a.
alcoholic
   a. cardiomyopathy
   a. cirrhosis
   a. hepatitis
   a. hyalin
alcoholism
ALD — aldolase
aldehyde
   a. dehydrogenase
   a. fuchsin
   a. oxidase
Alder-Reilly anomaly
Alder's anomaly
aldicarb
aldimine
aldofuranose
aldohexose
aldolase
   allothreonine a.
aldonolactonase
aldopentose
aldopyranose
aldose
   a. 1-epimerase
   a. mutarotase
   a. reductase
aldosterone
   a. stimulation test
   a. suppression test
aldosteronism
aldotransferase
aldotriose
aldrin
aleukemia
aleukemic
   a. granulocytic leukemia
   a. leukemia
   a. lymphocytic leukemia
   a. monocytic leukemia
   a. myelosis
aleukocytosis
aleuriospore
Alexander's disease
alexia
alexin
ALG — antilymphocyte globulin
      axiolinguogingival
alga
algae
algebra
   Boolean a.
algin
alginate
alginic acid
Alginobacter
Alginomonas
algorithm
algor mortis

ALH — anterior lobe hormone
    anterior lobe of the
      hypophysis
alicyclic
    a. hydrocarbon
aliesterase
alignment
alimentary
    a. tract
alimentation
aliphatic
    a. saturated hydrocarbon
    a. unsaturated hydrocarbon
alizarin
    a. red
alk — alkaline
alkalemia
alkalescence
Alkalescens-dispar
alkali
    caustic a.
    a. denaturation test
    fixed a.
    volatile a.
alkalimetry
alkaline
    a. phosphatase
alkalinuria
alkaloid
alkalosis
    compensated a.
    hypokalemic a.
    metabolic a.
    nonrespiratory a.
    potassium a.
    respiratory a.
alkane
alkapton
alkaptonuria
alkene
alkenyl
alkoxide ion

alkoxyaryl hydroxylase
alk phos — alkaline phosphatase
alkyl
    a. alcohol
    a. aryl ammonium bromide
    a. aryl ammonium chloride
    a. aryl polyether sulfate
    a. aryl polyether sulfonate
    a. dimethyl benzyl
      ammonium bromide
    a. dimethyl benzyl
      ammonium chloride
    a. dimethyl-3, 4-dichloro-
      benzene ammonium
      chloride
    a. dimethyl ethyl
      ammonium bromide
    a. dimethyl ethyl
      ammonium chloride
    a. dimethyl ethylbenzyl
      ammonium bromide
    a. dimethyl ethylbenzyl
      ammonium chloride
    a. hydroxyethyl imidazol-
      inium chloride
    a. mercuric chloride
    a. mercuric phosphate
    a. naphthyl methyl
      pyridium chloride
    a. peroxide
    a. phenol polyglycol ether
    a. quaternary ammonium
      bromide
    a. quaternary ammonium
      chloride
    a. sodium-*N*-methyltaurate
    a. sodium sulfate
    a. sodium sulfonate
    a. toluyl methyl trimethyl
      ammonium chloride
    a. trimethyl ammonium
      bromide

alkyl *(continued)*
    a. trimethyl ammonium
        chloride
alkylate
alkylation
alkylbenzene sulfonate
alkylhalidase
alkyne
ALL — acute lymphoblastic
       leukemia
       acute lymphocytic
       leukemia
allantoic
allantoicase
allantoin
allantoinase
allantois
allele
    multiple a's
allelic
    a. exclusion
allergen
allergic
    a. dermatitis
    a. encephalitis
    a. encephalomyelitis
    a. granulomatosis
    a. granulomatous angiitis
    a. neuritis
    a. purpura
    a. reaction
    a. rhinitis
allergoid
allergy
Allescheria
    A. boydii
allescheriosis
allethrin
alligator boy
alloagglutinin
alloalbuminemia
alloantibody
alloantigen
allobarbital
Allodermanyssus
    A. sanguineus
allogeneic
allogenic
allograft
alloimmunization
allometric
allometry
allophanamide
alloploidy
allopolyploidy
allopurinol
allosteric
allothreonine aldolase
allotoxin
allotropism
allotype
alloxan
    a.-Schiff reaction
alloy
allyl
    a. aldehyde
    a. isothiocyanate
    a. sulfide
    a. sulfocarbamide
    a. thiocarbamide
    a. tribromide
ALME — acetyl-lysine methyl
       ester
ALMI — anterior lateral myo-
       cardial infarct
ALN — anterior lymph node
ALO — axiolinguo-occlusal
aloin
alopecia
    a. areata
    a. mucinosa
    a. universalis
ALP — alkaline phosphatase
       antilymphocyte plasma

alpha
- a. acid glycoprotein
- a.-adrenergic receptor
- a. amino acids
- a. amino nitrogen
- a.-amylase
- a.-amylose
- a. antichymotrypsin
- a.-antiplasmin
- a.-antitrypsin
- a. band
- a.-beta variation
- a. cells
- a. chain
- a. decay
- a.-delta sleep pattern
- a.-dinitrophenol
- a.-estradiol
- a.-fetoglobin
- a.-fetoprotein
- a. globulin antibodies
- A_1 globulins
- A_2 globulins
- a-1-4 glucosidase
- a. granules
- a.-hypophamine
- a.-ketoglutarate
- a.-lipoproteins
- a. lobeline
- a. macroglobulin
- a. melanocytic-stimulating hormone
- a.-methyldopa
- a. motor neuron
- a.-naphthol thiourea
- a.-naphthyl thiourea
- a. nephthyl acetate esterase reaction
- a. particles
- a. protease inhibitor
- a. receptors
- a. rhythm

alpha *(continued)*
- a. seromucoid
- a. streptococcus
- a. thalassemia
- a.-tocopherol
- a.-trypsin
- a. variant rhythm

alphameric
alphaprodine hydrochloride
alphavirus
alphazurine
Alport's syndrome
ALS — amyotrophic lateral sclerosis
 antilymphatic serum
 antilymphocyte serum
alseroxylon
ALT — alanine aminotransferase
ALTEE — acetyl-L-tyrosine ethyl ester
alteration
- cytoplasmic a.
- extracellular fibril a.
- Golgi's a.
- Golgi's cavity a.
- Golgi's membrane a.
- Golgi's vacuole a.
- Golgi's vesicle a.
- Nissl substance a.
- predecidual a.

alternans
- electrical a.
- a. of the heart
- pulsus a.

Alternaria
alternation
- cardiac a.
- a. of generations

altitude
- a. anoxia
- a. sickness

alum
    a. carmine
alumina
aluminosis
aluminum
    a. acetate
    a. carbonate
    a. chloride
    a. compound
    a. dihydroxyaminoacetate
    a. hydroxide
    a. hydroxide gel
    a. oxide
    a. phosphate
alveolar
    a. abscess
    a. adenocarcinoma
    a. carcinoma
    a. cyst
    a. duct
    a. epithelium
    a. fenestra
    a. hydatid
    a. macrophage
    a. proteinosis
    a. rhabdomyosarcoma
    a. sac
    a. soft part sarcoma
alveolitis
alveolus (alveoli)
    dental a.
    pulmonary a.
alveus
ALW — arch-loop-whorl
alymphocystic
alymphocytosis
Alzheimer's disease
AM — alveolar macrophage
    ametropia
    amperemeter
    anovular menstruation

AM *(continued)*
    axiomesial
    myopic astigmatism
Am — americium
amacrine cells
Amanita
    A. muscaria
    A. pantherina
    A. phalloides
    A. rubescens
    A. verna
    A. virosa
amantadine
amaurosis
amaurotic familial idiocy
ambenonium chloride
ambient
    a. air
    a. temperature
Amblyomma
amblyopia
amboceptor
    bacteriolytic a.
    Bordet's a.
    hemolytic a.
ambutonium
AMC — axiomesiocervical
AMD — alpha-methyldopa
    axiomesiodistal
ameba
    coprozoic a.
amebiasis
amebic
    a. colitis
    a. dysentery
    a. granuloma
    a. meningoencephalitis
ameboflagellate
ameboma
amelanotic melanoma
amelia

ameloblast
ameloblastic
   a. fibroma
   a. hemangioma
   a. neurilemoma
   a. odontoma
   a. sarcoma
ameloblastoma
   calcifying a.
amelogenesis imperfecta
amenorrhea
American Academy of Microbiology
American Association for Clinical Chemistry
American Association for Clinical Immunology and Allergy
American Association for the Advancement of Science
American Association of Immunologists
American Association of Neuropathologists
American Association of Pathologist Assistants
American Association of Pathologists
American Association of Pathologists and Bacteriologists
American Blood Commission
American Cancer Society
American Chemical Society
American Clinical Laboratory Association
American hookworm
American Joint Committee on Cancer Staging
American Medical Technologists
American rat flea
American Society for Clinical Investigation
American Society for Experimental Pathology
American Society for Medical Technology
American Society for Microbiology
American Society of Bacteriologists
American Society of Clinical Laboratory Technicians
American Society of Clinical Pathologists
American Society of Cytology
American Society of Hematology
American Society of Parasitologists
americium
Ames Lab-Tek cryostat
Ames test
amethyst violet
AMG — antimacrophage globulin
       axiomesiogingival
Amh — mixed astigmatism with myopia predominating
AMI — acute myocardial infarction
      amitriptyline
      axiomesioincisal
amidase
   omega-a.
amide
   niacin a.
   a. synthetase
amidinotransferase
amidobenzene
amidophosphoribosyltransferase

amikacin sulfate
amine
   a. oxidase
   a. precursor uptake and decarboxylation
aminergic nervous system
aminoacetic acid
amino acid
   a. a. activating enzyme
   glucogenic a. a.
   ketogenic a. a.
   modified a. a.
aminoacidemia
aminoacidopathy
D-aminoacid oxidase
L-aminoacid oxidase
aminoaciduria
aminoacridine
aminoacyl-histidine dipeptidase
aminoacyl-*t*RNA hydrolase
aminoanthraquinone
aminobenzene
aminobenzoic acid
aminobutyrate aminotransferase
aminocaproic acid
aminodeoxyglucose
   a. acetyltransferase
   a. kinase
aminodeoxyglucosephosphate
   a. acetyltransferase
   a. isomerase
aminodimethylaniline
aminoglutaric acid
aminoglutethimide
aminoglycoside
aminohippurate
aminoisobutyric acid
2-aminoisovaleric acid
aminoketone dye
aminolevulinate dehydratase
aminolevulinic acid
aminomalonate decarboxylase
aminometradine
2-amino-5-nitrothiazole
aminopenicillanic acid
aminopentamide
aminopeptidase
   leucine a.
alpha-aminopeptide aminoacidohydrolase
p-aminophenol
aminophylline
aminopropionitrile
aminopterin
aminopurine
aminopyridine
aminopyrine
aminosalicylic acid
aminosuccinic acid
aminotransferase
aminotriazole
aminotripeptidase
amiphenazole
amisometradine
amitosis
amitriptyline
amitrole
AML — acute monocytic leukemia
       acute myelocytic leukemia
AMLS — antimouse lymphocyte serum
AMM — agnogenic myeloid metaplasia
       ammonia
ammeter
AMML — acute myelomonocytic leukemia
ammonemia
ammonia
   a. hemate
   a. nitrogen

ammoniated mercury
ammonium
  a. carbonate
  a. hydroxide
  a. oxalate
  a. salt, quaternary
  a. sulfamate
  a. sulfate
ammonium bromide
  a. b. alkyl aryl
  a. b. alkyl dimethyl benzyl
  a. b. alkyl dimethyl ethyl
  a. b. alkyl dimethyl ethylbenzyl
  a. b. alkyl quaternary
  a. b. alkyl trimethyl
ammonium chloride
  a. c. alkyl aryl
  a. c. alkyl dimethyl benzyl
  a. c. alkyl dimethyl 3,4-dichlorobenzene
  a. c. alkyl dimethyl ethyl
  a. c. alkyl dimethyl ethylbenzyl
  a. c. alkyl quaternary
  a. c. alkyl toluyl methyl trimethyl
  a. c. alkyl trimethyl
  a. c. dialkyl dimethyl
  a. c. di-isobutyl cresolyl ethoxy ethyl dimethyl benzyl
  a. c. di-isobutyl phenoxy ethoxy ethyl dimethyl benzyl
Ammon's horn
amnesia
  hysterical a.
  transient global a.
amniocentesis
amnion
  a. nodosum
amnionitis
amniorrhea
amniotic
  a. adhesion
  a. band
  a. fluid
  a. sac
  a. villi
AMO — axiomesio-occlusal
amobarbital
A-mode — amplitude modulation
amodiaquine hydrochloride
Amoeba
  A. buccalis
  A. cachexica
  A. coli
  A. coli mitis
  A. dentalis
  A. dysenteriae
  A. histolytica
  A. limax
  A. meleagridis
  A. urinae granulata
  A. urogenitalis
  A. verrucosa
AMoL — acute monocytic (monoblastic) leukemia
amolanone
amorph
amorphous
amoxapine
amoxicillin
AMP — acid mucopolysaccharide
      adenosine monophosphate
      ampicillin
      average mean pressure
amp — ampere
ampere

amphetamine
   a. adipate
   a. phosphate
   a. sulfate
amphiarkyochrome
amphiarthrosis
amphibian
amphibolia
amphicyte
Amphimerus
amphipath
amphiprotic
amphitrichous
amphixenoses
ampholyte
amphomycin
amphophil cell
amphophilic
amphoteric
amphotericin B
ampicillin
amplification
   gene a.
amplifier
amplitude
amprotropine
AMPS — abnormal mucopolysacchariduria
         acid mucopolysaccharides
ampule
ampulla (ampullae)
   membranaceous a.
   osseous a.
   rectal a.
   uterine tube a.
   a. of vas deferens
   a. of Vater
amputation
AMS — antimacrophage serum
        automated multiphasic screening

amsacrine
AMT — alpha-methyltyrosine
        American Medical Technologists
   amethopterin
amt — amount
amu — atomic mass unit
AMY — amylase
amyelia
amygdalase
amygdaloid nucleus
amyl
   a. acetate
   a. nitrite
amylase
   alpha-a.
   beta-a.
   pancreatic a.
   salivary a.
   serum a.
   urinary a.
amylasuria
amyloclast
amylo-1,6-glucosidase
amyloid
   a. degeneration
   a. of immunoglobulin origin
   a. tumor
amyloidosis
   diffuse a.
   familial primary systemic a.
   focal a.
   primary a.
   secondary a.
amylomaltase
amylopectin
amylopectinosis
amylorrhea
amylose
   alpha a.
   crystalline a's
amyoplasia congenita

amyotonia congenita
amyotrophic lateral sclerosis
amyotrophy
   diabetic a.
   neuralgic a.
An — anisometropia
      anodal
      anode
ANA — acetylneuraminic acid
       antinuclear antibodies
       aspartyl naphthylamide
anabasine
anabolic
anabolism
anabolite
anacidity
anaerobe
   facultative a's
   obligate a's
anaerobia
anaerobian
anaerobiase
anaerobic
   a. bacteria culture
   a. diphtheroids
   a. neisseria
   a. streptococcus
anaerobiosis
anaerogenic
anal — analysis
anal
analbuminemia
analeptic
analgesia
analgesic
   a. nephropathy
   a. neuropathy
analog
analogue
analysis (analyses)
   Fourier a.
   qualitative a.

analysis (analyses) *(continued)*
   quantitative a.
   semiquantitative a.
   a. of variance
analyzer
anamnesis
anaphase
anaphoresis
anaphylactic
   a. shock
anaphylactoid
   a. purpura
   a. reaction
anaphylatoxin
anaphylaxis
   generalized a.
   passive a.
anaplasia
Anaplasma
Anaplasmataceae
anaplastic
   a. adenocarcinoma
   a. carcinoma
anaplerotic
anasarca
anastalsis
anastomosis
   arteriovenous a.
   crucial a.
   postcostal a.
   precapillary a.
   precostal a.
anat — anatomical
anatomic
anatomically patent foramen
   ovale
anatomy
Anatrichosoma
AnCC — anodal-closure contraction
anconeus muscle
ancrod

anechoic lesion

Ancylidae
Ancylostoma
   A. braziliense
   A. caninum
   A. duodenale
Andersen's disease
androblastoma
androgen
androgenesis
androgenic
androgenization
andropathy
androstanediol
androstene
androstenedione
androsterone
AnDTe — anodal-duration tetanus
anemia
   achrestic a.
   acute posthemorrhagic a.
   Addison's a.
   aplastic a.
   aregenerative a.
   autoimmune hemolytic a.
   Biermer's a.
   chronic a.
   congenital dyserythropoietic a.
   congenital hypoplastic a.
   congenital nonspherocytic hemolytic a.
   Cooley's a.
   Diamond-Blackfan a.
   dyserythropoietic a.
   Estren-Damashek a.
   familial hemolytic a.
   Fanconi's a.
   folic acid a.
   glucose-6-phosphate dehydrogenase deficiency a.
   Heinz body hemolytic a.

anemia *(continued)*
   hemolytic a.
   hypochromic a.
   hypochromic microcytic a.
   hypoplastic a.
   iatrogenic a.
   icterohemolytic a.
   iron deficiency a.
   leukoerythroblastic a.
   macrocytic a.
   Mediterranean a.
   megaloblastic a.
   microangiopathic hemolytic a.
   microcytic a.
   microdrepanocytic a.
   myelophthisic a.
   normochromic a.
   normocytic a.
   nosocomial a.
   pernicious a.
   posthemorrhagic a.
   primaquine-sensitive a.
   protein deficiency a.
   refractory a.
   sickle cell a.
   sideroachrestic a.
   sideroblastic a.
   sideropenic a.
   spherocytic a.
   thrombopenic a.
   vitamin deficiency a.
anemic
anencephalic
anencephaly
anergic
anergy
anes — anesthesia
anesthesia
anetoderma
   a. erythematosum
aneucentric

aneuploid
aneuploidy
aneurysm
    abdominal a.
    aortic arch a.
    aortic sinusal a.
    arteriosclerotic a.
    arteriosclerotic thrombosed a.
    arteriovenous a.
    axial a.
    berry a.
    cardiac a.
    cirsoid a.
    congenital a.
    congenital ruptured a.
    cylindroid a.
    cystogenic a.
    dissecting a.
    ectatic a.
    embolic a.
    embolomycotic a.
    endogenous a.
    erosive a.
    exogenous a.
    false a.
    fusiform a.
    luetic a.
    miliary a.
    mycotic a.
    Park's a.
    popliteal a.
    Pott's a.
    racemose a.
    Rasmussen's a.
    Richet's a.
    Rodrigues' a.
    ruptured a.
    saccular a.
    syphilitic a.
    thoracic a.
    thrombosed a.

aneurysm *(continued)*
    traumatic a.
    ventricular a.
aneurysmal
    a. bone cyst
    a. dilatation
aneusomatic
ANF — alpha-naphthoflavone antinuclear factor
ang — angiogram
angiectasis
angiitis (angiitides)
    allergic granulomatous a.
angina
    Ludwig's a.
    a. pectoris
    Prinzmetal's a.
    Vincent's a.
anginal
angioataxia
angiocardiography
angioedema
angiofibroma
    juvenile a.
angiogenesis
angiogram
angiography
angioimmunoblastic lymphadenopathy
angioinvasive adenoma
angiokeratoma
    a. corporis diffusum
angiolipoma
angioma
    serpiginosum a.
    spider a.
angiomatosis
angiomatous meningioma
angiomyolipoma
angioneurotic edema
angiopathy
angiosarcoma

Angiostrongylus
   A. cantonensis
angiotensin I, II
angiotensinase
angiotensinogen
angstrom
Ångström's law
angulation
anhidrosis
anhydrase
anhydride
Anichkov's (Anitschkow's)
   cell
   myocyte
anileridine
aniline
anilinism
animal
   a. cell culture
   a. control
anion
anionic
anionotropy
aniridia
anisakiasis
Anisakis
   A. marina
anisindione
anisochromia
anisocytosis
anisohypercytosis
anisohypocytosis
anisokaryosis
anisoleukocytosis
anisonucleolinosis
anisonucleosis
anisotropic
anisotropine
ankle
   a. joint
   a. ligament
ankyloblepharon
ankyloglossia
ankylosing spondylitis
ankylosis
   cricoarytenoid joint a.
   extracapsular a.
   fibrous a.
   intracapsular a.
   osseous a.
   stapedial a.
anlage (anlagen)
ANLL — acute nonlymphocytic leukemia
Annelida
annular
annulus (annuli)
AnOC — anodal-opening contraction
anococcygeal
anode
anodic stripping voltammetry
anodontia
anomalous
   a. muscle band
   a. origin
   a. vascular distribution
   a. venous connection
   a. venous drainage
anomaly
   Alder-Reilly a.
   Alder's a.
   Chédiak-Higashi a.
   congenital a.
   Ebstein's a.
   May-Hegglin a.
   Pelger-Huët nuclear a.
   Uhl's a.
   Undritz a.
   vascular a.
anomer
anonymous mycobacterium
Anopheles
   A. maculipennis

anophthalmia
Anoplocephalidae
Anoplura
anorectic
anorexia
    a. nervosa
anosmia
ANOVA — analysis of variance
anovular
anovulation
anovulatory
anoxemia
anoxemic
anoxia
    altitude a.
    anemic a.
    anoxic a.
    fulminating a.
    histotoxic a.
    hypoxic a.
    myocardial a.
    neonatorum a.
    a. reaction
    stagnant a.
anoxic
    a. encephalopathy
ANS — antineutrophilic serum
        arteriolonephrosclerosis
        autonomic nervous
            system
ansa (ansae)
    a. cervicalis
    a. hypoglossi
    a. lenticularis
    a. peduncularis
    a. subclavia
ansaparamedian fissure
anserine
ansiform
ant — anterior
Antabuse
antacid

antagonism
    bacterial a.
    metabolic a.
    microbial a.
    salt a.
antagonist
    competitive a.
    enzyme a.
    insulin a.
    metabolic a.
    narcotic a.
    sulfonamide a.
antazoline
antebrachial
antebrachium
antecedent
    plasma thromboplastin a.
antecubital
    a. region
    a. space
anteflexion
antegrade
antemortem
antenatal
antepartum
anterior
    a. acute poliomyelitis
    a. axillary line
    a. complete dislocation
    a. displacement
    a. superior iliac spine
    a. synechia
anterodorsal
anterograde
anterolateral
anteromedial
anteroposterior
anteroventral
anthelix
anthelmintic
anthelmycin
anthocyanin

Anthomyia
  A. canicularis
  A. incisura
  A. manicata
  A. salatrix
  A. scalaris
Anthomyiidae
anthracene
anthracometer
anthracosilicosis
anthracosis
  a. linguae
anthralin
anthrapurpurin
anthraquinone
anthrarobin
anthrax
  a. bacillus
anthropoid
anthropozoonosis
antiandrogen
antibacterial
antibiosis
antibiotic
  a.-associated pseudomembranous colitis
  bactericidal a.
  bacteriostatic a.
  broad-spectrum a.
  macrolide a.
  oral a.
  polyene a.
antibody
  ABO a's
  alloantin-D a.
  antimicrosomal a's
  antimitochondrial a.
  antinuclear a.
  antitubular basement membrane a's
  Donath-Landsteiner a.

antibody *(continued)*
  Duffy a's, Fy^a, Fy^b
  Lewis a's, Le^a, Le^b
antibody-dependent cell-mediated cytotoxicity
antibody reaction
  blocking a. r.
  endogenous antigen-cell bound a. r.
  endogenous antigen-circulating a. r.
  endogenous antigen-transferred a. r.
  endogenous antigen-transferred cell-bound a. r.
  heterophil a. r.
  transferred antigen cell-bound a. r.
  transferred antigen-transferred a. r.
anticholinergic
anticholinesterase
anticoagulant
anticoagulative
anticoagulin
anticodon
anticolibacillary
anticollagenase
anticolloidoclastic
anticonvulsant
anti-D
antidiuretic hormone
anti-DNA
anti-DNase
antidote
antidromic
antiestrogen
anti-factor
  I disorder
  II disorder

anti-smooth-muscle antibody

ANTI-FACTOR – ANTISTREPTOCOCCIN

anti-factor *(continued)*
    III disorder
    V disorder
    VIII disorder
    IX disorder
antifibrinogen
antifolic
antifungal
anti-GBM (glomerular basement membrane) disease
antigen
    ABO a's
    Australia a.
    carcinoembryonic a.
    Diego a.
    E a.
    erythrocyte a. La
    H a.
    HLA a's
    Ia a. Ro
    Kell a's
    Kveim a.
    Rh a.
    SD a.
    Vi a.
    von Willebrand's a.
    Wassermann a.
antigen-antibody reaction
antigenic
    a. determinant
    a. modulation
antigenicity
antigenotherapy
antiglobulin
antihemagglutinin
antihemolysin
antihemolytic
antihemophilic
    a. factor
    a. globulin
antiheterolysin
antihistamine

antihyaluronidase
    a. titer
antihypercholesterolemic
antihypertensive
anti-infective
anti-inflammatory
anti-invasin
    a. I
    a. II
anti-isolysin
antilewisite
    British a.
antilymphocyte serum — my book
antimatter
antimetabolite
antimicrobial
antimony
    a. dimercaptosuccinate
    a. hydride
    a. potassium tartrate
    a. trichloride
antimorph
antimutagen
antineoplastic
antineutrino
antinuclear
    a. antibodies
    a. factor
antioxidant
antiparticle
antiphylaxis
antiplasmin
antiport
antiproaccelerin
antiprothrombin
antipyrine
antisepsis
antiseptic
antiserum
antistaphylolysin
antistreptococcic
antistreptococcin

antistreptokinase
antistreptolysin
    a. O
antithrombin III
antithromboplastin
antithymocyte
    a. globulins
    a. serum
antitoxin
antitragus
antitrypsin
antivenin
antiviral
Anton test
ANTR — apparent net transfer rate
antral
antrum (antrums, antra)
    ethmoid a.
    mastoid a.
    maxillary a.
    pyloric a.
    tympanic a.
ANTU — alpha-naphthylthiourea
anuclear
anucleated
anulus (anuli)
anuresis
anuria
anus
    imperforate a.
    melanocarcinoma of a.
    a. of Rusconi
    a. vesicalis
    a. vestibularis
AO — acridine orange
    anodal opening
    anterior oblique
    aorta
    aortic opening

AO *(continued)*
    axio-occlusal
    opening of the atrioventricular valves
AOC — anodal-opening contraction
AOCl — anodal-opening clonus
AOD — arterial occlusive disease
AOP — anodal-opening picture
aorta
    abdominal a.
    anulus fibrosus of a.
    ascending a.
    descending thoracic a.
    thoracic a.
aortic
    a. aneurysm
    a. arch
    a. arch syndrome
    a. bodies
    a. body tumor
    a. cusp
    a. dissection
    a. internal elastic membrane
    a. isthmus
    a. lymph node
    a. plexus
    a. pulmonary window
    a. regurgitation
    a. ring
    a. septal defect
    a. stenosis
    a. tunica adventitia
    a. tunica intima
    a. tunica media
    a. valve
aorticorenal
    a. ganglion
    a. plexus

aortitis
    bacterial a.
    Döhle-Heller a.
    luetic a.
    rheumatoid a.
    syphilitic a.
aortography
    abdominal a.
    catheter a.
    selective visceral a.
    thoracic a.
    translumbar a.
AOS — anodal-opening sound
AOTe — anodal-opening tetanus
AP — acid phosphatase
    acute proliferative
    alkaline phosphatase
    aminopeptidase
    angina pectoris
    antepartum
    anterior pituitary
    anteroposterior
    appendix
    arterial pressure
    association period
    axiopulpal
A & P — anterior and posterior
    auscultation and percussion
APA — aldosterone-producing adenoma
    aminopenicillanic acid
    antipernicious anemia factor
apallic syndrome
apathy
Apathy's gum syrup medium
apatite
APB — atrial premature beat
    auricular premature beat

APC — acetylsalicylic acid, phenacetin, caffeine
    adenoidal-pharyngeal-conjunctival
    aspirin, phenacetin, caffeine
    atrial premature contraction
APC-C — aspirin, phenacetin, caffeine; with codeine
APC virus
APD — action-potential duration
    atrial premature depolarization
APE — aminophylline, phenobarbital, ephedrine
    anterior pituitary extract
aperture
    Key-Retzius lateral a.
    orbital a.
    piriform a.
apeu virus
apex (apexes, apices)
APF — anabolism-promoting factor
    animal protein factor
Apgar score
APGL — alkaline phosphatase activity of the granular leukocytes
APH — antepartum hemorrhage
    anterior pituitary hormone
aphagia
aphakia
aphasia
    motor a.
    sensory a.
aphasmid

aphonia
APHP — anti-*Pseudomonas* human plasma
aphtha (aphthae)
aphthous
    a. fever
    a. stomatitis
    a. ulceration
aphthovirus
apiamine
apical
    a. abscess
    a. canaliculi
    a. granuloma
APL — acute promyelocytic leukemia
    anterior pituitary-like
aplanatic
aplasia
    congenital thymic a.
    erythroid a.
    germinal a.
    gonadal a.
    granulocytic a.
    hematopoietic a.
    megakaryocytic a.
    nuclear a.
    pure red cell a.
    retinal a.
    thymic-parathyroid a.
aplasmic
aplastic
    a. anemia
    a. bone marrow
    a. crisis
APN — acute pyelonephritis
apnea
    deglutition a.
    posthyperventilation a.
    sleep a.
apneusis

apochromatic
apocodeine
apocrine
    a. adenoma
    a. carcinoma
    a. metaplasia
    a. sweat gland
apoenzyme
apoferritin
apolipoprotein
apomorphine
    a. hydrochloride
aponeurosis (aponeuroses)
apophyseal
    a. joint
apophysis (apophyses)
apophysitis
apoplasmatic
apoplexy
apoprotein
    a. CII
apoptosis
aposiderin
apothecium
APP — alum-precipitated pyridine
app — appendix
apparatus
    absorption a.
    chromidial a.
    ciliary a.
    Horsley-Clarke a.
    respiratory a.
    subneural a.
    urogenital a.
    vasomotor a.
appendage
appendiceal
    a. artery
    a. crypt
    a. lymphoid muscle

appendiceal *(continued)*
   a. mucous membrane
appendicitis
   acute gangrenous a.
   acute suppurative a.
   catarrhal a.
   focal a.
   gangrenous a.
   healed a.
   healing a.
   suppurative a.
appendix (appendices, appendixes)
   a. epididymis
   a. epiploic
   fibrous a.
   a. testis
   vermiform a.
appetite
appliqué form
apposition
approx. — approximately, approximation
approximately
approximation
APR — amebic prevalence rate
apraxia
aprobarbital
apronalide
aprotic
APT — alum-precipitated toxoid
APTT — activated partial thromboplastin time
Apt test
aptyalism
APUD — amine precursor uptake and decarboxylation
aqua (aquae)
   a. regia

aqueduct
   cerebral a.
   a. of cochlea
   a. of Cotunnius
   a. of Fallopius
   a. of Sylvius
   vestibular a.
aqueous
AR — alarm reaction
      aortic regurgitation
      Argyll Robertson (pupil)
      artificial respiration
Ar — argon
ara-A — adenine arabinoside
L-arabinose dehydrogenase
D-arabitol dehydrogenase
L-arabitol dehydrogenase
ara-C — cytosine arabinoside
arachidonate
arachidonic acid
Arachis
   A. hypogaea
Arachnia
   A. propionica
Arachnida
arachnodactyly
arachnoid
   a. cap cell
   a. granulation
   intracranial a.
   a. mater
   spinal a.
   a. villi
arachnoidea
arachnoidism
arachnoiditis
aramite
Aran-Duchenne disease
Arantius
   duct of A.
arborescent

arborization
arborvirus
arbovirus
    Group A
    Group B
    Group C
    Group unclassified
ARC — anomalous retinal
      correspondence
arceau rhythm
arch
    aortic a.
    branchial a.
    hyoid a.
    mandibular a.
    zygomatic a.
archencephalon
archiblast
archicerebellum
archil
arcuate
    a. artery
    a. fasciculus
    a. fibers
    a. nucleus
    a. nucleus, medulla
      oblongata
    a. periventricular nucleus
arcus senilis
ARD — acute respiratory
      disease
      anorectal dressing
ARDS — acute respiratory
      distress syndrome
area (areae, areas)
    Broca's a.
    a. cribrosa
    a. postrema
    a. striata
arecoline
areflexia
aregenerative

Arenaviridae
arenavirus
areola (areolae)
areolar
    a. connective tissue
    a. gland
ARF — acute renal failure
      acute respiratory
      failure
Arg — arginine
arg — argentum
Argas
    A. persicus
    A. reflexus
argentaffin cell
argentaffinoma
Argentinian hemorrhagic fever
    virus
argentum
arginase
arginine
    a. deiminase
    a. glutamate
    a. hydrochloride
    a. monohydrochloride
    suberyl a.
    a. vasopressin
argininemia
argininosuccinase
argininosuccinate
    a. lyase
    a. synthetase
argininosuccinic
    a. acidemia
    a. aciduria
arginyl
Argo corn starch test
argon
Argyll Robertson pupil
argyremia
argyria
arhinencephaly

Arias-Stella
    cells
    effect
Arias syndrome
ariboflavinosis
Arizona
    A. arizonae
    A. hinshawii
ARM — artificial rupture of the membranes
Armanni-Ebstein
    cells
    kidney
Armed Forces Institute of Pathology
Armigeres
    A. obturbans
Armillifer
    A. armillatus
    A. moniliformis
Arneth's
    count
    formula
Arnold-Chiari malformation
aromatic
    a. acid
    a. amine
    a. compound
    a. hydrocarbon
    a. ring
aromatization
arrector (arrectores)
    a. pili muscle
arrest
    cardiac a.
    deep transverse a.
    developmental a.
    epiphyseal a.
    maturation a.
    sinus a.
    spermatogenic a.
    spermatogenic maturation a.

arrhenoblastoma
arrhinencephaly
arrhythmia
ARS — antirabies serum
arsanilic acid
arsenate
arsenic
    a. keratosis
    a. poisoning
    a. trioxide
    a. trisulfide
arsenite
arsine
arsphenamine
arsthinol
ART — absolute retention time
      automated reagin test
art — artery
arterial
    a. anastomosis
    a. blood
    a. cone
    a. pressure
arteriola (arteriolae)
arteriolar
    a. nephrosclerosis
    a. thrombonecrosis
arteriole
    afferent a.
    efferent a.
arteriolitis
arteriolonephrosclerosis
arteriolosclerosis
arterionephrosclerosis
arteriopathy
    hypertensive a.
arteriosclerosis
    Mönckeberg's a.
    a. obliterans
arteriosclerotic
    a. aneurysm
    a. aortic aneurysm

arteriosclerotic *(continued)*
    a. cardiovascular disease
    a. heart disease
    a. thrombosed aneurysm
arteriovenous
    a. aneurysm
    a. communication
    a. fistula
    a. malformation
arteritis (arteritides)
    giant cell a.
    rheumatic a.
    rheumatoid a.
    temporal a.
artery
    anterolateral striate a's
    anteromedial perforating a's
    Cohnheim's a.
    Huebner's recurrent a.
    lenticulostriate a's
    Mueller's a's
    perforating anterolateral a's
    pre-rolandic a.
    striate a's
    Zinn's a.
arthralgia
    rheumatic a.
    a. saturnina
arthritis (arthritides)
    atrophic a.
    chronic proliferative a.
    chronic villous a.
    a. deformans
    degenerative a.
    exudative a.
    gouty a.
    hypertrophic a.
    a. mutilans
    navicular a.
    neuropathic a.
    psoriatic a.

arthritis *(continued)*
    rheumatoid a.
    rheumatoid a., juvenile
    suppurative a.
    vertebral a.
arthrochondritis
Arthroderma
arthrodesis
    Moberg's a.
Arthrographis
    A. langeroni
arthrogryposis
arthrolith
arthropathy
    Charcot's a.
    neurogenic a.
    osteopulmonary a.
Arthropoda
arthrospore
arthrosynovitis
Arthus's reaction
articular
    a. capsule
    a. cartilage
    a. disc
articularis
    a. cubiti muscle
    a. genus muscle
articulated
articulation
artifact
artificial
    a. abortion
    a. dialyzer
    a. kidney
    a. respiration
Artyfechinostomum
aryepiglottic
    a. fold
arylamine acetyltransferase
arylaminopeptidase

arylesterase
aryl-ester hydrolase
aryl 4-hydroxylase
arylsulfatase
aryl-sulfotransferase
arytenoid
   a. cartilage
arytenoiditis
AS — acetylstrophanthidin
   Adams-Stokes (disease)
   alveolar sac
   androsterone sulfate
   antistreptolysin
   aortic stenosis
   arteriosclerosis
   astigmatism
   atherosclerosis
As — arsenic
ASA — acetylsalicylic acid
   Adams-Stokes attack
   argininosuccinic acid
   arylsulfatase-A
ASB — American Society of
   Bacteriologists
asbestosis
ascariasis
ascaricidal
ascaricide
ascarid
ascarides
Ascaridoidea
Ascaris
   A. alata
   A. canis
   A. lumbricoides
   A. mystax
   A. pneumonitis
   A. suum
ascending
   a. aorta
   a. cervical artery

ascending *(continued)*
   a. colon
   a. degeneration
   a. limb, Henle's loop
   a. pharyngeal artery
ascertainment
   complete a.
   incomplete a.
   multiple a.
   single a.
   truncate a.
Aschheim-Zondek
   hormone
   test
Aschoff-Rokitansky sinus
Aschoff's
   body
   nodule
Aschoff-Tawara node
ASCI — American Society for
   Clinical Investigation
ascites
   chylous a.
   hemorrhagic a.
Ascit. Fl. — ascitic fluid
ascitic fluid
ASCLT — American Society of
   Clinical Labora-
   tory Technicians
ascocarp
ascomycete
Ascomycetes
Ascomycotina
ascorbate
ascorbic acid
ascorbic reductase
ascospore
ascotrophosome
ASCP — American Society of
   Clinical Pathologists
ascus (asci)

ASCVD — arteriosclerotic cardiovascular disease
atherosclerotic cardiovascular disease
ASD — aldosterone secretion defect
atrial septal defect
ASEP — American Society for Experimental Pathology
asepsis
aseptic
asexual
ASF — aniline, sulfur, formaldehyde
ASH — American Society of Hematology
asymmetrical septal hypertrophy
AsH — hypermetropic astigmatism
Ashby's differential agglutination method
ASHD — arteriosclerotic heart disease
asialia
asialoglycoprotein
Asiatic cholera
asiderosis
ASIS — anterior superior iliac spine
ASK — antistreptokinase
Askanazy's cell
ASL — antistreptolysin
ASLO — antistreptolysin-O
ASM — American Society for Microbiology
AsM — myopic astigmatism
ASMI — anteroseptal myocardial infarct

ASMT — American Society for Medical Technology
ASN — alkali-soluble nitrogen
Asn — asparagine
ASO — antistreptolysin-O
arteriosclerosis obliterans
ASO titer — antistreptolysin-O titer
ASP — American Society of Parasitologists
area systolic pressure
Asp — aspartic acid
asparagic acid
asparaginase
asparagine-ketoacid aminotransferase
asparaginic acid
asparaginyl
aspartate
   a. aminotransferase
   a. carbamoyltransferase
   a. kinase
   a. transaminase
D-aspartate oxidase
aspartic acid
aspartokinase
aspartyl
aspartylacetylglucosaminidase
aspartylglucosaminuria
aspect
   dorsal a.
   ventral a.
aspergilloma
aspergillosis
Aspergillus
   A. amsteloidami
   A. auricularis
   A. barbae
   A. bouffardi
   A. candidus
   A. carneus

Aspergillus (continued)
  A. clavatus
  A. concentricus
  A. fisherii
  A. flavus
  A. fumigatus
  A. giganteus
  A. glaucus
  A. gliocladium
  A. mucoroides
  A. nidulans
  A. niger
  A. niveus
  A. ochraceus
  A. oryzae
  A. parasiticus
  A. pictor
  A. repens
  A. restrictus
  A. sulphureus
  A. sydowi
  A. terreus
  A. versicolor
aspermatism
aspermatogenesis
  induced a.
aspermia
aspheric
asphyxia
asphyxial
asphyxiation
aspidium oleoresin
aspirate
aspiration
  foreign body a.
  a. pneumonia
  tracheal a.
aspirin toxicity
asplenia
asplenic
asporogenic
asporous

ASR — aldosterone secretion rate
  aldosterone secretory rate
ASS — anterior superior spine
assay
  biologic a.
  ELISA (enzyme-linked immunosorbent a.)
  hemagglutination a.
  immune a.
  immunofluorescent a.
  leukotactic a.
assimilation
association
  a. constant
  a. fibers
Association for the Advancement of Medical Instrumentation
Association of Clinical Scientists
assortative mating
  negative a. m.
  positive a. m.
assortment
  independent a.
AST — aspartate aminotransferase
Ast — astigmatism
astasia
  a.-abasia
astatine
asteatosis
aster
asterixis
Asterococcus
asteroid
  a. body
Asth — asthenopia
asthenia
  neurocirculatory a.

asthma
    allergic a.
    alveolar a.
    bronchial a.
    cotton dust a.
    emphysematous a.
    essential a.
    grinders' a.
    intrinsic a.
    millers' a.
    miners' a.
    potters' a.
    steam-fitters' a.
    stone-strippers' a.
asthmatic
    a. bronchitis
astigmatism
ASTO — antistreptolysin-O
astomatous
Astra Blue
Astracyanine
astragaloid joint
astroblastoma
astrocyte
    fibrillary a.
    fibrous a.
    protoplasmic a.
astrocytoma
    anaplastic a.
    fibrillary a.
    fibrous a.
    gemistocytic a.
    Grades I–IV a's
    pilocytic a.
    piloid a.
    protoplasmic a.
astroglia
ASV — anodic stripping voltammetry
    antisnake venom
asymmetric
    a. carbon atom

asymmetric *(continued)*
    a. septal hypertrophy
asymmetry
asymptote
asynapsis
asynchronism
asynergia
asystole
AT — antitrypsin
AT-III — antithrombin III
AT_{10} — dihydrotachysterol
At — astatine
ATA — anti-*Toxoplasma* antibodies
    atmosphere absolute
    aurintricarboxylic acid
ataxia
    familial cerebellar a.
    Friedreich's a.
    hereditary cerebellar a.
    hereditary spinal a.
    a.-telangiectasia
ATD — asphyxiating thoracic dystrophy
ATE — adipose tissue extract
ATEE — acetyltyrosine ethyl ester
atelectasis
    a. neonatorum
    obstructive a.
Atelosaccharomyces
ATG — antithyroglobulin
atheroma
atheromatosis
atheromatous
    a. embolus
    a. plaque
atherosclerosis
atherosclerotic heart disease
athetoid
athetosis
athetotic

athlete's foot
ATL — antitension line
atlas
ATN — acute tubular necrosis
at. no. — atomic number
atocia
atom
atomic
- a. absorption spectrophotometry
- a. mass
- a. mass unit
- a. number
- a. spectrum
- a. weight

atony
atopen
atopic
- a. allergen
- a. dermatitis
- a. keratoconjunctivitis

atopy
ATP — adenosine triphosphate
ATPase — adenosinetriphosphatase
ATPase
- calcium-activated A.
- magnesium-activated A.
- A. stain

ATP pyrophosphohydrolase
ATPS — ambient temperature and pressure, saturated
atransferrinemia
Atrax
- *A. robustus*

atresia
- anal a.
- aortic a.
- biliary a.
- congenital a.
- duodenal a.

atresia *(continued)*
- esophageal a.
- follicular a.
- intestinal a.
- mitral a.
- prepyloric a.
- pulmonary a.
- tricuspid a.
- valvular a.

atretic
- a. follicle

atr fib — atrial fibrillation
atrial
- a. anomalous bands
- a. appendage
- a. arrhythmia
- a. fibrillation
- a. flutter
- a. premature beat
- a. premature contraction
- a. premature depolarization
- a. septal defect
- a. septum

atrichous
atrioventricular
- a. block
- a. bundle
- a. canal cushion
- a. node
- a. valve

atrium
atrophia maculosa varioliformis cutis
atrophic
- a. arthritis
- a. chronic gastritis
- a. endometrium
- a. fenestration
- a. gastritis
- a. glossitis
- a. lichen planus
- a. rhinitis

atrophoderma
- a. maculatum
- a. neuriticum
- a. reticulatum

atrophy
- acquired a.
- acute yellow a.
- brown a.
- Charcot-Marie-Tooth muscular a.
- circumscribed a.
- cystic a.
- disuse a.
- essential a.
- exhaustion a.
- fatty a.
- focal a.
- gelatinous a.
- granular a.
- infantile muscular a.
- Leber's optic a.
- lobar cerebral a.
- macular a.
- marantic a.
- mucinous a.
- muscular a., Charcot-Marie-Tooth
- muscular a., hypertrophic polyneuritic type
- muscular a., peroneal
- neuritic a.
- neurotrophic a.
- olivocerebellar a.
- olivopontocerebellar a.
- optic a.
- pressure a.
- progressive muscular a.
- progressive spinal muscular a.
- senile a.
- serous a.
- simple a.

atrophy *(continued)*
- Sudeck's a.
- traction a.
- traumatic a.

atropine

ATS — antitetanic serum
antithymocyte serum
arteriosclerosis

attack
- Adams-Stokes a.

attapulgite

at. vol. — atomic volume

at. wt. — atomic weight

atypia
- koilocytotic a.

atypical
- a. hyperplasia
- a. lymphocytes
- a. mycobacterium
- a. pneumonia
- a. primary pneumonia
- a. regeneration
- a. repetitive spike-and-slow waves
- a. verrucous endocarditis

AU — Angström unit
antitoxin unit
arbitrary units
azauridine

Au — Australia antigen
gold

Au Ag — Australia antigen

Auchmeromyia
- *A. luteola*

auditory
- a. artery
- a. canal
- a. evoked potential
- a. meatus
- a. nerve
- a. ossicle
- a. projection

auditory *(continued)*
  a radiation
  a. stimulation
  a. tube
  a. vein
  a. vesicle
Auerbach's plexus
Auer's bodies
Auger
  effect
  electron
AUL — acute undifferentiated leukemia
AUO — amyloid of unknown origin
aural
auramine
  a.-rhodamine stain
aurantiasis
Aureobasidium
  A. pullulans
aur fib — auricular fibrillation
auricle
  cervical a.
  left a. of heart
  right a. of heart
auricular
  a. appendage
  a. artery, posterior
  a. branch, tenth cranial nerve
  a. branch, vagus nerve
  a. cartilage
  a. fibrillation
  a. line
  a. lymph node, anterior
  a. lymph node, posterior
  a. nerve, greater
  a. point
  a. region
  a. tachycardia, paroxysmal
auricularis

auriculotemporal
aurintricarboxylic acid
aurochromoderma
Aurococcus
aurothioglucose
Austin Flint murmur
Australia antigen
Australian
  A. X disease
  A. X encephalitis virus
Australorbis
  A. glabratus
autacoid
autoadsorption
autoagglutination
autoagglutinin
autoallergy
autoantibody
autoanticomplement
autoantigen
autoantitoxin
autocatalysis
autochthonous
autoerythrophagocytosis
autofluorescence
autogenic
  a. graft
autogenous
autograft
autohemagglutination
autohemagglutinin
autohemolysin
autohemolysis
autohemotherapy
autoimmune
  a. hemolytic anemia
  a. leukopenia
  a. pancytopenia
  a. reaction
  a. thrombocytopenic purpura
  a. thyroiditis

autoimmunity
autoinfection
autoinoculation
autoisolysin
autologous
    a. graft
    a. transfusion
autolysis
autolysosome
automated immunoprecipitation
Automeris io
automutagen
autonomic
    a. nervous system
    a. plexus
autophagic
    a. vacuole
autophagosome
autophagy
autoplast
autoploidy
autoprothrombin
autopsy
autoradiography
autoradiolysis
autoregulation
autosensitization
autosomal
    a. dominant disorders
    a. recessive disorders
autosome
    a. translocation
autosplenectomy
autotroph
    facultative a.
    obligate a.
autotrophic
auxanography
auxesis
auxochrome
auxocyte
auxotroph
auxotrophic
AV — alveolar duct
    arteriovenous
    atrioventricular
AV or A-V — arteriovenous
    atrioventricular
A-V
    A-V (arteriovenous) aneurysm
    A-V (atrioventricular) block
Av — average
    avoirdupois
AV/AF — anteverted, anteflexed
AVCS — atrioventricular conduction system
average
    Walsh's a.
AVF — arteriovenous fistula
AVH — acute viral hepatitis
aviadenovirus
avidin
avidity
avipoxvirus
avirulence
avirulent
avitaminosis
AVM — arteriovenous malformation
AVN — atrioventricular node
Avogadro's number
AVP — arginine vasopressin
AVR — aortic valve replacement
AVRP — atrioventricular refractory period
A-V shunt — arteriovenous shunt
avulsion
AW — anterior wall

AWI — anterior wall infarction
AWMI — anterior wall myocardial infarction
awu — atomic weight unit
axenic
axial
axilla (axillae)
axillary
   a. artery
   a. fascia
   a. line
   a. lymph node
   a. nerve
   a. projection
   a. region
   a. vein
axiolateral
axis (axes)
   a. cylinder
   a. of rotation
axolemma
axon
   a. hillock
   unmyelinated a.
axonal
   a. degeneration
   a. demyelination
   a. reaction
   a. spheroid
axoneme
axonotmesis
axoplasm
axoplasmic
   a. flow
Ayerza's disease
Ayoub-Shklar method
Az — azote (French for nitrogen)
azacyclonol hydrochloride
azacytidine
azaguanine
azamethonium bromide
azanator maleate
azanidazole
azapetine phosphate
azaserine
azatadine maleate
azathioprine
6-azauridine
azeotropic
azeotropy
azg — azaguanine
azide
azine dye
azinphosmethyl
azo — (indicates presence of the group) —N:N—
azobenzene
   a. reductase
azobilirubin
azo dye
azoic dye
azoospermia
azoprotein
azote
azotemia
   chloropenic a.
   extrarenal a.
   hypochloremic a.
   postrenal a.
   prerenal a.
   renal a.
Azotobacter
azotorrhea
azoturia
AZT — Aschheim-Zondek test
AZ test — Aschheim-Zondek test
azul
AZUR — azauridine
azure
azure-eosin stain

54 AZURESIN – *BACILLUS*

azuresin
azygos
  a. lobe
  a. vein

azygous
azymia

B

B – bacillus
  Baumé's scale
  Benoist's scale
  bicuspid
  boron
  buccal
  whole blood
B. – *Brucella*
BA – bacterial agglutination
  betamethasone acetate
  blocking antibody
  bovine albumin
  branchial artery
  bronchial asthma
  buccoaxial
Ba – barium
Babès-Ernst granules
Babesia
  B. microti
babesiosis
Babinski's
  reflex
  sign
  syndrome
BAC – blood alcohol concentration
  buccoaxiocervical
bacampicillin hydrochloride
Bachman test
Bacillaceae
bacillary
  b. dysentery
bacilli
  acid-fast b.

bacilli *(continued)*
  gram-negative b.
  gram-positive b.
bacilliform
Bacillus
  B. acidi lactici
  B. aerogenes capsulatus
  B. aertrycke
  B. alvei
  B. ambiguus
  B. anthracis
  B. botulinus
  B. brevis
  B. bronchisepticus
  B. cereus
  B. circulans
  B. coli
  B. diphtheriae
  B. dysenteriae
  B. enteritidis
  B. faecalis alcaligenes
  B. influenzae
  B. larvae
  B. leprae
  B. licheniformis
  B. mallei
  B. megatherium
  B. necrophorus
  B. oedematiens
  B. oedematis maligni No. II
  B. pertussis
  B. pestis
  B. pneumoniae
  B. polymyxa

Bacillus (continued)
  B. proteus
  B. pseudomallei
  B. pumilus
  B. pyocyaneus
  B. sphaericus
  B. stearothermophilus
  B. subtilis
  B. suipestifer
  B. tetani
  B. tuberculosis
  B. tularense
  B. typhi
  B. typhosus
  B. welchii
  B. whitmori
bacillus (bacilli)
  b. abortivus equinus
  anthrax b.
  Bang's b.
  Battey bacilli
  Boas-Oppler b.
  Bordet-Gengou b.
  Calmette-Guérin b.
  coliform b.
  colon b.
  Döderlein's b.
  Ducrey's b.
  dysentery bacilli
  enteric b.
  Escherich's b.
  Fick's b.
  Flexner's b.
  Flexner-Strong b.
  Friedländer's b.
  fusiform b.
  Gärtner's b.
  Ghon-Sachs b.
  glanders b.
  Hansen's b.
  Hofmann's b.
  Johne's b.

bacillus (bacilli) *(continued)*
  Klebs-Löffler b.
  Klein's b.
  Koch's b.
  Koch-Weeks b.
  leprosy b.
  Morax-Axenfeld b.
  Morgan's b.
  Newcastle-Manchester b.
  Nocard's b.
  paracolon bacilli
  Pfeiffer's b.
  plague b.
  Preisz-Nocard b.
  pseudotuberculosis b.
  rhinoscleroma b.
  Schmitz's b.
  Schmorl's b.
  Shiga's b.
  smegma b.
  Sonne-Duval b.
  Strong's b.
  swine rotlauf b.
  tetanus b.
  timothy b.
  tubercle b.
  typhoid b.
  vole b.
  Welch's b.
  Whitmore's b.
bacitracin
back
  b. fascia
  functional b.
  b. pressure
  saddle b.
  b. subcutaneous tissue
backbone
backcross
backflow
background
  b. interference

background *(continued)*
   b. radiation
backscatter
   b. peak
baclofen
bact — bacterium
Bactec system
bacteremia
bacteria
   gram-negative b.
   gram-positive b.
   intermediate coliform b.
   monocytogenes b.
bacterial
   b. adherence
   b. agar method
   b. endaortitis
   b. endocarditis
   b. genetics
   b. opsonin
   b. susceptibility testing
   b. virus
bactericidal
bactericide
bacterid
   pustular b.
bacteriemia
bacterin
bacterioagglutinin
bacteriocin
bacteriocinogen
bacterioclasis
bacteriogenic
bacterioid
bacteriologic
bacteriologist
bacteriology
bacteriolysin
bacteriolysis
bacteriolytic
Bacterionema matruchotii
bacterio-opsonin

bacteriopexy
bacteriophage
   b. genetics
bacteriopsonic
bacteriostasis
bacteriostat
bacteriostatic
   b. agent
bacteriotherapy
bacteriotoxic
bacteriotropic
bacteriotropin
Bacterium
   B. aerogenes
   B. aeruginosum
   B. anitratum
   B. cholerae suis
   B. cloacae
   B. coli
   B. dysenteriae
   B. mirabilis
   B. pestis bubonicae
   B. sonnei
   B. subgroup B
   B. tularense
   B. typhosum
bacterium
   acid-fast b.
   aerobic b.
   anaerobic b.
   autotrophic b.
   beaded b.
   bifid b.
   chemoautotrophic b.
   chemoheterotrophic b.
   chromogenic b.
   denitrifying b.
   facultative b.
   gram-negative b.
   gram-positive b.
   heterotrophic b.
   hydrogen b.

BACTERIUM – BALL 57

bacterium *(continued)*
   lysogenic b.
   mesophilic b.
   nitrifying b.
   organotropic b.
   psychrophilic b.
   pyogenic b.
   rough b.
   smooth b.
   sulfur b.
   thermophilic b.
   toxigenic b.
   water b.
bacteriuria
bacteroid
Bacteroidaceae
Bacteroides ureolyticus
   B. corrodens
   B. fragilis
   B. funduliformis
   B. fusiformis
   B. melaninogenicus
   B. ochraceus
   B. oralis
   B. pneumosintes
   B. ruminicola
   B. serpens
bacteroides
bacteruria
Bactometer
Bactrim
BAEE – benzoyl arginine ethyl ester
     benzylarginine ethyl ester
BAEP – brain stem auditory evoked potential
BAG – buccoaxiogingival
bagassosis
bag-box circuit
Baggenstoss change

BAL = bronchoalveolar lavage

BAIB – beta-aminoisobutyric acid
Bainbridge reflex
Baker's
   acid hematein test
   cyst
   formol calcium
   pyridine extraction test
   Sudan black method
BAL – British antilewisite
     dimercaprol
Balamuth's
   buffer solution
   culture medium
balance
   acid-base b.
   calcium b.
   enzyme b.
   fluid b.
   genic b.
   microchemical b.
   nitrogen b.
   semimicro b.
balanitis
   b. xerotica obliterans
balanoposthitis
balantidiasis
Balantidium
   B. coli
Balbiani's
   body
   chromosome
   nucleus
   ring
baldness
Balkan nephropathy
ball
   chondrin b.
   fungus b.
   hair b.
   pleural fibrin b's

ballismus
ballistocardiogram
ballistocardiography
balloon
    Shea-Anthony antral b.
    sinus b.
ballooning degeneration
ballottement
ball-valve obstruction
bals — balsam
balsam
    Canada b.
    friars' b.
    peruvian b.
    silver b.
    tolu b.
BAME — benzoylarginine methyl ester
Bancroft's filariasis
band
    A b.
    Büngner's b's
    b. cell
    b. form
    H b.
    I b.
    b. keratopathy
    b. neutrophil
    b. spectrum
banding
    C b.
Bandl's ring
bandpass
    b. filter
bandwidth
Bang's bacillus
Banti's
    disease
    spleen
BAO — basal acid output
BAP — blood agar plate
bar
    chromatoidal b.
    hyoid b.
    labial b.
    lingual b.
    median b.
    Passavant's b.
    sternal b.
    terminal b's
baragnosis
barbital
barbiturate
Bargen's streptococcus
barium
    b. fluosilicate
    b. sulfate
    b. test
Barlow's syndrome
barn
Barnett-Bourne acetic alcohol silver nitrate
barometer
barometric
    b. pressure
baroreceptor
baroreflex
barosinusitis
Barr bodies
barreling distortion
Barrett's
    epithelium
    esophagus
    ulcer
barrier-layer cell
Barrnett-Seligman
    dihydroxydinaphthyl disulfide method
    indoxyl esterase method
Barroso-Moguel and Costero silver method
bartholinitis

Bartholin's
  abscess
  cyst
  gland
Bartonella
  B. bacilliformis
Bartonellaceae
bartonellosis
Bart's hemoglobin
Bartter's syndrome
basal
  b. acid output
  b. body
  Bruch's b. membrane
  b. feet
  b. ganglia
  b. granule
  b. lamina
  b. metabolic rate
  b. metabolism
  b. nuclei
  b. plate
  b. projection
  b. region
  b. vein
basal cell
  b. c. carcinoma
  b. c. hyperplasia
  b. c. nevus syndrome
  b. c. papilloma
basaloid carcinoma
base
  Brönsted-Lowry b.
  b. excess
  b. ionization constant
  b. pair
  b. pairing
  purine b's
  pyrimidine b's
  b. ratio
  Schiff b.

Basedow's disease
baseline
  b. steady state
basement membrane
bas-fond
BASH — body acceleration given synchronously with the heartbeat
basic
  b. anhydride
  b. dye
basicaryoplastin
Basidiobolus
  B. haptosporus
Basidiomycetes
basidium (basidia)
basilar
  b. artery
  b. membrane
  b. region, pons
  b. white matter
basilic vein
basipetal
basis (bases)
  b. cerebri
  b. pedunculi
  b. pulmonis
basket
  b. cell
  fiber b's
Baso — basophil
basophil
  b. adenoma
  b. cell
  b. chemotactic factor
basophilia
basophilic
  b. degeneration
  b. erythroblast
  b. granular degeneration
  b. granule

basophilic *(continued)*
   b. hyperplasia
   b. leukemia
   b. leukocyte
   b. leukocytosis
   b. megakaryocyte
   b. metamyelocyte
   b. myelocyte
   b. normoblast
   b. promyelocyte
   b. stippling
basophilism
   Cushing's b.
   pituitary b.
basosquamous
Bassen-Kornzweig syndrome
bassorin
batch processing
bath
   antipyretic b.
   carbon dioxide b.
   foam b.
   immersion b.
   sedative b.
bathochrome
bathochromic
   b. shift
bathophenanthroline
bathrocephaly
bathycardia
Batten's disease
Battey
   bacilli
   -type mycobacterium
battledore placenta
baud
Bauer reaction
Baumé's scale
Baumgartner method
Bayes's theorem
BB — blood bank
   blood buffer base

BB *(continued)*
   blue bloaters (emphysema)
   breakthrough bleeding
   breast biopsy
   buffer base
BBB — blood-brain barrier
   bundle branch block
BBT — basal body temperature
BC — bactericidal concentration
   bone conduction
   buccocervical
BCB — brilliant cresyl blue
BCD — binary coded decimal
BCE — basal cell epithelioma
B cells
BCF — basophil chemotactic factor
BCG — bacille Calmette-Guérin (vaccine)
   ballistocardiogram
   bicolor guaiac (test)
   bromocresol green
BCNU — bischloroethylnitrosourea
   bischloronitrosourea
BCP-D — bromcresol purple desoxycholate
BD — base deficit
   bile duct
   buccodistal
Bdellonyssus bacoti
BDG — buffered desoxycholate glucose
BE — bacillary emulsion (tuberculin)
   bacterial endocarditis
   base excess
   bovine enteritis
Be — beryllium
Beard test

beat
- apex b.
- capture b's
- dropped b.
- ectopic b.
- fusion b.
- premature b.
- reciprocal b's

Beau's lines
beauvariosis
Beaver direct smear method
Becker's dystrophy
Beckmann thermometer
Beck's triad
Beckwith-Wiedemann syndrome
beclomethasone dipropionate
becquerel
Bedsonia
Beer's law
Behçet's syndrome
behenic acid
BEI — butanol-extractable iodine
bejel
bel
Belascaris
belladonna
Bellini's papillary duct
Bell-Magendie law
Bell's palsy
bemegride
benactyzine hydrochloride
Bence Jones
- albumin
- albumosuria
- protein
- protein test
- proteinuria
- reaction

Benditt hypothesis
bendroflumethiazide
bends
Benedict's test
Bengston's method
benign
- b. monoclonal gammopathy
- b. nephrosclerosis

Bennett's sulfhydryl method
Bennhold's Congo red method
benoxinate hydrochloride
Benoy scale
Bensley's
- aniline-acid fuchsin-methyl green method
- osmic dichromate fluid
- safranin acid violet

bentonite
- b. flocculation test

benzaldehyde
- b. dehydrogenase

benzalkonium chloride
benzene
- b. hexachloride

benzestrol
benzethonium
benzidine
benzoate
benzocaine
benzodepa
benzodiazepine
benzoflavine
benzoic acid
benzoin
benzol
benzomethamine
benzonatate
benzopurpurine
benzopyrene
benzo sky blue method
benzoyl
- b. chloride
- b. oil red
- b. peroxide

benzoylaminoacetic acid

benzoylation
benzoylcholinesterase
benzoylecgonine
benzoylglycine
benzphetamine hydrochloride
benzpyrene
benzpyrinium bromide
benzthiazide
benztropine mesylate
benzydroflumethiazide
benzyl
    b. alcohol
    b. benzoate
    b. bromide
    b. carbinol
    b. fumarate
    b. mandelate
    b. succinate
benzylamine
o-benzyl-parachlorophenol
benzylpenicillin
bephenium hydroxynaphthoate
berberine
Bereitschaftspotential
bergamot oil
Berger's
    disease
    rhythm
Bergey's classification
Berg's chelate removal method
beriberi
Berkefeld filter
berkelium
Bernstein test
Bernthsen's methylene violet
berry
    b. aneurysm
    b. cell
Berthelot reaction
Bertiella
    B. mucronata
    B. studeri

Bertini's renal columns
berylliosis
beryllium
    b. granulomatosis
Besnier-Boeck disease
Bessey-Lowry unit
Bessey-Lowry-Brock unit
Best's
    carmine stain
    disease
beta
    b.-aminoisobutyric acid
    b.-aminoisobutyricaciduria
    b. band
    b. basophil
    b. blocker
    b.-butoxy-beta-thiocyano-
        diethyl ether
    b. cell
    b.-cholestanol
    b. decay
    b. emitter
    b.-endorphin
    b.-globulin
    b. hemolysis
    b.-hemolytic streptococcus
    b.-hypophamine
    b.-lactamase
    b.-lactose
    b.-lipoprotein
    b.-lysin
    b.-microglobulin
    b. particles
    b.-phenylisopropylamine
    b.-pyridyl-carbinol
    b. radiation
    b. ray
    b. receptor
    b. streptococcus
    b. thalassemia
    b.-thiocyanoethyl
    b.-thromboglobulin

beta-adrenergic
   b. antagonist
   b. blocking agent
   b. receptor
betaine
   b. aldehyde dehydrogenase
   b. homocysteine methyltransferase
betamethasone
betanaphthol
beta-oxybutyria
betatron
betazole hydrochloride
bethanechol chloride
Bethesda-Ballerup group of *Citrobacter*
Bethesda unit
Betke-Kleihauer test
Betke stain
Betz cells
BeV — billion electron volts
bezoar
Bezold-Jarisch reflex
BF — blastogenic factor
      blood flow
B/F — bound-free ratio
bf — bouillon filtrate (tuberculin)
BFC — benign febrile convulsion
BFP — biologic false-positive
BFR — biologic false-positive reactor
       blood flow rate
       bone formation rate
BFT — bentonite flocculation test
BFU-E — burst-forming unit-erythroid
BG — blood glucose
     bone graft
     buccogingival

BGG — bovine gamma globulin
BGH — bovine growth hormone
BGP — beta-glycerophosphatase
BGSA — blood granulocyte-specific activity
BGTT — borderline glucose tolerance test
BH — benzalkonium and heparin
BHA — butylated hydroxyanisole
BHC — benzene hexachloride
BHI — brain-heart infusion
BHS — beta-hemolytic streptococcus
BHT — butylated hydroxytoluene
BH/VH — body hematocrit-venous hematocrit ratio
BI — bacteriological index
     burn index
Bi — bismuth
biallylamicol
Bial's reagent
bibulous
bicameral
bicarbonate
   blood b.
   plasma b.
   b. of soda
biceps
   b. brachii muscle
   b. femoris muscle
   b. femoris superior muscle
   b. tendon
bichloride
bicipital
bicipitoradialis
biconcave
biconvex
bicornuate

bicuspid
- b. aortic valve

BIDLB — block in the postero-inferior division of the left branch

Biebrich scarlet
Bielschowsky-Jansky disease
Bielschowsky's method
Biermer's anemia
bifascicular
- b. block

bifid
- b. tongue
- b. ureter
- b. uterus

Bifidobacterium
- *B. bifidum*
- *B. eriksonii*
- *B. infantis*

bifurcation
bigeminal
bigeminy
- ventricular b.

BIH — benign intracranial hypertension
BIL — bilirubin
bil — bilateral
bilat — bilateral
bilateral
bile
- b. acids
- b. canaliculi
- capillary b.
- b. cast
- b. extravasation
- b. infarct
- b. lake
- b. nephrosis
- b. pigment demonstration in tissue
- b. pigments

bile *(continued)*
- b. salts
- b. solubility test
- b. stasis

bile duct
- b. d. adenoma
- b. d. canaliculus
- b. d. carcinoma
- common b. d.
- cystic b. d.
- extrahepatic b. d.
- hepatic b. d.
- interlobular b. d.
- intrahepatic b. d.

bile ductule
- intralobular b. d.
- periportal b. d.

Bilharzia
bilharzial
bilharziasis
biliary
- b. achalasia
- b. atresia
- b. cirrhosis
- b. fistula
- b. obstruction

biliousness
bilirubin
- b. encephalopathy

bilirubinemia
- hereditary nonhemolytic b.

bilirubinuria
biliverdin
billion electron volts
Billroth's
- cords
- operation

bilobate
bilobed
Bilopaque
bimodal

bimolecular
binary
    b. acid
    b. addition
    b. code
    b. coded decimal
    b. digit
    b. fission
    b. variate
binasal hemianopsia
binding energy
binomial
    b. coefficient
    b. distribution
    b. nomenclature
binuclear
binucleate
bioaccumulation
bioassay
bioavailability
biochemical
    b. energetics
biochemistry
biodegradability
biodegradable
bioenergetics
bioequivalence
biofeedback
biogenesis
biogenetic
biohazard
    b. sign
    b. symbol
biologic
    b. false-positive
biological
Biological Stain Commission
biology
    population b.
bioluminescence
biomass
biomechanics

biomedical engineering
biometry
Biomphalaria
    B. glabrata
bionics
biophysics
biopsy
    aspiration b.
    cone b.
    excisional b.
    fine-needle b.
    incisional b.
    punch b.
    thin-needle b.
biopterin
biosynthesis
biotin
biotinidase
biotransformation
biotype
BIP — bismuth iodoform paraffin
biparietal
    b. hump
biperiden
biphasic
biphenamine
biphenyl
bipolar
    b. cell
    b. neuron
bipyridyl
birefringence
    crystalline b.
    flow b.
    form b.
    strain b.
birefringent
birthmark
    vascular b.
bisacodyl
    b. tannex

bisalbuminemia
bis(2-chloroethyl) sulfide
bis-(*p*-chlorophenoxy) methane
bis-(*p*-chlorophenyl) ethanol
1-1-bis-(*p*-chlorophenyl)-2-
 nitrobutane
1-1-bis(*p*-chlorophenyl)-2-
 nitropropane
bis-(*p*-chlorophenyl) trichloroethanol
bis-(diethylthiocarbamyl) disulfide
bis-(dimethylamino)-phospho-
 rus anhydride
bis-(dimethylthiocarbamyl)
 disulfide
bisection
bishydroxycoumarin
bismuth
    b. aluminate
    b. pigmentation
    b. subcarbonate
    b. subgallate
    b. subsalicylate
    b. violet
bisphosphatidylglycerol
bisphosphoglycerate
    b. phosphatase
bisphosphoglyceromutase
bis-trimethylsilylacetamide
bisulfate
bisulfite
bitemporal hemianopsia
bithionol
Bithynia
Bitot's spots
biundulant milk fever virus
biuret
    b. reaction
bivalent
BJ — Bence Jones

BJP — Bence Jones protein
Bk — berkelium
BL — baseline
    Bessey-Lowry (units)
    bleeding
    blood loss
    buccolingual
    Burkitt's lymphoma
black
    b. fly
    b. hairy tongue
    b. lung disease
    b. tongue
    b. widow spider
blackbody
    b. radiation
bladder
    neurogenic b.
    urinary b.
blast
    b. cell
    b. cell leukemia
    b. crisis
blastema
blastic
    b. transformation
blastocyst
Blastocystis
    B. hominis
blastocyte
blastoderm
blastogenesis
blastoma
    pluricentric b.
    unicentric b.
blastomere
Blastomyces
    B. brasiliensis
    B. coccidioides
    B. dermatitidis
blastomycin

blastomycosis
    European b.
    North American b.
    South American b.
blastospore
blastula (blastulae)
blastulation
Blattidae
BLB unit — Bessey-Lowry-Brock unit
bl cult — blood culture
bleaching
bleb
    emphysematous b.
bleeding
    functional b.
    implantation b.
    occult b.
    placentation b.
bleeding time
    Duke's method of b. t.
    Ivy's method of b. t.
blennorrhagia
blennorrhagic
blennorrhea
    b. adultorum
    inclusion b.
    b. neonatorum
bleomycin
    b. sulfate
blepharitis
    b. ulcerosa
blepharoplast
blepharoptosis
BLG — beta-lactoglobulin
blighted ovum
blindness
    color b.
    night b.
    word b.
blink responses

blister
    blood b.
    fever b.
    Marochetti's b's
BLN — bronchial lymph nodes
block
    adrenergic b.
    alveolar-capillary b.
    bundle-branch b.
    caudal b.
    epidural b.
    intercostal b.
    intraspinal b.
    methadone b.
    nerve b.
    paracervical b.
    parasacral b.
    paravertebral b.
    perineural b.
    sacral b.
    sinoatrial b.
    stellate b.
    subarachnoid b.
    sympathetic b.
    tubal b.
    uterosacral b.
    vagal b.
    ventricular b.
    Wenckebach b.
blockade
    adrenergic b.
    adrenergic neuron b.
    alpha b.
    alpha-adrenergic b.
    beta-adrenergic b.
    cholinergic b.
    narcotic b.
    renal b.
    virus b.
blocker
    beta b.

blocking
- adrenergic b.
- b. antibody

blood
- b.-air barrier
- anticoagulated b.
- arterial b.
- b. bank
- b.-brain barrier
- b. buffering capacity
- b.-cerebral barrier
- citrated b.
- b. clot
- b. coagulation disorder
- b. component
- cord b.
- b. culture
- defibrinated b.
- b. dyscrasia
- b. extravasation
- b. film
- b. fluke
- b. gas analysis
- b. gases
- b. glucose
- b. groups (ABO)
- b. island
- b. lancet
- b. loss anemia
- occult b.
- peripheral b.
- b. poisoning
- b. pool scan
- b. pressure
- b. smear
- splanchnic b.
- b. sugar
- b. typing
- b. urea clearance
- b. urea nitrogen
- venous b.
- b. vessel

blood *(continued)*
- b. volume measurements
- whole b.

blood cell(s)
- b. c. count
- erythrocytic b. c.
- granulocytic b. c.
- lymphocytic b. c.
- megakaryocytic b. c.
- monocytic b. c.
- plasma b. c.
- plasmacytic b. c.

Bloodgood's disease

blood serum
- Löffler's b. s.

blood urea nitrogen

blood vessel
- embryonic b. v.
- vitelline b. v.

Bloom's syndrome

Bloor's test

Blount's disease

blowback

Bloxam's test

BLP — Boothby, Lovelace, Bulbulian (mask)

bl pr — blood pressure

BLT — blood-clot lysis time

BLU — Bessey-Lowry units

blue
- b. baby
- b. diaper syndrome
- b. dome cyst
- b. nevus
- b. rubber bleb disease
- Turnbull b.

Blumberg's sign

blunt duct adenosis

BM — basement membrane
body mass
bone marrow
bowel movement

BM *(continued)*
    buccomesial
BMG — benign monoclonal gammopathy
bmk — birthmark
B-mode
BMR — basal metabolic rate
BN — branchial neuritis
BNO — bladder neck obstruction
BNPA — binasal pharyngeal airway
BNS — benign nephrosclerosis
BO — bucco-occlusal
B & O — belladonna and opium
Boas-Oppler
    bacillus
    lactobacillus
Boas' test
BOBA — beta-oxybutyric acids
Bochdalek's foramen
Bodansky unit
Bodian's method
Bodo
    B. caudatus
    B. saltans
    B. urinaria
Bodonidae
body (bodies)
    Aschoff's b.
    asteroid b's
    Auer's b's
    Balbiani's b.
    Barr b's
    Cabot's ring b's
    Call-Exner b's
    b. cavity
    chromatin b's
    Civatte's b.
    conchoidal b.
    contact b.
    Councilman's b's

body (bodies) *(continued)*
    Cowdry b's
    Döhle's inclusion b's
    Donné's b's
    Donovan's b's
    F b.
    fibrin b.
    fibrous b.
    b. fluids
    foreign b.
    Gall B.
    Gordon's b.
    Guarnieri's b's
    Heinz b's
    Heinz-Ehrlich b's
    Herring b's
    Howell-Jolly b's
    Howell's b's
    inclusion b's
    b. joint
    Jolly's b's
    ketone b's
    Lafora's b's
    Leishman-Donovan b's
    Lewy b.
    louse b.
    Mallory's b's
    Maragiliano b.
    melon seed b.
    Michaelis-Gutmann b's
    Negri b's
    Nissl b's
    Pappenheimer b.
    Pick's b's
    psammoma b's
    rice b.
    Russell's b.
    Schaumann's b's
    b.-section radiography
    spiculated b's
    b. surface area
    thermostable b.

70 BODY (BODIES) – BONE

body (bodies) *(continued)*
    Todd b's
    Verocay b.
    b. wall
    Weibel-Palade b.
    Wesenberg-Hamazaki b.
    X chromatin b's
BOEA – ethyl biscoumacetate
Boeck-Drbohlav-Locke egg-serum medium
Boeck's
    disease
    sarcoid
Boettcher cells
Bogaert's disease
Bohr
    effect
    equation
    magneton
Bol. – pill (*bolus*)
Boletus
Boltzmann constant
bolus
    b. alba
    alimentary b.
BOM – bilateral otitis media
Bombay phenotype
bombesin
Bombidae
Bombus californicus
Bonanno's test
bond
    coordinate covalent b.
    covalent b.
    electron pair b.
    b. energy
    high-energy b.
    hydrogen b.
    ionic b.
    metallic b.
    peptide b.
    pi b.

bond *(continued)*
    sigma b.
bonding
bone
    capitate b.
    carpal b.
    b. cell
    b. conduction
    cortex b.
    cranial b.
    b. crystal alteration
    b. cyst
    ethmoid b.
    facial b.
    frontal b.
    hamate b.
    hyoid b.
    innominate b.
    lunate b.
    b. marrow
    b. marrow abnormality
    b. marrow aspiration
    b. marrow biopsy
    b. marrow differential count
    b. marrow embolus
    b. marrow scan
    b. matrix alteration
    occipital b.
    palatine b.
    parietal b.
    pelvic b's
    pisiform b.
    b. resorption
    b. scan
    scaphoid b.
    b. sclerosis
    sesamoid b.
    sphenoid b.
    b. spur
    tarsal b.
    temporal b.

bone *(continued)*
    trabecular b.
    trapezial b.
    trapezoidal b.
    triangular b.
    b. tumor
    zygomatic b.
bongkrekic acid
Bonnet's plexus
Bonnevie-Ullrich syndrome
bony
    b. ankylosis
    b. callus
Boolean
    algebra
    function
Boophilus
    B. annulatus
booster
bootstrap loader
borate
borax
Borchgrevink method
border
Bordetella
    B. bronchiseptica
    B. parapertussis
    B. pertussis
Bordet-Gengou
    agar
    bacillus
Bordet's amboceptor
boric acid
borism
borneol
Bornholm disease
bornyl
    b. chloride
boroglycerin
boron
    b. carbide
    b. trifluoride-methanol

boron *(continued)*
    b. trioxide
borosilicate glass
Borrelia
    B. aegyptica
    B. anserina
    B. berbera
    B. buccalis
    B. carteri
    B. caucasica
    B. duttonii
    B. hermsii
    B. hispanica
    B. kochii
    B. neotropicalis
    B. novyi
    B. parkeri
    B. persica
    B. recurrentis
    B. refringens
    B. theileri
    B. turicatae
    B. venezuelensis
    B. vincentii
Borst-Jadassohn intraepidermal
    basal cell epithelioma
boss
    parietal b's
Boston exanthem
bothridium
bothrium
Bothrops atrox serine
    proteinase
botryoid
    b. rhabdomyosarcoma
    b. sarcoma
botryomycosis
botulin
botulinum toxin
botulism
Bouchard's nodes
bougie

bougienage
Bouguer's law
Bouin's fluid
Bourneville's disease
bouton
    b. en passant
    terminal b.
    b's termineaux
boutonneuse fever
bovine
    b. gamma globulin
    b. serum albumin
bowel
bowel sounds
    hyperactive b. s.
    hypoactive b. s.
Bowen's disease
Bowers-McComb unit
Bowie's stain
Bowman's
    capsule
    glands
    lamina
    membrane
Boyden chamber
Boyle's law
BP — back pressure
    benzpyrene
    blood pressure
    bronchopleural
    buccopulpal
    bypass
bp — base pair
    boiling point
BPH — benign prostatic hypertrophy
BPL — beta-propiolactone
BPO — benzylpenicilloyl
Bq — becquerel
BR — bilirubin
Br — bromine
Br. — Brucella

brachial
    b. artery
    b. fascia
    b. lymph node
    b. neuritis
    b. plexus
    b. vein
brachialis muscle
brachiocephalic
    b. artery
    b. vein
brachioradialis muscle
brachium
    b. conjunctivum
    b. pontis
brachycephalic
brachydactyly
brachytherapy
Bradshaw's
    albumosuria
    test
bradyarrhythmia
bradycardia
    junctional b.
    nodal b.
    sinus b.
    b.-tachycardia syndrome
bradykinin
Bragg
    curve
    reflection
brain
    b. artery
    b. death syndrome
    olfactory b.
    respirator b.
    b. sand
    b. scan
    b. stem
    b. stem auditory evoked potential
    b. waves

braking radiation
branch
branched
    b. chain
    b.-chain aminoaciduria
    b.-chain ketoacid decarboxylase
    b.-chain ketoacid dehydrogenase
    b.-chain ketoaciduria
brancher
    b. deficiency
    b. enzyme
branchial
    b. arch
    b. cleft cyst
    b. cleft sinus
    b. cyst
    b. region
branching
    b. decay
    b. enzyme
    b. fraction
    b. ratio
Branhamella
    B. catarrhalis
Brasil's fixative
brazilin
BRBC — bovine red blood cells
BrdU — 5-bromodeoxyuridine
breakdown
    Zener's b.
breast
    Cooper's irritable b.
    funnel b.
    shotty b.
    b. specimen radiography
    b. tumors
breathing
    b. frequency
    b. zone
Brecher-Cronkite method

Brecher's new methylene blue technique
breech presentation
breeder reactor
Breed smear
bregma
bremsstrahlung
Brenner tumor
Breus mole
brevicollis
bridge
    conjugation b.
bridging
    b. hepatic necrosis
    b. vein
brilliant
    b. cresyl blue
    b. crocein
    b. green
    b. purpurin
Brill's disease
Brill-Symmers disease
Brill-Zinsser disease
British
    B. antilewisite
    B. thermal unit
BRM — biuret-reactive material
broad
    b.-beta disease
    b. fish tapeworm
    b.-spectrum
Broca's area
Broders' index
Brodie's abscess
broken cell preparation
bromate
brombenzyl cyanide
bromcresol purple desoxycholate
bromelain
bromide
bromination

bromine
- b. isotope

brominism

bromism

bromisovalum

bromocresol
- b. green
- b. purple

bromocriptine
- b. mesylate
- b. suppression test

bromodeoxyuracil

bromodeoxyuridine

bromoderma

bromodiphenhydramine hydrochloride

bromoiodism

bromomethane

bromophenol blue

2-bromo-4-phenyl phenol

bromothymol blue

brompheniramine
- b. maleate

Bromsulphalein

bronchial
- b. adenoma
- b. artery
- b. asthma
- b. branch
- b. breathing
- b. carcinoma
- b. cartilage
- b. lumen
- b. lymph node
- b. mucous gland
- b. mucus
- b. submucosa
- b. tree
- b. vein

bronchiectasis
- cylindrical b.
- fusiform b.

bronchiectasis *(continued)*
- saccular b.

bronchiolar
- b. adenocarcinoma
- b. carcinoma
- b. cell

bronchiole
- respiratory b.
- terminal b.

bronchiolectasis

bronchiolitis
- b. fibrosa obliterans

bronchiolization

bronchitis
- acute b.
- asthmatic b.
- chronic b.

bronchium

bronchoaspergillosis

bronchoblastomycosis

bronchocandidiasis

bronchoconstriction

bronchoconstrictor

bronchodilatation

bronchodilator

bronchoesophageal

bronchoesophagoscopy

bronchogenic
- b. carcinoma
- b. cyst

bronchography
- Cope method of b.

broncholithiasis

bronchomalacia

bronchomycosis

bronchopathy

bronchopleural

bronchopneumonia
- acute b.
- acute hemorrhagic b.
- confluent b.
- diffuse b.

bronchopneumonia *(continued)*
    focal b.
    hemorrhagic b.
    necrotizing b.
    sequestration b.
    subacute b.
    virus b.
bronchopneumopathy
bronchopulmonary
    b. lavage
    b. segment
bronchoscopy
    fiberoptic b.
bronchospasm
bronchospirometry
bronchostenosis
bronchotracheal
    b. aspirate
bronchus
Brönsted-Lowry
    acid
    base
bronzed diabetes
Brooke's tumor
broth
    brain-heart infusion b.
    chopped meat b.
    gram-negative b.
    hippurate b.
    indole-nitrate b.
    Middlebrook's b.
    Mueller-Hinton b.
    nutrient b.
    selenite b.
    sodium chloride b.
    thioglycollate b.
    Todd-Hewitt b.
    trypticase soy with agar b.
    Voges-Proskauer b.
brown
    b. atrophy
    b. fat

brown *(continued)*
    b. recluse spider
    b. tumor
Brown-Brenn technique
brownian movement
Brown-Séquard syndrome
BRP — bilirubin production
brth — breath
Brucella
    B. abortus
    B. bronchiseptica
    B. canis
    B. melitensis
    B. suis
brucella
    b. agglutination test
Brucellaceae
brucellin
brucellosis
Bruch's basal membrane
brucine
Brudzinski's sign
Brugia
    B. malayi
    B. microfilariae
bruise
bruising
bruit
Brunhilde virus
Brunner's glands
Brunn's epithelial nests
brush border
Bruton's
    agammaglobulinemia
    disease
BS — blood sugar
       breath sounds
BSA — bismuth-sulfite agar
        body surface area
        bovine serum albumin
BSAP — brief short-action
         potential

76 BSB – BULLOUS

BSB – body surface burned
BSDLB – block in the antero-superior division of the left branch
BSE – bilateral symmetrical and equal
BSF – back scatter factor
BSI – bound serum iron
BSO – bilateral salpingo-oophorectomy
BSP – Bromsulphalein
BSR – basal skin resistance
BSS – balanced salt solution
 buffered saline solution
BT – bladder tumor
 bleeding time
 brain tumor
BTB – breakthrough bleeding
BTPS – body temperature, ambient pressure, saturated
BTR – Bezold-type reflex
BTU – British thermal unit
BU – Bodansky units
bubo
bubonic plague
buccal
 b. branch
 b. cavity
 b. gland
 b. mucosa
 b. nerve
 b. region
Bucky grid
buclizine hydrochloride
Budd-Chiari syndrome
budding
BUDR – bromodeoxyuracil
BUDU – bromodeoxyuridine
Buerger's disease
buffer
 b. base

buffer *(continued)*
 bicarbonate b.
 cacodylate b.
 b. capacity
 Holmes' alkaline b.
 phosphate b.
 protein b.
 b. system
 b. value
 veronal b.
buffered desoxycholate glucose
buffy coat smear
Bulan
bulb
 duodenal b.
 end b.
 Krause's end b.
 olfactory b.
 sinovaginal b.
 vaginal b.
bulbar
 b. conjunctiva
 b. palsy
bulbocapnine
bulbopontine
bulbospongiosus
bulbourethral
bulbus (bulbi)
 b. cordis
 b. oculi
 b. penis
bulimia
Bulimus
 B. fuchsianus
Bulinus
bulla (bullae)
Bullis fever
bullosis
 b. diabeticorum
bullous
 b. emphysema
 b. inflammation

bullous *(continued)*
    b. lichen planus
    b. pemphigoid
BUN — blood urea nitrogen
bunamiodyl
bundle
    b. bone
    b. branch block
    b. of His
Büngner's bands
bunion
Bunsen
    burner
    coefficient
Bunyamwera virus
Bunyaviridae
bunyavirus
buoyant density
buphthalmos
bupivacaine hydrochloride
Burdach's tract
buret, burette
Burkitt's tumor
burn
    first degree b.
    fourth degree b.
    second degree b.
    third degree b.
    ultraviolet b.
burner
    Bunsen b.
Burnett's syndrome
Burow's solution
burr cell
bursa
    anserine b.
    b. of biceps femoris superior muscle
    b. of bicipitoradialis
    b. of calcaneal tendon
    b. of extensor carpi radialis brevis muscle

bursa *(continued)*
    b. of Fabricius
    iliac b.
    infrahyoid b.
    infrapatellar b.
    intermuscular b.
    ischial b.
    omental b.
    b. of piriformis muscle
    retrohyoid b.
    retromammary b.
    sacral b.
    b. of semimembranosus muscle
    subacromial b.
    subcutaneous b.
    subdeltoid b.
    subfascial b.
    submuscular b.
    subtendinous b.
    suprapatellar b.
    b. of tensor veli palatini muscle
    trochanteric b.
bursitis
burst-suppression
BUS — Bartholin's, urethral, Skene's (glands)
Buschke-Löwenstein giant condyloma
Busse-Buschke disease
Busse's saccharomyces
busulfan, busulphan
    b. lung
butabarbital sodium
butadiene
butane
butanoic acid
butanol
    b.-extractable iodine
2-butanone
butaperazine

78 BUTENE – c.

butene
butethamine hydrochloride
butopyronoxyl
butorphanol tartrate
butoxypolypropylene glycol
buttock
butyl
    b. acetate
    b. alcohol
    b. aminobenzoate
    b. carbitol
    b. chloride
    b. methacrylate
N-butyl acetanilide
butyleneglycol dehydrogenase
butylidene chloride
butylmethyl ketone
butylphenamide
butyrate coenzyme A transferase
Butyribacterium
butyrophenone
butyryl-coenzyme A dehydrogenase

BV — biologic value
    blood vessel
    blood volume
    bronchovesicular
BVH — biventricular hypertrophy
BVI — blood vessel invasion
BVV — bovine vaginitis virus
BW — birth weight
    body water
    body weight
Bwamba
    B. fever
    B. virus
BX — biopsy
BYE — Barile-Yaguchi-Eveland (culture medium)
Byler's disease
bypass
    b. capacitor
byssinosis
byte

C

C — calculus
    calorie (large)
    carbohydrate
    carbon
    cervical
    chest
    clonus
    complement
    compound
    contracture
    curie
C. — cathodal
    cathode
    Celsius

C. *(continued)*
    centigrade
    cervical
    clearance
    clonus
    closure
    color sense
    congius (gallon)
    contraction
    cylinder
C. — *Clostridium*
    Cryptococcus
c. — calorie (small)
    contact

c. *(continued)*
   curie
C_{alb} — albumin clearance
C_{am} — amylase clearance
C_{cr} — creatinine clearance
C_{in} — insulin clearance
C_{pah} — para-aminohippurate clearance
C_u — urea clearance
C1q immunoradioassay
c' — coefficient of partage
CA — carcinoma
   cardiac arrest
   cathode
   cervicoaxial
   chronological age
   cold agglutinin
   common antigen
   coronary artery
   corpora amylacea
   croup-associated (virus)
Ca — calcium
   cancer
   cathodal
   cathode
caapi
CAB — coronary artery bypass
CABG — coronary artery bypass graft
Cabot's ring bodies
cacao oil
CACC — cathodal closure contraction
cachectic anergy
cache memory
Cache Valley virus
cachexia
   cancerous c.
   c. exophthalmica
   c. hypophysiopriva
   malarial c.
   c. strumipriva

cachexia *(continued)*
   c. suprarenalis
   thyroid c.
   uremic c.
cacodylic acid
cactinomycin
cacumen
CAD — coronary artery disease
cadaver
cadaverine
cadmium
   c. assays
   c. sulfide
   c. telluride detector
CADTe — cathodal-duration tetanus
café au lait spots
caffeine sodium benzoate
CAG — chronic atrophic gastritis
CAH — chronic active hepatitis
   congenital adrenal hyperplasia
CAHD — coronary atherosclerotic heart disease
CAHEA — Committee on Allied Health Education and Accreditation
caisson disease
Cajal's
   formol ammonium bromide solution
   gold-sublimate method
   uranium silver method
Cal — large calorie
cal — small calorie
calabar swelling
calamine
calamus
   c. scriptorius
calcaneal
calcaneus

calcar
   c. avis
   c. femorale
   c. pedis
calcareous
calcarine
   c. artery
   c. fissure
calcemia
calcicosis
calciferol
calcific
   c. aortic stenosis
   c. concretions
   c. nodular stenosis
   c. stenosis
calcification
   dystrophic c.
   focal c.
   medial c.
   metastatic c.
   Mönckeberg's medial c.
calcified
   c. granuloma
   c. granulomatous inflammation
calcifying
   c. ameloblastoma
   c. epithelial odontogenic tumor
   Malherbe's c. epithelioma
calcinosis
   c. circumscripta
   c. universalis
calciorrhachia
calciotropism
calcipenia
calcipexy
calciphilia
calciphylaxis
   systemic c.

calciphylaxis *(continued)*
   topical c.
calcite
calcitonin
calcitriol
calcitropic
calcium
   c. acetate formalin
   c. aminosalicylate
   c. arsenate
   c. arsenite
   c. assays
   Baker's formol c.
   c. calculus
   c. carbimide, citrated
   c. carbonate
   c. caseinate
   c. caustic alkali
   c. chloride
   c. compound
   c. cyanamide
   c. cyanide
   c. deposit demonstration
   c. deposition
   c. disodium edathamil
   c. gluconate
   c. ion
   c. isotope
   c. lactate
   c. leucovorin
   c. orotate
   c. oxalate
   c. oxalate test
   c. pantothenate
   c. phosphate
   c. polysulfide
   c. red
   c. undecylenate
calciuria
calcivirus
calcoglobulin

calcospherite
calculosis
calculus
    articular c.
    biliary c.
    calcium oxalate c.
    calcium phosphate c.
    cholesterol c.
    cystine c.
    dental c.
    joint c.
    lacrimal c.
    mixed c.
    pigment c.
    renal c.
    salivary c.
    struvite c.
    urate c.
    uric acid c.
    urinary c.
    vesical c.
Caldwell-Moloy
    classification
    method
Caldwell projection
calefacient
calentura, calenture
calf
calibrate
calibration
    c. curve
    c. materials
caliculus
California encephalitis
    C. e. virus
californium
calix (calices)
Call-Exner bodies
calling sequence
Calliphora
    C. vomitoria

Callitroga
callosal
callosity
callosomarginal
callosum
callus
    bony c.
    central c.
    definitive c.
    ensheathing c.
    myelogenous c.
    provisional c.
Calmette-Guérin bacillus
calmodulin
calomel
calor
    c. febrilis
    c. fervens
    c. innatus
    c. mordicans
calorie
calorigenesis
calorigenic
calorimeter
calorimetry
calotte
calsequestrin
calusterone
calutron
calvacin
calvaria
Calvatia
    C. gigantea
Calvé-Perthes disease
Calymmatobacterium
    C. donovania
    C. granulomatis
calyx (calyces)
    c. chlorata
    major c.
    minor c.

calyx (calyces) *(continued)*
    c. sulfurata
CAM — chorioallantoic membrane
        contralateral axillary metastasis
camera
    c. lucida
    c. oculi
    c. pulpi
    scintillation c.
cAMP — adenosine 3′,5′-cyclic phosphate
        cyclic adenosine monophosphate
Campbell's cruciate sulcus
Camp-Gianturco method
camphene
camphor
camphorism
CAMP test
camptocormia
Campylobacter
    C. fetus
    C. fetus intestinalis
    C. fetus jejuni
    C. sputorum
Canada balsam
Canada-Cronkhite syndrome
canal
    adductor c.
    anal c.
    auditory c.
    cervical c.
    Cloquet's c.
    endocervical c.
    femoral c.
    Hering's c.
    Hunter's c.
    hyaloid c.
    inguinal c.
    internal auditory c.

canal *(continued)*
    Nuck's c.
    Schlemm's c.
    semicircular c.
    spiral c.
    Sucquet-Hoyer c.
    Volkmann's c.
canaliculus (canaliculi)
    apical c.
    bile canaliculi
    innominate c.
    intercellular c.
    mastoid c.
    secretory c.
    tympanic c.
canalization
canavalin
canavaninosuccinic acid
cancellous
    c. bone
cancer
    c. alternate therapies
    c.-free white mouse
    c. management therapy
    c. promoter
    c. staging
candela
candicidin
Candida
    C. albicans
    C. albidus
    C. guilliermondi
    C. krusei
    C. laurentii
    C. lusitaniae
    C. luteolus
    C. parakrusei
    C. parapsilosis
    C. pseudotropicalis
    C. stellatoidea
    C. tropicalis
    C. viswanathii

candidal
candida precipitin test
candidemia
candidiasis
candidid
candidin
candidosis
canescent
canities
canker
   c. sore
cannabinoid
cannabis
cannabism
cannon wave
cannula
cannulation
   venous c.
canrenoate potassium
canrenone
cantharidin
canthomeatal
   c. line
canthus (canthi)
   inner c.
   outer c.
CAO – chronic airway obstruction
CAP – capsule
   cellulose acetate phthalate
   chloramphenicol
   College of American Pathologists
   cystine aminopeptidase
cap
   c. cell
   cradle c.
   head c.
   knee c.
   phrygian c.
   pyloric c.

cap *(continued)*
   skull c.
capacitance
   membrane c.
capacitation
capacitor
   ceramic c.
   disk c.
   electrolytic c.
   junction c.
   Mylar c.
   paper c.
   variable c.
capacity
Capillaria
   C. hepatica
   C. philippinensis
capillariasis
capillaropathy
capillary (capillaries)
   arterial c's
   basement membrane c's
   bile c's
   continuous c's
   endothelial c's
   erythrocytic c's
   fenestrated c's
   c. fragility
   glomerular c's
   c. hemangioma
   lymphatic c's
   secretory c's
   sinusoidal c's
   venous c's
capillus
capistration
capitate
Caplan's syndrome
capneic
Capnocytophaga
capnohepatography
capobenate sodium

capotement
capping
capreomycin
capric acid
caproic acid
caprylic acid
capsicum
capsid
capsomer
capsular
    c. cell
    c. space
capsule
    adrenal c.
    articular c.
    Bowman's c.
    c. cell
    external c.
    extreme c.
    Glisson's c.
    hepatic c.
    internal c.
    kidney c.
    lens c.
    lymph node c.
    ovarian c.
    pituitary c.
    prostate c.
    salivary gland c.
    splenic c.
    thymic c.
    thyroid c.
    tonsillar c.
capsulitis
    adhesive c.
captamine hydrochloride
captodiamine hydrochloride
caput (capita)
    c. medusae
    c. succedaneum
Carazzi's hematoxylin
carbachol

carbamate
    ethyl c.
    c. kinase
carbamazepine
    c. assay
carbamide
carbaminocarbon dioxide
carbaminohemoglobin
carbamoyl
    c. phosphate
    c.-phosphate synthetase
carbamoyltransferase
carbamylurea
carbanion
carbarsone
    c. oxide
carbaryl
carbaspirin calcium
carbazochrome salicylate
carbenicillin
    c. disodium
    c. indanyl sodium
    c. phenyl sodium
    c. potassium
    c. sodium
carbenoxolone sodium
carbetapentane citrate
carbide
carbimazole
carbinol
carbinoxamine maleate
Carbitol
carbohydrate
    c. identification test
carbol-fuchsin
    c. methylene blue staining method
carbolic acid
carbolineum
carbolism
carbolxylene
carbomycin

carbon
- c. bisulfide
- c. dioxide
- c. dioxide absorbent
- c. dioxide combining power
- c. dioxide combining power measurements
- c. dioxide concentration
- c. dioxide concentration assays
- c. dioxide dissociation curve
- c. dioxide fixation
- c. dioxide output
- c. dioxide production
- c. dioxide response curve
- c. dioxide tension
- c. disulfide
- c. disulfide assays
- c. gelatin mass
- c. inorganic compound
- c. isotope
- c. monoxide
- c. monoxide assays
- c. monoxide fractional uptake
- c. oxysulfide
- radioactive c.
- c. tetrachloride
- c. tetrachloride assays
- c. trichloride

carbonate
- c. dehydratase
- ferrous c.

carbonic
- c. acid
- c. anhydrase
- c. anhydrase inhibitor

carbonuria
- dysoxidative c.

carbonyl
- c. chloride

carbonyl *(continued)*
- c. hemoglobin

carbophenothion
carboprost
Carborundum
Carbowax
carboxydismutase
Carboxydomonas
carboxyglutamate
carboxyhemoglobin
carboxyhemoglobinemia
carboxyhemoglobinuria
carboxyl
carboxylase
carboxylate ion
carboxylesterase
carboxylic
- c. acid
- c. ester hydrolase

carboxyl terminal
carboxyltransferase
carboxymethylcellulose sodium
carboxypeptidase
alpha-carboxypeptide amino-acidohydrolase
carboxypolypeptidase
carbromal
carbuncle
- malignant c.
- renal c.

carbunculosis
carcinelcosis
carcinemia
carcinoembryonic
- c. antigen

carcinogen
carcinogenesis
carcinogenic
carcinoid
- c. heart disease
- c. syndrome

carcinoid *(continued)*
   c. tumor
carcinoma(s)
   acinar cell c.
   adenoid cystic c.
   adenosquamous c.
   adnexal c.
   adrenal cortical c.
   alveolar c.
   anaplastic c.
   basal cell c.
   basaloid c.
   basosquamous c.
   bile duct c.
   bile duct c., hepatocellular
   bronchial c.
   bronchiolar c.
   bronchogenic c.
   ceruminous c.
   cloacogenic c.
   colloid c.
   embryonal c.
   epidermoid c.
   follicular c.
   gelatinous c.
   giant cell c.
   granulosa cell c.
   hepatocellular c.
   Hürthle cell c.
   infiltrating duct c.
   infiltrating lobular c.
   inflammatory c.
   intraductal c.
   intraepidermal c.
   islet cell c.
   liver cell c.
   lobular c.
   medullary c.
   mesometanephric c.
   metastatic c.
   mixed hepatocellular c.
   mucinous c.

carcinoma(s) *(continued)*
   mucoepidermoid c.
   oat cell c.
   papillary c.
   papillary transitional cell c.
   pleomorphic c.
   recurrent c.
   renal cell c.
   reserve cell c.
   residual c.
   scirrhous c.
   sebaceous c.
   secondary c.
   signet ring c.
   simplex c.
   c. in situ
   small cell c.
   solid c.
   spindle cell c.
   squamous cell c.
   superficial multicentric
     basal cell c.
   sweat gland c.
   thymic c.
   trabecular c.
   transitional cell c.
   undifferentiated c.
   verrucous c.
   wolffian duct c.
carcinomatosis
carcinomatous
carcinosarcoma
   embryonal c.
carcinosis
card
   c. punch
   c. reader
cardia
cardiac
   c. arrest
   c. catheterization
   c. cirrhosis

cardiac *(continued)*
    c. conduction alteration
    c. conduction system
    c. cycle
    c. decompensation
    c. dilation
    c. edema
    c. enlargement
    c. failure
    c. fibrillation
    c. glycoside
    c. index
    c. massage
    c. murmur
    c. muscle
    c. nerve
    c. output
    c. plexus
    c. rate alteration
    c. rhythm alteration
    c. sclerosis
    c. shunt detection
    c. silhouette
    c. sound alteration
    c. standstill
    c. tamponade
    c. valve
    c. valvular malformation
    c. valvular regurgitation
    c. vein
cardiasthenia
cardiectasis
cardinal
cardioangiography
Cardiobacterium
    C. hominis
cardiocentesis
cardiochalasia
cardioesophageal
cardiogenesis
cardiogenic
Cardiografin
cardiogram
cardiography
cardiolipin
    c. natural lecithin
    c. synthetic lecithin
cardiology
cardiomegaly
cardiomyopathy
cardiopathy
cardioplegia
cardiopulmonary
    c. resuscitation
cardiospasm
cardiosphygmograph
cardiotachometer
cardiothoracic (ratio)
cardiotocography
cardiotoxic
cardiovascular
    c. malformation
    c. murmur
    c. system
cardiovascular disease
    arteriosclerotic c. d.
    hypertensive c. d.
cardioversion
cardioverter
cardiovirus
carditis
    rheumatic c.
    streptococcal c.
    verrucous c.
Carey's Ranvier technique
caries
carina (carinae)
    c. of trachea
    c. of vagina
carinate
cariogenesis
carious
carisoprodol
carmalum

carmine
  alizarin c.
  chrome alum c.
  c. gelatin mass
  indigo c.
  lithium c.
carminic acid
carmustine
carnaceous
carnification
carnitine acetyltransferase
Carnivora
carnosinase
carnosine
carnosinemia
carnosinuria
Carnoy's fixative
carotenase
carotene
  c. assays
carotenemia
carotenoid
carotic
caroticotympanic
carotid
  c. artery
  c. body
  c. body tumor
  c. nerve
  c. plexus
  c. sheath
  c. sinus
  c. sinus nerve
  c. sinus stimulation
  c. sinus syncope
  c. sinus syndrome
  c. tracing
carpal
  c. bone
  c. tunnel
  c. tunnel decompression
  c. tunnel syndrome

carphenazine maleate
carphology
Carpoglyphus
  C. passularum
carpometacarpal
carpophalangeal
carpoptosis
carprofen
carpus
carrier
  c.-free
  c. gas
  c.-mediated transport
  c. protein
Carrión's disease
cartilage
  articular c.
  arytenoid c.
  auricular c.
  bronchial c.
  corniculate c.
  costal c.
  cricoid c.
  cuneiform c.
  epiglottic c.
  fibroelastic c.
  greater alar c.
  hyaline c.
  laryngeal c.
  lateral nasal c.
  c. matrix alteration
  Meckel's c.
  nasal c.
  nasal septal c.
  Santorini's c.
  thyroid c.
  tracheal c.
  vomeronasal c.
cartilaginous
  c. exostosis
  c. metaplasia
  c. rest

caruncle
    amniotic c's
    hymenal c's
    lacrimal c.
    sublingual c.
    urethral c.
carvacrol
casanthranol
cascade
    electron c.
cascara sagrada
case
    c.-control study
    c. history
caseating
    c. granuloma
    c. granulomatous inflammation
    c. inflammation
caseation
casein
    c. agar
    c.-calcium
    c. hydrolysate
    serum c.
caseous
    c. inflammation
    c. necrosis
    c. tubercle
Casoni's intradermal test
cassette
cast
    bile c.
    decidual c.
    endometrial c.
    granular c.
    hemoglobin c.
    hyaline c.
    mucous c.
    urinary c's
    waxy c.

Castellanella
    C. castellani
Castellani's test
casting
castor
    c. bean
    c. oil
castrate
castration
    c. cells
    female c.
    male c.
    parasitic c.
CAT — chlormerodrin accumulation test
    computed axial tomography
    computerized axial tomography
catabolic
catabolism
    antibody c.
catabolite
cataclysm
catacrotism
catalase
    c. test
catalepsy
Catalpa
catalysis
catalyst
    negative c.
catalytic
catalyze
catalyzer
catamenia
catamnesis
cataphasia
cataphoresis
cataphoretic
cataphylaxis

cataplectic
cataplexy
catapophysis
cataract
catarrh
catarrhal
    c. appendicitis
    c. conjunctivitis
    c. inflammation
catatonia
catatonic
    c. schizophrenia
cat-bite fever
cat-cry syndrome
catechol
    c.-*O*-methyl transferase
    c. oxidase
catecholamine
    c. assays
categorical data
Catenabacterium
cath — cathartic
      catheter
      catheterize
catharsis
cathemoglobin
cathepsin
catheter
    Swan-Ganz c.
catheterization
cathexis
cathodal
    c. opening tetanus
cathode
    c. ray
    c.-ray tube
cathodoluminescence
cation
    c.-exchange resin
    c. interference
cationic
    c. dye

cationogen
cat liver fluke
cat-scratch disease
cauda (caudae)
    c. equina
    c. nuclei caudati
caudad
caudal
    c. area
    c. dipygus duplication
    c. displacement
    c. duplication
    c. myotome
caudate
    c. lobe
    c. nucleus
    c. vein
cauliflower ear
Caulobacter
caumesthesia
causalgia
causative
cause
    constitutional c.
    predisposing c.
    proximate c.
caustic
cauter
cauterant
cauterization
cautery
CAV — congenital absence of vagina
      congenital adrenal virilism
cave-in
caveola (caveolae)
cavernous
    c. hemangioma
    c. plexus
    c. sinus
cavitation

cavity
    accessory sinus c.
    amniotic c.
    chorionic c.
    cranial c.
    endometrial c.
    exocelomic c.
    glenoid c.
    inflammatory c.
    laryngeal c.
    nasal c.
    nasopharyngeal c.
    oral c.
    pelvic peritoneal c.
    pericardial c.
    peritoneal c.
    pharyngeal c.
    pleural c.
    renal pelvic c.
    c. resonator
    serous c.
    thoracic c.
    tympanic c.
    upper respiratory tract c.
    urinary bladder c.
cavography
cavum (cava)
    c. septi pellucidi
    c. vergae
cavus
CB – chronic bronchitis
Cb – columbium
CBA – chronic bronchitis with asthma
C banding
CBC – complete blood count
CBD – common bile duct
CBF – cerebral blood flow
    coronary blood flow
CBG – corticosteroid-binding globulin
    cortisol-binding globulin
CBS – chronic brain syndrome
CBV – central blood volume
    circulating blood volume
    corrected blood volume
CC – cardiac cycle
    chief complaint
    compound cathartic
    cord compression
    costochondral
    creatinine clearance
cc – cubic centimeter
CCA – chick-cell agglutination
    chimpanzee coryza agent
    common carotid artery
CCAT – conglutinating complement absorption test
CCC – cathodal-closing contraction
    chronic calculous cholecystitis
CCCl – cathodal-closure clonus
C cells
CCF – cephalin-cholesterol flocculation
    compound comminuted fracture
    congestive cardiac failure
CCK – cholecystokinin
CCK-PZ – cholecystokinin-pancreozymin
c. cm. – cubic centimeter
C3 convertase
CCP – ciliocytophthoria
CCTe – cathodal-closure tetanus
CCU – Cherry-Crandall units
    Coronary Care Unit
CCV – conductivity cell volume

CCW — counterclockwise
CD — cadaver donor
    cardiac disease
    cardiac dullness
    cardiovascular disease
    circular dichroism
    common duct
    conjugata diagonalis
    consanguineous donor
    curative dose
    cystic duct
Cd — cadmium
    caudal
    coccygeal
cd — candela
CDA — congenital dyserythropoietic anemia
CDC — Centers for Disease Control
    chenodeoxycholate
CDE — canine distemper encephalitis
    chlordiazepoxide
    common duct exploration
CDH — ceramide dihexoside
    congenital dislocation of the hip
CDL — chlorodeoxylincomycin
cDNA — complementary DNA
CDP — continuous distending pressure
    cytidine diphosphate
CE — California encephalitis
    cardiac enlargement
    chick embryo
    cholesterol esters
    contractile element
Ce — cerium
CEA — carcinoembryonic antigen

CEA *(continued)*
    crystalline egg albumin
ceanothus extract
cebocephalus
cebocephaly
cecal
cecum
cedar oil
CEEV — Central European encephalitis virus
CEF — chick embryo fibroblast
cefaclor
cefadroxil
cefamandole
cefaparole
cefatrizine
cefazaflur sodium
cefazolin
cefoperazone
cefaranide
cefotaxime
cefoxitin
Cel — Celsius
Celebes vibrio
celestin blue B
celiac
    c. artery
    c. disease
    c. ganglion
    c. lymph node
    c. plexus
    c. sprue
celiocentesis
celioma
celioparacentesis
celiopathy
celioscopy
cell
    acanthoid c's
    accessory c's
    acidophilic c's

CELL – CELL 93

cell *(continued)*
   alpha c's
   aneuploid c's
   Anichkov's (Anitschkow's) c.
   argentaffin c's
   argyrophilic c's
   Arias-Stella c's
   Armanni-Ebstein c's
   Askanazy's c.
   B c's
   band c's
   beta c's
   Betz c's
   Boettcher c's
   buffy-coated c's
   burr c.
   C c's
   chromaffin c's
   Clara c's
   columnar c.
   comet c.
   Conway c.
   crenated c's
   decidual c's
   delta c's
   c. differentiation
   c. division
   Dorothy Reed c's
   Downey c's
   endothelial c's
   ependymal c's
   epithelial c's
   erythroid c's
   Ferrata's c's
   gamma c's
   Gaucher's c.
   granulosa c's
   granulosa-lutein c's
   $H-2^b$ mouse c's
   Hargraves' c.
   HeLa c's

cell *(continued)*
   helmet c.
   hilar c's
   Hofbauer c's
   Hürthle c's
   interstitial c's
   islet c's
   c. kinetics
   Kupffer's c's
   lacunar c's
   Langerhans' c.
   Leydig's interstitial c's
   lutein c's
   lymphoid c's
   mast c's
   c.-mediated immunity
   Merkel's c.
   mesothelial c's
   metallophil c's
   migratory c's
   monosomic c's
   Mott c.
   null c's
   olfactory c's
   packed c's
   Paneth's c's
   parafollicular c's
   pathologic c.
   Pick's c's
   plasma c's
   progenitor c's
   Purkinje's c's
   Reed-Sternberg c.
   Renshaw c.
   reticulum c's
   Rouget's c.
   Russell-Crooke c.
   sarcogenic c's
   Schwann's c.
   serous c.
   Sertoli's c.
   sickle c.

cell *(continued)*
- stem c's
- Sternberg-Reed c.
- suppressor c's
- sustentacular c's
- T c's
- target c's
- tart c.
- theca c's
- Touton giant c.
- trisomic c's
- Türk's c.
- tympanic c's
- zymogenic c's

Cellfalcicula
cellobiase
cellobiose
celloidin
cellophane
- c. tape method

cellular
- c. adaptation
- c. atypia
- c. blue nevus
- c. immunity
- c. immunity deficiency syndrome
- c. inclusions
- c. swelling

cellulase
cellulitis
- streptococcal c.

cellulose
- c. acetate phthalate
- c. caprate
- microcrystalline c.
- oxidized c.
- c. phosphate
- tetranitrate c.

cellulosity
Cellvibrio
- C. flavescens

Cellvibrio (continued)
- C. fulvus
- C. ochraceus
- C. vulgaris

celosomia
Celsius
- scale
- thermometer

cement
- intercellular c.
- c. line
- c. substance

cementification
cementifying fibroma
cementoblast
cementoblastoma
cementoma
cementum
cenobium
censored observation
Cent — centigrade
cent — centimeter
Centers for Disease Control
centigrade temperature scale
centigram
centiliter
centimeter
- c.-gram second system

centimorgan
centipede
centipoise
centistoke
central
- c. canal
- c. core disease
- c. hemorrhagic necrosis
- c. limit theorem
- c. necrosis
- c. nervous system
- c. retinal artery

Central European encephalitis virus

centralis
centric
    c. fusion
centrifugal
    c. analyzer
    c. flotation
    c. force
centrifugalization
centrifugation
centrifuge
centrilobular
    c. emphysema
    c. necrosis
centriole
centripetal
    c. force
centroacinar cells
centromere
    c. interference
centromeric bands
centronuclear
    c. myopathy
centroplasm
centrosome
centrosphere
centrum (centra)
Centruroides
cenurosis
cephacetrile sodium
cephalad
cephalexin
cephalgia
cephalhematoma
cephalic
    c. index
    c. vein
cephalin
    c.-cholesterol flocculation test
cephaloglycin
cephalometer

cephalometry
    fetal c.
    roentgen c.
    ultrasonic c.
cephalonia
cephalopathy
cephalopelvic
cephalopelvimetry
Cephalopoda
cephaloridine
cephalosporin
Cephalosporium
    C. falciforme
    C. granulomatis
cephalostat
cephalothin
cephalothoracopagus
cephamycin
cephapirin
Ceph floc — cephalin flocculation
cephradine
cera
ceramidase
ceramide
    galactosyl c.
    c. glucoside
    c. hexoside
    c. lactoside
    c. lactoside lipidosis
    c. trihexosidase
Ceratophyllus
cercaria (cercariae)
cercarial dermatitis
Cercomonas
Cercospora apii
cercosporamycosis
cerebellar
    c. artery
    c. ataxia, familial
    c. ataxia, hereditary

cerebellar *(continued)*
    c. biventral lobule
    c. ciliary body
    c. cortex
    c. declive
    c. dentate nucleus
    c. dyssynergia
    c. emboliform nucleus
    c. fasciculus uncinatus
    c. fastigial nucleus
    c. fimbriate nucleus
    c. fissure
    c. folium
    c. globose nucleus
    c. gracile lobule
    c. lenticular nucleus
    c. lobe
    c. motor tectal nucleus
    c. peduncle
    c. posterior inferior ansiform lobule
    c. posterior lobe
    c. pressure cone
    c. pyramis
    c. region
    c. roof nucleus
    c. sarcoma
    c. tonsil
    c. tuber
    c. vein
    c. vermis
    c. white matter
cerebellomedullary cistern
cerebello-olivary
cerebellopontine
cerebellorubrospinal
cerebellum
    c. agenesis
cerebral
    c. arcuate fibers
    c. artery thrombosis

cerebral *(continued)*
    c. atrophy
    c. cortex
    c. dorsum
    c. edema
    c. fissure
    c. gray matter
    c. hemisphere
    c. hemorrhage
    c. herniation
    c. infarct
    c. medial surface
    c. palsy
    c. peduncle
    c. superolateral surface
    c. thrombosis
    c. vascular accident
    c. vein
    c. ventricle
    c. white matter
cerebritis
cerebrocuprein
cerebronic acid
cerebrosclerosis
cerebroside
    c.-galactosidase
    c.-glucosidase
    c. lipidosis
    c. sulfatide
cerebrosidosis
cerebrospinal
    c. fluid
    c. fluid assays
    c. fluid culture
    c. fluid electrophoresis
    c. fluid pressure
    c. meningitis
cerebrotendinous
    c. xanthomatosis
cerebrovascular
    c. accident

cerebrum
cerium
    c. oxalate
ceroid
    c. storage disease
cerous oxalate
Certificate in Industrial Health
certified
    c. stains
    c. standards
Certified Reference Materials
cerulein
ceruloplasmin
    c. assays
cerumen
ceruminal
ceruminous
    c. adenoma
    c. carcinoma
    c. gland
cerveau isolé
cervical
    c. artery
    c. branch
    c. canal
    c. culture
    c. cutaneous nerve
    c. esophagus
    c. fascia
    c. ganglion
    c. gland
    c. intraepithelial neoplasia
    c. lamina propria
    c. lymphatics
    c. lymph node
    c. mucous membrane
    c. mucus
    c. myotome
    c. nerve
    c. plexus
    c. polyp
    c. rib

cervical *(continued)*
    c. rib syndrome
    c. scraper
    c. secretion
    c. somatosensory evoked
        potential
    c. spinal cord
    c. vein
    c. vertebra
cervicitis
cervicoaxial
cervix (cervices)
    incompetent c.
    c. uteri
CES — central excitatory state
cesarean section
cesium
C1 esterase inhibitor
Cestoda
cestode
cestodiasis
cetaben sodium
cetalkonium chloride
cetiedil citrate
cetocycline hydrochloride
Cetraria
cetrimonium bromide
cetyl
cetylpyridinium chloride
cetyltrimethylammonium
    bromide
cevadine
CF — carbolfuchsin
    cardiac failure
    carrier-free
    chemotactic factor
    chest and left leg
    Chiari-Frommel syn-
        drome
    Christmas factor
    citrovorum factor
    complement fixation

CF *(continued)*
    complement-fixing
    contractile force
    cystic fibrosis
CF antibody titer
Cf — californium
cf — confer
CFA — complement-fixing antibody
    complete Freund adjuvant
CFF — critical flicker fusion test
c.f.f. — critical fusion frequency
CFP — chronic false-positive
    cystic fibrosis of the pancreas
CFT — complement-fixation test
CFU-C — colony-forming unit–culture
CFU-E — colony-forming unit–erythroid
CFU/mL — colony forming units/mL
CFU-S — colony-forming unit–spleen
CFWM — cancer-free white mouse
CG — cardiogreen
    chorionic gonadotropin
    chronic glomerulonephritis
    colloidal gold
    phosgene (choking gas)
Cg or **cg** — centigram
CGD — chronic granulomatous disease
CGL — chronic granulocytic leukemia
cgm — centigram
cGMP — cyclic guanosine monophosphate
CGN — chronic glomerulonephritis
CG/OQ — cerebral glucose oxygen quotient
CGP — choline glycerophosphatide
    chorionic growth hormone prolactin
    circulating granulocyte pool
CGS or **cgs** — centimeter-gram-second
CGT — chorionic gonadotropin
CGTT — cortisone glucose tolerance test
CH — cholesterol
    crown-heel
CHA — congenital hypoplastic anemia
    cyclohexylamine
Chaddock's sign
Chaetoconidium
Chaetomium
chafe
Chagas' disease
chagoma
chain
    branched c.
    J c.
    kappa c.
    lambda c.
    nuclear c.
    c. reaction
    sympathetic c.
chaining
chalasia
chalazion
chalcogen
chalcogenide

chalcone
chalcosis
chalicosis
challenge
chalone
chamaecephaly
chamber
    Boyden c.
    hyperbaric c.
    vitreous c.
Chamberland filter
chancre
chancroid
change
    Baggenstoss c.
    harlequin color c.
Chang's aniline-acid fuchsin method
channel
    blood c's
    lymph c's
    perineural c.
    thoroughfare c.
character
    acquired c.
    c. density
    dominant c.
    mendelian c.
    monogenic c.
    primary sex c.
    recessive c.
    secondary sex c.
    sex-conditioned c.
    sex-limited c.
    sex-linked c.
    X-linked c.
    Y-linked c.
characteristic
    c. curve
    c. fluorescent ray
    c. ray

charcoal
    activated c.
Charcot-Böttcher crystalloids
Charcot-Leyden crystals
Charcot-Marie-Tooth
    disease
    muscular atrophy
Charcot's
    arthropathy
    joint
charge
    c.-transfer complex
charged particle
Charles' law
charring
chart
    c. recorder
    Snellen c.
chassis
chaulmoogra oil
CHB — complete heart block
CHD — congestive heart disease
         coronary heart disease
ChE — cholinesterase
check
    c. bit
    c. digit
Chediak-Higashi
    anomaly
    syndrome
Chediak's test
cheek
    cleft c.
cheese washer's disease
cheilitis
cheilosis
cheiragra
cheirarthritis
chelate
chelating agent
chelation

Chem — chemotherapy
chemical
    c. bond
    incompatible c.
    c. interference
    c. mediators
    c. pneumonia
    c. shift
    c. waste
cheminosis
chemiosmotic
    c. hypothesis
chemisorption
chemistry
    analytical c.
    inorganic c.
    organic c.
    physical c.
chemoattractant
chemoautotroph
chemoautotrophic
chemocoagulation
chemodectoma
chemodifferentiation
chemoheterotroph
chemoimmunology
chemokinesis
chemolithotroph
chemoluminescence
chemoorganotroph
chemoreceptor
    central c.
    peripheral c.
chemoresistance
chemostat
chemosterilant
chemosynthesis
chemotactic
    c. activity
    c. factor
chemotactin

chemotaxis
    c. assays
chemotherapy
chemotransmitter
chemotroph
chemotropism
chemstrip
chenodeoxycholate
chenodeoxycholic acid
chenodeoxycholylglycine
chenopodium oil
cherry red spot
cherubism
chest
    alar c.
    barrel c.
    blast c.
    foveated c.
    pterygoid c.
    tetrahedron c.
    c. tube
Cheyletiella
    C. parasitovorax
Cheyne-Stokes respiration
CHF — congestive heart failure
CHH — cartilage-hair hypoplasia
Chiari-Frommel syndrome
Chiari's
    network
    syndrome
chiasm
chiasma (chiasmata)
chickenpox
    c. virus
chief cell adenoma
Chievitz's organ
Chiffelle and Putt method
chigger
chikungunya
    c. fever
    c. fever virus

chilblain
childbed fever
Chilomastix
   C. mesnili
chilopod
Chilopoda
chimera
   blood group c.
   dispermic c.
   heterologous c.
   homologous c.
   isologous c.
   radiation c.
chimerism
chin
   galoche c.
Chinese liver fluke
Chinese restaurant syndrome
chiniofon
chip
   bone c.
   c. fracture
chiral
   c. center
chirality
Chiroptera
chi-squared
   c. distribution
   c. test
chitin
CHL — chloramphenicol
Chlamydia
   C. oculogenitalis
   C. psittaci
   C. trachomatis
Chlamydiaceae
chlamydiosis
Chlamydobacteriaceae
Chlamydobacteriales
Chlamydophrys
chlamydospore
Chlamydozoaceae
Chlamydozoon
chloasma
chlophedianol hydrochloride
chloracne
chloral
   c. betaine
   c. hydrate
chlorambucil
chloramine-T
chloramphenicol
chloranil
chloranilate method
chlorasol
chlorate
   c. assays
chlorazanil hydrochloride
chlorazol
   c. black E
   c. black E stain
chlorbenside
chlorcyclizine hydrochloride
chlordane
chlordantoin
chlordiazepoxide
   c. hydrochloride
chlorhexidine
chloride
   c. methods
   c. shift
chloridometer
chlorinated
   c. hydrocarbon pesticide assays
   c. hydrocarbon pesticides
chlorine
   c. isotope
chlorisondamine chloride
chlormerodrin
   c. Hg 197
   c. Hg 203
chlormezanone
chloroacetic acid

chloroacetone
chloroacetophenone
chloroallyl diethyldithiocarbamate
chloroaniline
Chlorobacteriaceae
Chlorobacterium
chlorobenzene
chlorobenzilate
Chlorobium
1-chloro-3-bromopropene-1
chlorobutanol
Chlorochromatium
chlorocresol
chlorodiallylacetamide
chlorodiethylacetamide
chlorodimethyl phenoxy
  ethanol
chloro-dinitrobenzene
chloroethanol
chlorofluorocarbon
chloroform
  c. assays
  c.-methanol
chloroguanide hydrochloride
chlorohydrocarbon
  c. assays
chloroleukemia
chlorolymphosarcoma
chloroma
p-chloromercuribenzoate
p-chlorometacresol
chloromethane
1-chloro-1-nitroethane
1-chloro-1-nitropropane
chloro-*o*-phenyl phenol
p-chlorophenol
chlorophenothane
chlorophenoxyacetic acid
chlorophenoxy herbicides
p-chlorophenyl-*p*-chlorobenzyl
  sulfide

3-(*p*-chlorophenyl)-1,1-
  dimethyl urea
chlorophenyl dimethylurea trichloroacetate
p-chlorophenyl phenyl sulfone
chlorophyll
chlorophyllase
chlorophyllin
chloropicrin
Chloropidae
chloroplast
chloroprocaine hydrochloride
chloropsia
chloroquine
chlorothen citrate
chlorothiazide
Chlorothion
chlorothymol
chlorotoloxyacetic acid
chlorotrianisene
chlorous
  c. acid reagent
chlorovinyldichloroarsine
chloroxine
chloroxylenol
chlorphenesin
  c. carbamate
chlorpheniramine
  c. maleate
chlorphenoxamine hydro-
  chloride
chlorphentermine hydro-
  chloride
chlorpromazine
  c. assays
chlorpropamide
chlorprothixene
chlorquinaldol
chlortetracycline
  c. hydrochloride
chlorthalidone
chlorthion

chlorzoxazone
CHN — central hemorrhagic
  necrosis
CHO — carbohydrate
choana (choanae)
choanal
chocolate
  c. agar
  c. cyst
choke
  ophthalmovascular c.
chol. — cholesterol
cholagogue
cholaneresis
cholangiectasis
cholangioadenoma
cholangiocarcinoma
cholangiogram
cholangiography
  delayed operative c.
  direct c.
  intravenous c.
  operative c.
  percutaneous transhepatic
    c.
  postoperative c.
cholangiole
cholangiolitic cirrhosis
cholangiolitis
cholangioma
cholangiotomogram
cholangitis
  sclerosing c.
  suppurative c.
cholanthrene
cholate
cholecalciferol
cholechromopoiesis
cholecyst
cholecystagogue
cholecystangiography
cholecystectasia

cholecystitis
  acute hemorrhagic c.
  emphysematous c.
  follicular c.
  glandularis proliferans c.
cholecystocholangiography
cholecystogram
cholecystography
  intravenous c.
  oral c.
cholecystokinase
cholecystokinin
cholecystolithiasis
cholecystosis
  hyperplastic c.
choledochal
choledochogram
choledochography
choledocholithiasis
choledochus
cholegraphy
cholelithiasis
cholemia
cholemic
  c. nephrosis
choleophosphatase
cholepathia
choleperitoneum
cholepoiesis
cholera
  Asiatic c.
  pancreatic c.
Choleraesuis
  C. salmonella
choleragen
choleraphage
choleresis
choleretic
cholescintigram
Chol est — cholesterol esters
cholestasis
cholesteatoma

cholesterohistechia
cholesterol
   c. assays
   c. calculus
   c. desmolase
   c. esterase
   c. ester storage disease
   c. oxidase
   c. staining methods
cholesterolemia
cholesterolestersturz
cholesterolopoiesis
cholesterolosis
cholesteroluria
cholesterosis
   extracellular c.
cholestyramine resin
cholic acid
choline
   c. acetyltransferase
   c. dehydrogenase
   c. kinase
cholinephosphate cytidylyltransferase
cholinephosphotransferase
cholinergic
   c. fibers
   c. receptors
cholinesterase
   c. assays
   c. inhibitors
cholinolytic
Cholografin
choloyl-coenzyme A synthetase
choluria
Chondodendron
chondralgia
chondritis
chondroblast
chondroblastoma
chondrocalcinosis

chondrocyte
   isogenous c's
chondrodermatitis
   c. nodularis chronica helicis
chondrodysplasia
chondrodystrophy
chondroectodermal
chondroid
   c. metaplasia
   c. syringoma
chondroitin
   c. sulfate
   c. sulfate A
   c. sulfate staining
chondroma
chondromalacia
chondromatosis
   synovial c.
chondromatous
   c. exostosis
   c. giant cell tumor
chondrometaplasia
chondromucoprotein
chondromyxoid
   c. fibroma
chondroporosis
chondrosarcoma
chondrosulfatase
chondrus
CHOP — cyclophosphamide, doxorubicin, vincristine and prednisone
chopped meat medium
chorda (chordae)
   c. tendineae cordis
   c. tympani
chordee
chorditis
chordoblastoma
chordoma

chorea
    Huntington's c.
    Sydenham's c.
choreic
choreiform
choreoathetosis
chorioadenoma
    c. destruens
chorioallantoic membrane
chorioamnionitis
chorioangioma
choriocarcinoma
chorioepithelioma
choriomeningitis
    lymphocytic c.
chorion
    c. frondosum
    c. laeve
    primitive c.
    shaggy c.
chorionic
    c. carcinoma
    c. cavity
    c. gonadotropin
    c. plate
    c. somatomammotropin
    c. villi
choristoma
choroid
    c. lamina basalis
    c. plexus
choroidal
choroideremia
choroiditis
Chr. – *Chromobacterium*
chr – chronic
Christeller reaction
Christensen's urea agar
Christmas
    disease
    factor

chromaffin
    c. body
    c. cells
    c. paraganglioma
    c. reaction
    c. tumor
chromaffinoma
    medullary c.
chromargentaffin
chromate
    c. method
chromatic
    c. aberration
chromatid
    c. interference
    nonsister c's
    sister c's
chromatin
    c.-negative
    nucleolar-associated c.
    c.-positive
    sex c.
chromatinic
    c. body
chromation
chromatofocusing
chromatogram
chromatograph
chromatography
    anion-exchange c.
    gel-filtration c.
chromatokinesis
chromatolysis
chromatophil
chromatophilic
    c. granules
chromatophore
chromatotaxis
chrome
    c. alum hematoxylin-
        phloxine method

chrome *(continued)*
    c. violet
chromic
    c. acid
    c. phosphate colloid
chromium
    c. assays
    c. sulfate
    c. trioxide
Chromobacterium
    C. amythistinum
    C. janthinum
    C. marismortui
    C. typhiflavum
    C. violaceum
chromoblastomycosis
chromocenter
chromocholoscopy
chromocystoscopy
chromocyte
chromogen
    Porter-Silber c's
chromogenesis
chromogenic
chromogranin
chromomere
chromomycosis
chromonar hydrochloride
chromonema (chromonemata)
chromophil
chromophobe
    c. adenoma
    c. cell
chromophore
chromoprotein
chromosomal
    c. aberration
    c. breakage syndrome
    c. derangement
    c. RNA
chromosome
    accessory c's
    c. alteration

chromosome *(continued)*
    Balbiani's c.
    c. banding
    c. complement
    gametic c.
    homologous c.
    c. map
    c. nomenclature
    Philadelphia c.
    ring c.
    sex c.
    somatic c.
    c. translocation
    c. trisomy
    X c.
    Y c.
chromotrope
chromotropic acid
chromoxane
    c. cyanin R
    c. pure blue B
    c. pure blue BLD
chronaxie, chronaxy
chronic
    c. active hepatitis
    c. bronchitis
    c. granulomatous disease
    c. interstitial nephritis
    c. lymphatic leukemia
    c. lymphocytic leukemia
    c. lymphosarcoma (cell) leukemia
    c. monocytic (monoblastic) leukemia
    c. myelocytic leukemia
    c. myelogenous leukemia
    c. obstructive pulmonary disease
    c. renal disease
    c. renal failure
    c. subdural hematoma
    c. thyroiditis
chronological age

chronotropic
chronotropism
chrotoplast
chrysiasis
Chrysomyia
chrysophoresis
Chrysops
Chrysosporium
chrysotile
CHS — Chédiak-Higashi syndrome
   cholinesterase
Chvostek's sign
chyle
chylocele
chylomicron
chylomicronemia
chylopericarditis
chylopericardium
chyloperitoneum
chylopleura
chylopneumothorax
chylorrhea
chylothorax
chylous
   c. ascites
   c. effusion
chyluria
chymase
chyme
chymodenin
chymosin
chymotrypsin
chymotrypsinogen
CI — cardiac index
   cardiac insufficiency
   cerebral infarction
   chemotherapeutic index
   colloidal iron
   color index
   coronary insufficiency
   crystalline insulin

Ci — curie
Ciaccio's
   fluid
   method
   stain
Cib. (cibus) — food
cicatrix (cicatrices)
Cicuta
cicutoxin
CID — cytomegalic inclusion disease
CIDS — cellular immunity deficiency syndrome
CIE — countercurrent immunoelectrophoresis
CIEP — counterimmunoelectrophoresis
CIF — clone-inhibiting factor
ciguatera
ciguatoxin
CIH — Certificate in Industrial Health
Ci-hr — curie-hour
ciliary
   c. artery
   c. body
   c. crown
   c. ganglion
   c. gland
   c. muscle
   c. nerve
   c. plicae
   c. process
   c. ring
Ciliata
ciliocytophthoria
Ciliophora
cilium (cilia)
Cillobacterium
cimetidine
Cimex
   C. lectularius

CIN — cervical intra-epithelial
    neoplasia
    chronic interstitial
    nephritis
cinchonidine sulfate
cinchophen
cinclisis
cineangiocardiography
cineangiography
    radionuclide c.
cinebronchography
cinedensigraphy
cinefluorography
cinemicrography
cinepazet maleate
cinephlebography
cineradiography
cinerea
cinerins
cineurography
cingulate
    c. fasciculus
    c. gyrus
    c. sulcus
cingulum (cingula)
cinoxacin
circ — circulation
circadian
    c. rhythm
circinate
circle
    c. of confusion
    c. of Willis
circuit
    c. breaker
    open c.
    reflex c.
    short c.
circuitry
circulating
    c. anticoagulants

circulating *(continued)*
    c. antithromboplastin disorder
    c. atypical lymphocytes
    c. cells
    c. reticuloendothelial cells
circulation
    c. time
circulatory
    c. failure
    c. overload
    c. system
circulus (circuli)
circumanal
circumarticular
circumaxillary
circumcallosal
circumcision
circumflex
    c. artery
    c. iliac vein
    c. radial artery
    c. ulnar artery
    c. vein
circumscribed
    c. atrophy
    c. inflammation
circumvallate
cirrhosis
    alcoholic c.
    biliary c.
    cardiac c.
    cholangiolitic c.
    Laennec's c.
    nutritional c.
    obstructive c.
    pigmentary c.
    pipestem c.
    portal c.
    posthepatic c.
    postnecrotic c.

cirrhosis *(continued)*
   toxic c.
cirrhotic
cirrus (cirri)
cirsoid
CIS — carcinoma in situ
      central inhibitory state
cis
   c. configuration
cisplatin
cistern
   basal c.
   great c.
   subarachnoidal c's
   terminal c's
cisterna (cisternae)
   c. ambiens
   c. cerebellomedullaris
   c. chiasmatica
   c. chyli
   c. corpus callosum
   c. fossae lateralis
   c. interpeduncularis
   c. lamina terminalis
   c. magna
   c. pontis
   c. superioris
cisternal
   c. puncture
cisternography
   radionuclide c.
cis-trans test
cistron
citrate
   c. agar gel electrophoresis
   c. condensing enzyme
   cupric c.
   ferric c.
   c.-phosphate-dextrose
   c.-phosphate-dextrose-
     adenine
   c. synthase

citrate *(continued)*
   c. test
citreoviridin
citric acid
   c. a. assays
   c. a. cycle
Citrobacter
   Bethesda-Ballerup group of *C.*
   C. diversus *koseri*
   C. freundii
citron
citrophosphate
citrovorum factor
citrulline
citrullinemia
citrullinuria
Civatte's
   body
   poikiloderma
CIXU — constant infusion
      excretory urogram
CK — creatine kinase
CL — chest and left arm
Cl — chlorine
Cl. — *Clostridium*
cl — centiliter
Cladosporium
   C. bantianum
   C. carrionii
   C. cladosporoides
   C. mansonii
   C. trichoides
   C. werneckii
clamoxyquin hydrochloride
Clara
   cells
   hematoxylin
clarificant
clarification
clarify
Clarke-Hadfield syndrome

Clarke's
- column
- fluid
- nucleus

Clark's
- oxygen electrode
- rule
- test

CLAS — congenital localized absence of skin

clasmatocyte
clasmatocytosis
clasmatosis
classical
- c. complement pathway

classification
- Bergey's c.
- Caldwell-Moloy c.
- Denver c.
- Duke's c.
- Jensen's c.
- Kauffman-White c.
- Lancefield c.
- Runyon's c.

clathrate
Clathrochloris
Clathrocystis
claudication
- intermittent c.
- venous c.

clause
- Delaney c.

claustrum (claustra)
clava
clavate
Claviceps
clavicle
clavicular
- c. region

claviculus
clavipectoral
clavus (clavi)

clawfoot
clawhand
CLBBB — complete left bundle branch block
CLD — chronic liver disease
chronic lung disease
clean-catch collection method
clearance
- blood urea c.
- creatinine c.
- immune c.
- interocclusal c.
- iron plasma c.
- plasma c.
- urea c.

clear cell
- c. c. adenocarcinoma
- c. c. adenoma
- c. c. carcinoma
- c. c. hidradenoma
- c. c. sarcoma

clearing
- c. factor lipase

cleavage
- c. cell

cleft
- c. leaflet, mitral valve
- c. leaflet, tricuspid valve
- c. lip
- c. nose
- c. palate
- c. tongue

cleistothecium
Cleland's reagent
clemastine
clemizole
- c. hydrochloride
- c. penicillin

click
- ejection c.
- midsystolic c.

clidinium bromide

climacteric
clindamycin
cline
clinical
    c. bacteriologic specimens
    c. chemistry
    c. chemistry automation
    c. chemistry quality control
    c. laboratory
    c. microbiology quality control
    c. spectrum
    c. toxicology
    c. trials
Clinical Laboratory Management Association
Clinical Laboratory Scientist
clinician
Clinilab
Clinistix
Clinitest
clinography
Clinoril
clinoscope
Clitocybe
clitoridal
    c. artery
    c. fascia
clitoris
    cavernous body of c.
    dorsal nerve of c.
    prepuce of c.
clivus
CLL — chronic lymphatic leukemia
    chronic lymphocytic leukemia
CLMA — Clinical Laboratory Management Association
cloaca (cloacae)

cloacal
    c. membrane
cloacogenic
    c. carcinoma
clock
    biological c.
clofibrate
clomiphene
    c. citrate
    c. test
clomipramine hydrochloride
clonal
clonazepam
clone
    c.-inhibiting factor
clonic
clonidine hydrochloride
cloning
    cellular c.
    molecular c.
clonorchiasis
Clonorchis
    C. sinensis
clonus
Cloquet's
    canal
    lymph node
clorazepate
clorexolone
cloroperone hydrochloride
clorophene
closed
    c. dislocation
    c. fracture
closing volume
clostridial
clostridiopeptidase
Clostridium
    C. bifermentans
    C. botulinum
    C. butyricum

Clostridium (continued)
   C. clostridiiforme
   C. difficile
   C. histolyticum
   C. histolyticum collagenase
   C. innocuum
   C. novyi
   C. perfringens
   C. ramosus
   C. septicum
   C. sordelli
   C. sphenoides
   C. tetani
   C. welchii
clostridium (clostridia)
clot
   c. lysis
   c. reaction
clotrimazole
clotting time
cloudy swelling
clove oil
cloxacillin sodium
cloxyquin
CLSL — chronic lymphosarcoma (cell) leukemia
CLT — clot-lysis time
clubbed
   c. fingers
   c. toes
clubbing
clubfoot
clubhand
clump
clumping
clysis
clyster
CM — capreomycin
   chloroquine-mepacrine
   cochlear microphonic
   costal margin

Cm — curium
cm — centimeter
cm^3 — cubic centimeter
CMB — carbolic methylene blue
CMC — carboxymethyl cellulose
   critical micelle concentration
CMF — chondromyxoid fibroma
   Cytoxan, methotrexate, 5-fluorouracil
CMGN — chronic membranous glomerulonephritis
CMI — carbohydrate metabolism index
   cell-mediated immunity
CMID — cytomegalic inclusion disease
c/min — cycles per minute
CML — chronic myelocytic leukemia
   chronic myelogenous leukemia
CMM — cutaneous malignant melanoma
cmm — cubic millimeter
CMN — cystic medial necrosis
CMN-AA — cystic medial necrosis of the ascending aorta
CMO — cardiac minute output
cMo — centimorgan
CMoL — chronic monocytic (monoblastic) leukemia
C-MOPP — cyclophosphamide, nitrogen mustard, vincristine (Oncovin), procarbazine, and prednisone

CMOS — complementary metal oxide semiconductor
CMP — cardiomyopathy
    cytidine monophosphate
CMR — cerebral metabolic rate
    crude mortality ratio
CMRG — cerebral metabolic rate of glucose
CMRO — cerebral metabolic rate of oxygen
CMRR — common mode rejection ratio
CMS — Clyde Mood Scale
CMU — chlorophenyldimethylurea
CMV — cytomegalovirus
CN — cyanide anion
    cyanogen
Cnephia
CNHD — congenital nonspherocytic hemolytic disease
CNL — cardiolipin natural lecithin
CNP — continuous negative pressure
CNS — central nervous system
CNV — conative negative variation
    contingent negative variation
CO — carbon monoxide
    cardiac output
    cervicoaxial
    coenzyme
    compound
    corneal opacity
CO_2 — carbon dioxide
CoA — coenzyme A
coacervate
coacervation
coag — coagulation
coagulant
coagulase
    c. test
coagulate
coagulation
    disseminated intravascular c.
    exogenous anticoagulant c.
    c. factor
    c. factor assays
    c. factor inhibitors
    fibrinolysin c.
    c. pathways
    plasmin c.
    c. time test
coagulative
    c. necrosis
coagulin
coagulogram
coagulum (coagula)
coal tar
coal workers' pneumoconiosis
coarctate
coarctation
    c. of aorta
    postductal c. of the aorta
    preductal c. of the aorta
coarsening
coat
    buffy c.
Coats' disease
cobalamin
cobalt
    c. assays
    c. isotope
    c. salipyrine
    c. 60
cobaltinitrite method
cobaltous chloride
cobbler's chest

cobra venom solution
COBS — cesarean-obtained barrier-sustained
COC — cathodal opening clonus
cathodal opening contraction
coccygeal
cocaine
    c. assays
    c. hydrochloride
    c. metabolite assay
cocarboxylase
cocarcinogen
cocarcinogenesis
coccal
cocci
    gram-negative c.
    gram-positive c.
Coccidia
coccidioidal
    c. granuloma
Coccidioides
    C. immitis
coccidioidin
coccidioidomycosis
coccidiosis
Coccidium
    C. hominis
coccidium (coccidia)
coccobacillus
coccobacteria
coccoid
coccus (cocci)
coccygeal
    c. glomus
    c. ligament
    c. plexus
coccygeus
coccygodynia
coccyx (coccyges)
cochlea

cochlear
    c. duct
    c. nerve
    c. nucleus
    c. root
    c. spiral canal
    c. window
cocillana
Cockayne's syndrome
cockscomb polyp
COCL — cathodal opening clonus
cocoa butter
Coct. (*coctio*) — boiling
coctoprecipitin
cocultivation
cocurrent
COD — cause of death
code
    genetic c.
    Hollerith c.
    triplet c.
coded aperture imaging
codeine
    c. assays
    c. phosphate
    c. sulfate
coding
    c. triplet
cod liver oil
Codman's
    triangle
    tumor
codocyte
codominance
codon
coefficient
    Bunsen c.
    creatinine c.
    c. of inbreeding
    osmotic c.

coefficient *(continued)*
    phenol c.
    sedimentation c.
    Spearman's rank correlation c.
    urohemolytic c.
    urotoxic c.
    c. of variation
    velocity c.
    volume c.
coelenterate
coeloblastula
coelom
    extraembryonic c.
    intraembryonic c.
coelomic
    c. cavity
coenurus
coenzyme
    c. A
    c. Q
    c. R
    c. I
    c. II
coenzymometer
coeur en sabot
cofactor
    platelet c. I
    platelet c. II
Cogan's syndrome
cognition
COGTT — cortisone-primed oral glucose tolerance test
cogwheel respiration
COHB — carboxyhemoglobin
coherent
cohesion
cohesive
    c. termini
Cohnheim's artery

cohort
    c. labeling
    c. study
coil
    paranemic c.
    plectonemic c.
    relational c.
    standard c.
coincidence
    c. correction
    c. error
    c. sum peak
coinlike
coinosite
coitus
Colcemid
Colcher-Sussman method
colchicine
COLD — chronic obstructive lung disease
cold
    c. agglutinin
    c. agglutinin syndrome
    c. agglutinin test
    c. hemagglutinin
    c. hemoglobinuria
    c. injury
    c. intolerance
    c.-knife conization
    c. lesion
    c.-reacting antibody
coldsore
Coleman-Schiff reagent
Coleoptera
Cole's hematoxylin
colestipol hydrochloride
Coley's toxin
colibacillary
colibacillemia
colibacilluria
colibacillus

colic
   biliary c.
   endemic c.
   intestinal c.
   menstrual c.
   pancreatic c.
   renal c.
   uterine c.
   verminous c.
colicin
colicinogen
coliform
colinearity
colipase
coliphage
colistimethate sodium
colistin
   c. sulfate
colitis
   acute ulcerative c.
   amebic c.
   balantidial c.
   chronic ulcerative c.
   granulomatous c.
   ischemic c.
   mucous c.
   pseudomembranous c.
   radiation c.
   regional c.
   spastic c.
   ulcerative c.
   uremic c.
colitose
solitoxemia
colitoxicosis
colitoxin
coliuria
collagen
   c. disease
   c. fibril alteration
   fibrous long-spacing c.
   segmental long-spacing c.

collagen *(continued)*
   c. staining method
collagenase
collagenoblast
collagenocyte
collagenous
   c. fibers
collapse
   circulatory c.
   massive c.
   c. therapy
collateral
   c. eminence
   c. sulcus
   c. ulnar artery
   c. ventilation
collecting tubule
College of American Pathologists
colliculus (colliculi)
   inferior c.
   superior c.
collidine
colligative
collimate
collimator
colliquation
   ballooning c.
   reticulating c.
collision
collodion
colloid
   c. adenocarcinoma
   c. adenoma
   c. body
   c. carcinoma
   c. cyst
   c. degeneration
   c. goiter
   c. milium
   c.-osmotic lysis
   thyroid c.

colloidal
- c. gold
- c. iron stain
- c. osmotic pressure

colloidoclasia

collum (colla)

coloboma (colobomas, colobomata)

colocynth

colon
- ascending c.
- descending c.
- mesenteric c.
- rectosigmoid c.
- sigmoid c.
- transverse c.
- c. tumor

colonic
- c. crypts of Lieberkühn
- c. lumen
- c. mucous membrane
- c. mucus
- c. muscularis propria
- c. serosa
- c. solitary lymphoid nodule
- c. submucosa
- c. subserosa
- c. vomitus

colonization

colonoscope

colonoscopy

colony
- bitten c.
- butyrous c.
- D c.
- daughter c.
- disgonic c.
- dwarf c.
- effuse c.
- c.-forming units
- H c.
- M c.

colony *(continued)*
- matte c.
- mucoid c.
- O c.
- R c.
- raised c.
- rough c.
- S c.
- satellite c.
- smooth c.
- c.-stimulating activity
- c.-stimulating factor

color
- c. blindness
- complementary c.
- c. index
- c. index number
- primary c.
- spectral c.
- c. vision

Colorado
- C. tick fever
- C. tick fever virus

colorectitis

colorimeter

colorimetric

colorimetry

colostrum

colpectasia

colpitis

colpocytogram

colpocytology

colpohyperplasia

colpomicroscope

colposcope

colposcopy

Columbia blood agar

Columbia-SK virus

columbium

columella (columellae)

column
- Bertini's renal c's

118 COLUMN – COMPARTMENTAL

column *(continued)*
    Clarke's c.
    fornix c.
    vertebral c.
columna (columnae)
columnar
    c. epithelium
coma
    alcoholic c.
    apoplectic c.
    c. dé passé
    diabetic c.
    hepatic c.
    irreversible c.
    metabolic c.
    uremic c.
    c. vigil
Comamonas terrigena
comatose
combination
combined
    c. immunodeficiency
    c. systems disease
comb rhythm
combustible
    c. gas
    c. gas detector
    c. liquid
    c. vapor
combustion
comedo (comedones)
comedocarcinoma
comedomastitis
comet cell
commensal
commensalism
comminuted
    c. fracture
commissura (commissurae)
commissure
    anterior c.
    aortic c.

commissure *(continued)*
    Forel's c.
    habenular c.
    hippocampal c.
    inferior colliculus c.
    laryngeal c.
    mitral valve c.
    posterior c.
    pulmonic valve c.
    superior colliculus c.
    tricuspid valve c.
Committee on Allied Health Education and Accreditation
common
    c. antigen
    c. bile duct
    c. carotid artery
    c. facial vein
    c. iliac artery
    c. iliac vein
    c. logarithm
    c. mode rejection ratio
    c. mode signal
    c. peroneal nerve
    c. reference
    c. storage
    c. tendon sheath
communicable
communicating
    c. hydrocephalus
commutator
compact
    c. bone
comparison
    c. film
    c. operation
compartment
    muscular c.
    vascular c.
compartmental
    c. analysis

compatibility
  ABO c.
  c. test
compatible
compensation
  broken c.
  dosage c.
  c. neurosis
compensatory
  c. emphysema
  c. hypertrophy
  c. regeneration
competence
  embryonic c.
  immunologic c.
competition
competitive
  c. inhibition
  c. protein-binding
compile
  c. time
compiler
complement
  c. activation
  c. assays
  c. components
  c. deficiency state
  dominant c.
  endocellular c.
  c. fixation
  c.-fixation test
  c.-fixing
  c. inactivation
  c. lysis sensitivity test
  c.-mediated cytotoxicity
complementary
  c. bases
  c. DNA
  c. genes
  c. metal oxide semiconductor logic
complementophil

complete
  c. anomalous venous drainage
  c. anterior dislocation
  c. antibody
  c. blood count
  c. heart block
  c. inferior dislocation
  c. penetrance
  c. posterior dislocation
  c. reaction of degeneration
  c. right bundle branch block
  c. superior dislocation
complex
  c. adrenal endocrine disorder
  antigen-antibody c.
  Eisenmenger's c.
  c. endocrine disorder
  Ghon c.
  Golgi's c.
  c. gonadal endocrine disorder
  HLA c.
  immune c.
  major histocompatibility c.
  Meyenburg's c.
  c. number
  c. odontoma
  c. pituitary endocrine disorder
  c. thyroid endocrine disorder
  von Meyenburg's c.
compliance
  dynamic c.
  specific c.
  static c.
complication
component
  M c.

component *(continued)*
    plasma thromboplastin c.
    splanchnic motor c.
    splanchnic sensory c.
composite tumor
compound
    acyclic c.
    aliphatic c.
    c. B
    binary c.
    condensation c.
    diazo c.
    c. dislocation
    endothermic c.
    exothermic c.
    c. F
    c. fracture
    c. granular corpuscle
    isocylic c.
    c. leukemia
    c. multiple fractures
    c. nevus
    nonpolar c's
    c. odontoma
    organometallic c.
    c. presentation
    c. S
    saturated c.
    substitution c.
    tertiary c.
    c. tumor
    c. X
compressed
    c. fracture
    c. gas storage
    c. spectral assay
compression
    c. injury
compromised
Compton
    edge
    effect

Compton *(continued)*
    photon
compulsion
computed
    c. tomography
computer
    general-purpose c.
    c. graphics
computerized
    c. axial tomography
    c. transaxial tomography
COMT — catechol-*O*-methyl
        transferase
ConA — concanavalin A
conc — concentration
concanavalin A
concatenation
Concato's disease
concave
concentrate
concentrated
concentration
    hydrogen ion c.
    ionic c.
    limiting isorrheic c.
    maximum urinary c.
    MC c.
    minimal isorrheic c.
    molar c.
    substance c.
concept
    second messenger c.
conception
conceptional age
concha (conchae)
conchoidal
concordance
concretio
    c. cordis
    c. pericardii
concretion
concussion

condensation
condenser
    Abbe's c.
    cardioid c.
    darkfield c.
    paraboloid c.
conditional
    c. jump
    c. probability
conditioned stimulus
conductance
conduction
    c. deafness
    c. defect
    c. electron
    c. system
    c. time
    c. velocity
conductivity
    c. cell volume
    water c.
conductometry
conductor
condyle
condyloma (condylomata)
    c. acuminatum
    giant c. of Buschke-Löwenstein
    c. latum
cone
    c. shell
confabulation
configuration
    trans c.
confluent
    c. bronchopneumonia
    c. inflammation
    c. pneumonia
conformation
conformer
confusion
congener
congenital
    c. adrenal hyperplasia
    c. nonspherocytic hemolytic disease
    c. thymic dysplasia
congestion
congestive
    c. cirrhosis
    c. edema
    c. heart failure
conglutination
Congo
    C. Corinth
    C. floor maggot
    C. red
    C. red stain
    C. red test
conical
conidial
Conidiobolus
conidiophore
conidiospore
conidium (conidia)
coniine
coniofibrosis
coniophage
coniosis
Coniosporium
coniosporosis
coniotoxicosis
Conium
conization
conjoined twins
conjugate
    c. acid
    c. base
    c. redox pair
conjugated protein
conjugation
conjunctiva (conjunctivae)
    c. and sclera
    bulbar c.

conjunctiva *(continued)*
   lymphatics of c.
   palpebral c.
conjunctival
conjunctivitis
   adult gonococcal c.
   allergic c.
   angular c.
   catarrhal c.
   follicular c.
   granular c.
   inclusion c.
   meningococcus c.
   c. neonatorum
   phlyctenular c.
   spring catarrhal c.
   swimming pool c.
   tularemic c.
   vernal c.
   welder's c.
conjunctivoma
connective tissue
   dense elastic c. t.
   dense fibrous c. t.
   endocervical c. t.
   exocervical c. t.
   loose areolar c. t.
   mammary interlobular c. t.
   mammary intralobular c. t.
   mucous c. t.
   c. t. nevus
connector
Conn's syndrome
Conray
consanguineous
   c. mating
consanguinity
consciousness
   c. disturbance
consensual
   c. light reflex
console
consolidation
   c. therapy
conspecific
constant
   Boltzmann c.
   Faraday's c.
   Planck's c.
   c. region
constipation
constitution
constitutional
   c. dwarf
   c. hyperbilirubinemia
   c. psychopathic inferiority
   c. thrombopathy
constitutive
   c. heterochromatin method
constriction
constrictive
constrictor pharyngeus muscle
constructable
constructive
   c. proof
consumption
   c. coagulopathy
contact
   c. catalysis
   c. dermatitis
   c. inhibition
   c. sensitivity
contagion
contagious
contagium
   c. animatum
   c. vivum
containment
contaminant
contamination
contents
   gastrointestinal c.
continence
continent

contingency table
contingent negative variation
continuous
    c. distending pressure
    c. flow culture
    c. function
    c. murmur
    c. negative pressure
    c. positive airway pressure
    c. spectrum
    c. x-ray spectrum
contour
contoured
contraception
contracted
    c. kidney
contractile
    c. force
    c. ring
contractility
contraction
    c. time
contracture
    congenital c.
    Dupuytren's c.
    ischemic c.
    Volkmann's c.
contraindication
contralateral
    c. axillary metastasis
contrast
    c. media
    c. media reaction
contrecoup
control
    c. group
    c. materials
    c. panel
    c. system
    c. unit
controlled substance
Controlled Substances Act
contuse
contusion
    contrecoup c.
conus (coni)
    c. arteriosus
    c. artery
    c. medullaris
    c. papillary muscle
    c. terminalis
convalescence
convallamarin
convallarin
convection
convergence
conversational mode
conversion
    c. coefficient
    c. electron
    c. hysteria
    Mantoux c.
    c. ratio
convertase
    C3 c.
converter
    D/A c.
convertin
convex
convoluted
    c. tubule
convolution
convulsant
convulsion
convulsive shock therapy
Conway cell
coolant
Cooley's anemia
Coombs' test
    direct
    indirect
Cooper's
    irritable breast
    suspensory ligament

coordinate
   cartesian c.
   polar c.
   spherical polar c.
coordination
   c. compound
   c. number
COP — colloid osmotic pressure
       Cytoxan, Oncovin, prednisone
coparaffinate
COPD — chronic obstructive pulmonary disease
Cope method bronchography
Copepoda
Coplin jar
copolymer
copper
   c. acetoarsenite
   c. arsenate
   c. assays
   c. deposit demonstration
   c. intoxication
   c. naphthenate
   c. oxidase
   c. oxychloride sulfate
   c. 3-phenyl salicylate
   c. storage protein
   c. sulfate
   c. undecylenate
copperhead
coprecipitin
copremesis
Coprinus
coproantibody
coprohematology
coprolith
Copromastix
   C. prowazeki
Copromonas
   C. subtilis
coprophagia
coprophil
coproporphyria
coproporphyrin
   c. assay
coproporphyrinogen
   c. oxidase
coproporphyrinuria
coprostanol
coprostasis
coprosterol
coprozoic
cor
   c. biloculare
   c. bovinum
   c. pseudotriloculare
   c. pulmonale
   c. triatriatum
   c. triloculare biatriatum
   c. triloculare biventriculare
CORA — conditioned orientation reflex audiometry
coracobrachialis muscle
coracoid
Corbin technique
cord
   Billroth's c's
   c. bladder
   c. blood
   c. factor
   spermatic c.
   spinal c.
   umbilical c.
   vocal c.
Cordylobia
   C. anthropophaga
core
   air c.
   c. antigen
   magnetic c.
   c. memory
corectasis

coremium
corepressor
Corinth
    Congo C.
coriphosphine O
Cori's
    cycle
    disease
corium
corn
cornea
corneal
    c. reflex
    c. vascularization
corniculate
cornification
corn meal agar
cornu (cornua)
corona (coronas, coronae)
    c. ciliaris
    c. of glans penis
    c. radiata
    c. veneris
coronal
    c. plane
    c. suture
coronary
    c. artery
    c. atherosclerotic heart
      disease
    c. heart disease
    c. insufficiency
    c. ligament
    c. sinus
    c. thrombosis
    c. vein
coronavirus
coroner
coronoid
coroscopy
corpora
    c. amylacea

corpora *(continued)*
    c. arenacea
    c. lutea
    c. quadrigemina
corps ronds
corpus (corpora)
    c. albicans
    c. atreticum
    c. callosum
    c. cavernosum clitoridis
    c. cavernosum penis
    c. coccygeum
    c. fimbriatum
    c. fornicis
    c. hemorrhagicum
    c. hemorrhagicum cyst
    c. luteum
    c. pancreatis
    c. striatum
    c. uteri
corpuscle
    compound granular c.
    Donné's c's
    Golgi-Mazzoni c.
    Golgi's c.
    Hassall's c.
    Meissner's c.
    Merkel's c.
    renal c.
    Ruffini's c.
    Vater-Pacini c.
corrected
    c. reticulocyte count
    c. sedimentation rate
    c. transposition
correction
correlation
    c. coefficient
corresponding ray
Corrigan's pulse
corrin
    c. ring

corrosion
    c. cast
corrosive
corrosivity
cort — cortex
cortex (cortices)
cortical
    c. bone
    c. DC potential
    c. defect
    c. necrosis
    c. stromal hyperplasia
corticifugal
corticipetal
corticobulbar
    c. tract
corticocollicular
corticoid
corticopontine
corticorubral
corticospinal
    c. tract
corticosteroid
    c.-binding globulin
corticosterone
corticothalamic
corticotrope
corticotropic
corticotropin
    c.-releasing factor
cortin
Cortinarius orellanus
Corti's
    ganglion
    organ
cortisol
    c. assays
    c. secretion rate
    urinary free c.
cortisone
    c. acetate
    c.-glucose tolerance test

cortisone *(continued)*
    c. reductase
cortol
cortolone
Cortrosyn
corymbiform
Corynebacteriaceae
Corynebacterium
    C. acnes
    C. belfantii
    C. diphtheriae
    C. enzymicum
    C. equi
    C. hemolyticum
    C. hoagii
    C. hofmannii
    C. infantisepticum
    C. minutissimum
    C. mycetoides
    C. necrophorum
    C. parvulum
    C. pseudodiphtheriticum
    C. pseudotuberculosis-ovis
    C. renale
    C. tenuis
    C. ulcerans
    C. vaginale
    C. xerosis
coryneform
coryza
coryzavirus
cosine
cosmic
    c. radiation
    c. rays
costa (costae)
costal
    c. cartilage
    c. element
    c. pleura
costochondral
costotransverse

costovertebral
    c. angle
    c. joint
cosyntropin
COTe — cathodal opening tetanus
cothromboplastin
cotinine
cotransport
cotton
    collodion c.
    salicylated c.
    c.-wool appearance
    c.-wool spot
Cotunnius' aqueduct
cot value
cotyledon
cough
    dry c.
    c. plate
    productive c.
    c. reflex
    whooping c.
coulomb
Coulomb's law
coulometer
coulometric
    c. titration
coulometry
Coulter counter
coumachlor
coumaric anhydride
coumarin
Councilmania
    C. dissimilis
    C. lafleuri
Councilman's bodies
count
    Addis c.
    Arneth's c.
    blood c.
    complete blood c.

count *(continued)*
    c. density
    differential c.
    c. information density
    c. rate
    c. rate meter
    reticulocyte c.
    Schilling blood c.
counter
    binary c.
    cell c.
    Coulter c.
    decade c.
    frequency c.
    Geiger c.
    Geiger-Müller c.
    proportional c.
    radiation c.
    ring c.
    ripple c.
    scintillation c.
    shift c.
    synchronous c.
countercurrent
    c. extraction
    c. immunoelectrophoresis
counterimmunoelectrophoresis
counterpulsation
counterstain
counting
    c. cadence
    c. chamber
    c. plate
coup
    c. de fouet
    en c. de sabre
    c. de sang
    c. de soleil
    c. sur coup
coupling
    c. capacitor
    excitation-contraction c.

coupling *(continued)*
    fixed c.
Courvoisier's law
covalence
covalent
covariance
coverglass
coverslip
Cowdry bodies
Cowper's gland
cowpox
    c. virus
coxa
    c. valga
    c. vara
coxal
    c. region
coxalgia
Coxiella
    C. burnetii
coxitis
coxodynia
coxsackievirus
    c. A
    c. B
Cox vaccine
cozymase
CP — cerebral palsy
    chemically pure
    chloropurine
    chloroquine and primaquine
    chronic pyelonephritis
    closing pressure
    cochlear potential
    coproporphyrin
    creatine phosphate
C/P — cholesterol-phospholipid ratio
cP — centipoise
CPA — cerebellar pontine angle
    chlorophenylalanine

CPAP — continuous positive airway pressure
CPB — cardiopulmonary bypass
    competitive protein-binding
CPC — cetylpyridinium chloride
    chronic passive congestion
    clinicopathologic conference
CPD — cephalopelvic disproportion
    citrate-phosphate-dextrose
CPDA — citrate-phosphate-dextrose-adenine
CPE — chronic pulmonary emphysema
    cytopathic effect
C-peptide
CPI — coronary prognostic index
CPIB — chlorophenoxyisobutyrate
CPK — creatine phosphokinase
cpm — counts per minute
CPN — chronic pyelonephritis
CPP — cyclopentenophenanthrene
CPPB — continuous positive-pressure breathing
CPPD — calcium pyrophosphate dihydrate
CPR — cardiopulmonary resuscitation
    cerebral cortex perfusion rate
    cortisol production rate
cps — cycles per second
CPZ — chlorpromazine
CQ — chloroquine-quinine
    circadian quotient

CR — chest and right arm
  chloride
  conditioned reflex
  creatinine
  crown rump
Cr — chromium
CRA — central retinal artery
Crabtree effect
Craigie's tube method
cramp
  c. discharge
cran — cranial
craniad
cranial
  c. arteritis
  c. bone
  c. cavity
  c. duplication
  c. dura mater
  c. epidural space
  c. monocephalus duplication
  c. nerve
  c. pia mater
  c. subarachnoid space
  c. subdural space
craniobuccal
craniocaudal
  c. projection
craniofenestria
craniolacunia
craniometry
craniopagus
craniopharyngioma
craniorachischisis
cranioschisis
cranioslerosis
cranioscopy
craniostenosis
craniosynostosis
craniotabes
craniotomy

cranium (craniums, crania)
crateriform
craw-craw
CRBBB — complete right bundle branch block
CRD — chronic renal disease
  complete reaction of degeneration
C-reactive protein
  C.-r. p. test
crease
  palmar c.
  simian c.
creat — creatinine
creatinase
creatine
  c. assays
  c. kinase
  c. kinase assay
  c. kinase isoenzyme electrophoresis
  c. kinase isoenzymes
  c. phosphate
  c. phosphokinase
creatininase
creatinine
  c. assays
  c. clearance
  c. coefficient
creatinuria
Credé's
  method
  ointment
creeping
  c. eruption
  c. substitution of bone
C region
cremaster muscle
cremasteric
  c. fascia
  c. reflex

crena (crenae)
crenate
crenated
    c. cell
crenation
crenulate
crepitation
crepitus
crescent
    c. cell
    epithelial c.
    sublingual c.
crescentic
    c. glomerulopathy
cresol
    c. assays
    c. red
crest
    iliac c.
    pubic c.
    c. time
cresyl
    c. blue
    c. fast violet
    c. violet acetate
cresylic acid
cretinism
Creutzfeldt-Jakob disease
CRF — chronic renal failure
        corticotropin-releasing
        factor
cribriform
    c. carcinoma
    c. plate
cricoid cartilage
cri du chat syndrome
Crigler-Najjer syndrome
Crimean hemorrhagic fever
    virus
crinin
crinophagy

Crippa's lead tetraacetate
    method
crisis (crises)
    addisonian c.
    adrenal c.
    anaphylactoid c.
    blast c.
    celiac c.
    thyroid c.
crista (cristae)
    c. ampullaris
    c. galli
    c. supraventricularis
    c. urethra
critical
    c. angle
    c. illumination
    c. mass
    c. micelle concentration
    c. path analysis
    c. region
    c. temperature
CRM — cross-reacting material
cRNA — chromosomal RNA
crocidolite
Crohn's disease
cromolyn sodium
Crooke's hyaline degeneration
cross
    c. activation
    c.-assembler
    c.-compiler
    c.-fire treatment
    c. product
    c.-reacting antigen
    c.-reacting material
    c. reaction
    c.-reactivity
    c.-sectional survey
    c. wall
crossmatching

crossover
    c. frequency
crotalin
crotamiton
crotin
crotonase
croton oil
crot value
croup
    c.-associated (virus)
Crouzon's
    craniofacial dysostosis
    disease
crowded cell index
crowding
    c. effect
CRP — C-reactive protein
CRS — Chinese restaurant syndrome
CRST — calcinosis cutis, Raynaud's phenomenon, sclerodactyly, and telangiectasia
CRT — cathode ray tube
cruciate
    c. lobe
    c. sulcus
crucible
cruor (cruores)
crural
crus (crura)
    c. cerebri
    c. fornix
    c. penis
crush
    c. injury
    c. kidney
    c. syndrome
CRV — central retinal vein
cryalgesia
cryoablation
cryobank
cryobiology
cryocautery
cryocrit
cryofibrinogen
cryofibrinogenemia
cryogammaglobulin
cryogenic
cryoglobulin
cryoglobulinemia
cryohydrocytosis
Cryokwik
cryopathic hemolytic syndrome
cryophile
cryoprecipitate
cryopreservation
cryoprobe
cryoprotectant
cryoprotein
cryoscope
cryostat
    Ames Lab-Tek c.
cryosurgery
cryotherapy
crypt
    anal c.
    appendiceal c.
    colonic c.
    Lieberkühn's c's
    Luschka's c's
    Morgagni's c.
    rectal c.
    small intestinal c.
    tonsillar c's
cryptenamine
cryptic
cryptitis
Cryptococcaceae
cryptococcal
    c. antigen
    c. meningitis
cryptococci
cryptococcosis

Cryptococcus
  C. albidus/albidus
  C. albidus/diffluens
  C. capsulatus
  C. epidermidis
  C. gilchristi
  C. histolyticus
  C. hominis
  C. laurentii
  C. luteolus
  C. meningitidis
  C. neoformans
  C. terreus
cryptomenorrhea
cryptophthalmos
cryptorchidism
cryptorchism
Cryptostroma
  C. corticale
cryptostromosis
cryptoxanthin
cryptozoite
crys – crystal
crystal
  asthma c's
  blood c's
  c. cell
  Charcot-Leyden c's
  c. deposition disease
  leukocytic c's
  liquid c's
  Lubarsch's c's
  Reinke c's
  rock c.
  sperm c's
  urine sediment c's
  c. violet
  whetstone c's
crystalline
  c. aggregate, nuclear
  c. macromolecule alteration
crystallization
crystallography
crystalloid
  Charcot-Böttcher c's
crystalluria
CS – cesarean section
  chondroitin sulfate
  chorionic somatomammotropin
  conditioned stimulus
  coronary sinus
  corticosteroid
  cycloserine
C & S – conjunctiva and sclera
  culture and sensitivity
Cs – cesium
CSA – canavaninosuccinic acid
  chondroitin sulfate A
  colony-stimulating activity
  compressed spectral assay
CSC – coup sur coup
CSF – cerebrospinal fluid
  colony-stimulating factor
CSH – chronic subdural hematoma
  cortical stromal hyperplasia
CSL – cardiolipin synthetic lecithin
CSM – cerebrospinal meningitis
CSN – carotid sinus nerve
CSR – Cheyne-Stokes respiration
  corrected sedimentation rate
  cortisol secretion rate
CSS – carotid sinus stimulation
CST – convulsive shock therapy

cSt — centistoke
CT — cardiothoracic (ratio)
    carotid tracing
    carpal tunnel
    cerebral thrombosis
    chlorothiazide
    circulation time
    clotting time
    coagulation time
    collecting tubule
    computed tomography
    computerized tomography
    connective tissue
    contraction time
    Coombs' test
    coronary thrombosis
    corrected transposition
    crest time
    cytotechnologist
CTA — chromotropic acid
CTAB — cetyltrimethylammonium bromide
CTAT — computerized transaxial tomography
CTBA — cetrimonium bromide
CTC — chlortetracycline
CTD — carpal tunnel decompression
    congenital thymic dysplasia
Ctenocephalides
    C. canis
C-terminal
ctetosome
CTFE — chlorotrifluoroethylene
CTH — ceramide trihexoside
CTL — cytologic T lymphocyte
CT number
CTP — cytidine triphosphate
CTR — cardiothoracic ratio
CTX — cytoxan
CTZ — chlorothiazide
Cu — copper
cubic
cubital
    c. fossa
    c. lymph node
    c. vein
cubitus
    c. valgus
    c. varus
cuboid
cuboidal
CUC — chronic ulcerative colitis
cu cm — cubic centimeter
cuffing
CUG — cystourethrogram
cul-de-sac
    conjunctival c.
    Douglas's c.
    dural c.
culdocentesis
culdoscope
culdoscopy
Culex
Culicidae
Culicoides
Cullen's sign
culling
culmen
cultivation
culture
    attenuated c.
    bacterial c.
    blood c.
    cell c.
    chorioallantoic c.
    continuous flow c.
    direct c.
    flask c.
    hanging-block c.

culture *(continued)*
    hanging-drop c.
    mixed c.
    needle c.
    plate c.
    primary c.
    pure c.
    radioisotopic c.
    secondary c.
    c. and sensitivity
    sensitized c.
    shake c.
    slant c.
    slope c.
    smear c.
    stab c.
    stock c.
    streak c.
    stroke c.
    synchronized c.
    thrust c.
    tissue c.
    tube c.
    type c.
culture media. *See* Appendix 3, Culture Media.
cu mm — cubic millimeter
cumulative
    c. distribution
cumulus (cumuli)
    c. oophorous
    ovarian c.
cuneate
cuneiform
    c. cartilage
    c. lobe
cuneus
Cunninghamella
    C. bertholletiae
    C. elegans
CuO — cupric oxide
cupping
cupremia
cupric
cuprous
curare
curariform
curarization
curet
curettage
    endometrial c.
curette
curie
    c.-hour
curietherapy
curium
Curling's ulcer
current
    c. gain
    c. regulator
Curschmann's spirals
cursor
curvature
    greater c. of stomach
    lesser c. of stomach
    spinal c.
curve
    Bragg c.
    c. fitting
    H and D c.
    Price-Jones c.
Curvularia
    C. geniculata
cushingoid
Cushing's
    basophilism
    disease
    reflex
    syndrome
    ulcer
cuspid
    deciduous c.
    mandibular c.
    maxillary c.

cutaneous
   c. branch
   c. fluids
   c. gland
   c. horn
   c. malformation
   c. mucous gland
   c. nerve
cutdown
cuticle
cuticulum
Cutie Pie
cutireaction
cutis
   c. anserina
   c. elastica
   c. laxa
   c. verticis gyrata
cutoff
   c. frequency
cuvet, cuvette
Cuvier's duct
CV – cardiovascular
   cell volume
   central venous
   cerebrovascular
   coefficient of variation
   color vision
   conjugate diameter of pelvic inlet
   corpuscular volume
   cresyl violet
CVA – cardiovascular accident
   cerebrovascular accident
   costovertebral angle
CVD – cardiovascular disease
   color vision deviant
CVH – combined ventricular hypertrophy
   common variable hypogammaglobulinemia
C virus – Coxsackie virus
CVO – conjugata vera obstetrica (obstetric conjugate diameter of pelvic inlet)
CVOD – cerebrovascular obstructive disease
CVP – cell volume profile
   central venous pressure
   cyclophosphamide, vincristine, prednisone
   Cytoxan, vincristine, prednisone
CVR – cardiovascular-renal
   cerebrovascular resistance
CVRD – cardiovascular renal disease
CVS – cardiovascular surgery
   cardiovascular system
C wave
CWDF – cell wall-deficient bacterial forms
CWI – cardiac work index
CWP – coal workers' pneumoconiosis
cwt – hundredweight
Cx or cx – convex
CXR – chest x-ray film
Cy – cyanogen
cyanamide
cyanate
cyanhemoglobin
cyanide
   c. anion
   c.-ascorbate test
   c. assays
   mercuric c.
cyanin
cyanmethemoglobin
Cyanobacteria
cyanocobalamin
   radioactive c.

cyanogen
  c. bromide
  c. chloride
cyanoketone
cyanol FF
cyanophil
cyanopia
cyanose tardive
cyanosis
cybernetics
cybrid
cyclacillin
cyclamate
cyclandelate
cyclase
  adenyl c.
  adenylate c.
cyclazocine
cycle
  anovulatory c.
  biliary c.
  carbon c.
  cardiac c.
  citric acid c.
  Cori's c.
  cytoplasmic c.
  Embden-Meyerhof c.
  estrous c.
  gastric c.
  Golgi's c.
  Hodgkin c.
  Krebs' c.
  Krebs-Henseleit c.
  menstrual c.
  nitrogen c.
  ovarian c.
  c's per second
  pregnancy c.
  Schiff's biliary c.
  tricarboxylic acid c.
  urea c.
  uterine c.

cycle *(continued)*
  vaginal c.
cyclic
  c. adenosine monophosphate
  c. alteration
  c. AMP
  c. GMP
  c. guanosine monophosphate
  c. neutropenia
  c. nucleotides
  c. tissue alteration
cyclitis
cyclitol
cyclization
cyclizine
  c. hydrochloride
Cyclo – cyclophosphamide
        cyclopropane
cycloalkane
cycloalkene
cyclobarbital
cyclobenzaprine hydrochloride
cyclobutane
cyclocryotherapy
cyclocumarol
cyclodimerization
cyclogeny
cyclogram
cyclohexane
cyclohexanol
cyclohexene oxide
cycloheximide
cyclohexylamine
2-cyclohexyl-4,6-dinitrophenol
cyclomethycaine sulfate
cyclonite
cyclopentamine hydrochloride
cyclopentane
cyclopentanoperhydrophenanthrene

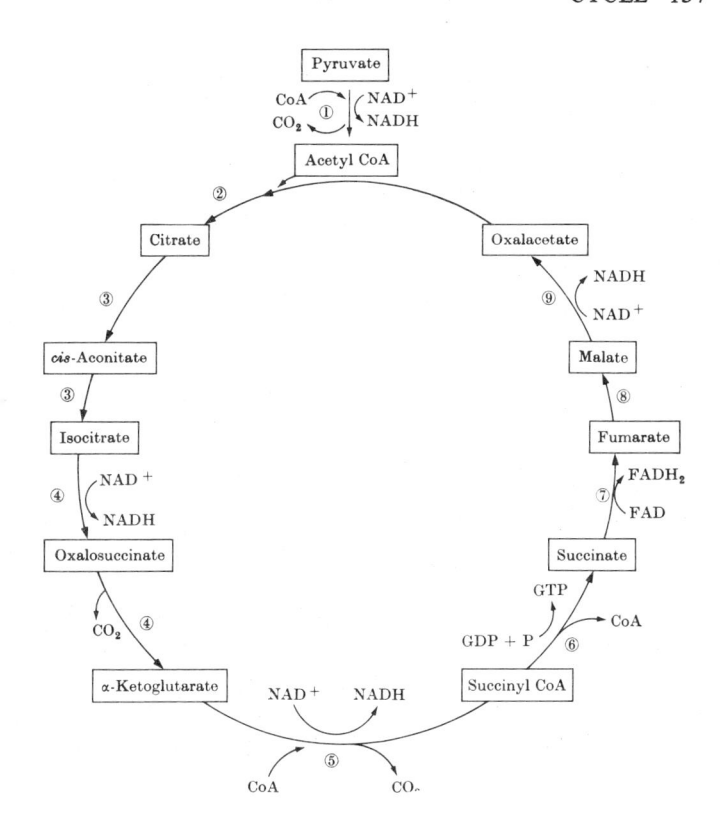

TRICARBOXYLIC ACID (KREBS') CYCLE

Representation of reactions by which carbon chains of sugars, fatty acids and amino acids are metabolized to yield carbon dioxide, water, and high-energy phosphate bonds. Key to enzymes (circled numbers): 1 = pyruvate dehydrogenase, 2 = citrate synthase, 3 = aconitrate dehydrogenase, 4 = isocitric dehydrogenase, 5 = α-ketoglutarate dehydrogenase, 6 = succinyl-CoA synthetase, 7 = succinate dehydrogenase, 8 = fumarate hydratase (furmarase), 9 = malate dehydrogenase. (Mazur and Harrow.)

(From Dorland's Illustrated Medical Dictionary. 26th ed. Philadelphia, W. B. Saunders Company, 1981.)

cyclopentolate hydrochloride
cyclophosphamide
Cyclophyllidea
cyclopia
cyclopropane
Cyclops
cyclops
    c. hypognathus
cycloscope
cycloserine
cyclosis
cyclothiazide
cyclothymic
cyclotron
cycrimine hydrochloride
cyesis
cylinder
cylindric
cylindrical
    c. bronchiectasis
    c. embryo
cylindroid
cylindroma
    dermal eccrine c.
cylindruria
cymarin
cynanche
    c. maligna
    c. tonsillaris
cyproheptadine hydrochloride
cyproterone acetate
cyrtometer
cys — cysteine
cyst
    aneurysmal bone c.
    Baker's c.
    Bartholin's c.
    blue dome c.
    branchial c.
    branchial cleft c.
    bronchial c.
    bronchogenic c.

cyst *(continued)*
    chocolate c.
    colloid c.
    congenital c.
    corpus hemorrhagicum c.
    corpus luteum c.
    dental follicular c.
    dentigerous c.
    dermoid c.
    embryonal duct c.
    epidermal c.
    epidermal inclusion c.
    epidermoid c.
    epidermoid inclusion c.
    epididymal c.
    epithelial c.
    epithelial inclusion c.
    follicle c.
    follicular c.
    ganglion c.
    Gartner's duct c.
    gas c.
    germinal epithelial inclusion c.
    germinal inclusion c.
    globulomaxillary c.
    hemorrhagic c.
    hydatid c.
    inclusion c.
    inflammatory c.
    keratinous c.
    Kobelt's c.
    luteal c.
    luteinized follicular c.
    meibomian c.
    mesonephric c.
    mesothelial c.
    milium c.
    Morgagni's c.
    mucinous c.
    mucous c.
    multilocular c.

cyst *(continued)*
    myxoid c.
    nabothian c.
    odontogenic c.
    paraphyseal c.
    parathyroid c.
    pericardial c.
    periodontal c.
    pilonidal c.
    radicular c.
    ranular c.
    renal c.
    retention c.
    sebaceous c.
    serous c.
    simple c.
    solitary c.
    tension c.
    theca lutein c.
    thyroglossal duct c.
cystadenocarcinoma
    mucinous c.
    papillary c.
    papillary serous c.
    pseudomucinous c.
    serous c.
cystadenofibroma
cystadenoma
    c. lymphomatosum
    mucinous c.
    oncocytic papillary c.
    papillary c.
    papillary serous c.
    pseudomucinous c.
    serous c.
cystalgia
cystathionase
cystathionine
    c. lyase
    c. synthase
cystathioninuria
cysteamine dehydrogenase

cystectasia
cystectomy
cysteic acid method
cysteine
    c. aminotransferase
    c. desulfhydrase
    c. synthase
    c. synthetase
cysteinesulfinate decarboxylase
cysteinyl
cysteinyl-glycine dipeptidase
cystic
    c. acute inflammation
    c. artery
    c. atrophy
    c. chronic cervicitis
    c. chronic inflammation
    c. corpus hemorrhagicum
    c. corpus luteum
    c. degeneration
    c. dermoid teratoma
    c. disease
    c. duct
    c. endometrial hyperplasia
    c. fibrosis
    c. granulomatous inflammation
    c. hygroma
    c. hyperplasia
    c. inflammation
    c. mastitis
    c. mastopathy
    c. medial necrosis
    c. medionecrosis
    c. ovarian follicle
    c. vein
cysticerci
cysticercoid
cysticercosis
Cysticercus
    C. acanthrotrias
    C. bovis

Cysticercus (continued)
  C. cellulosae
  C. fasciolaris
  C. ovis
  C. tenuicollis
cysticercus (cysticerci)
cystine
  c. calculus
  c. reductase
cystinemia
cystinosis
cystinuria
cystitis
  acute hemorrhagic c.
  c. cystica
  c. follicularis
  c. glandularis
  hemorrhagic c.
  Hunner's c.
  c. pneumatoides
  ulcerative c.
cysto — cystoscopic examination
cystoblast
cystocele
cystogram
  voiding c.
cystography
  radionuclide c.
  retrograde c.
cystoid
Cystokon
cystolith
cystoma
  serous c.
cystometer
cystometrography
cystopyelitis
cystosarcoma
  c. phyllodes
  c. phylloides
cystoscope

cystoscopy
cystostomy
cystoureteritis
cystoureterogram
cystoureterography
cystourethroscope
cystyl
cytarabine
  c. hydrochloride
cytase
cytidine
  c. deaminase
  c. diphosphate
  c. monophosphate
  c. phosphate
  c. triphosphate
cytidylic acid
cytidylyl
cytisine
cytisism
cytoanalyzer
cytoblast
cytoblastema
cytocentrifugation
cytocentrifuge
cytochalasin
  c. B
cytochemical
cytochemistry
cytochrome
  c. oxidase
  c. peroxidase
  c. reductase
  c. reductase assays
cytoclasis
cytoclastic
cytode
cytodegenerative
cytodiagnosis
  exfoliative c.
cytodifferentiation
cytofluorography

cytogene
cytogenetic map
cytogenetics
    clinical c.
    population c.
cytoid
cytokine
cytokinesis
cytokinetic
cytokinin
cytolipin H
cytologic
    c. alteration
    c. degeneration
    c. engulfment
    c. T lymphocyte
cytology
    aspiration-biopsy c.
    exfoliative c.
cytolysate
    blood c.
cytolysin
cytolysis
    immune c.
cytolysosome
cytomegalic
    c. inclusion disease
    c. inclusion disease virus
cytomegalovirus
cytomegaly
cytometer
cytometry
cytopathic
    c. effect
cytopathogenesis
cytopathogenic
cytopathology
cytopenia
cytophilic
cytophotometer
cytophotometry
cytophylaxis
cytoplasm
cytoplasmic
    c. aggregate
    c. crystalline aggregate
    c. fiber alteration
    c. fibril alteration
    c. filament alteration
    c. inclusion
    c. lipid aggregate
    c. lipid droplet alteration
    c. macromolecule aggregate
    c. matrix alteration
    c. membrane
    c. vacuolization
cytoplast
cytorrhyctes
cytoscopy
cytosiderin
cytosine
    arabinoside c.
    hydroxymethyl c.
cytoskeleton
cytosol
cytosome
cytostasis
cytostatic
cytostome
cytotaxin
cytotaxis
cytotechnologist
cytotoxic
    c. necrosis
    c. T cells
cytotoxicity
cytotoxin
cytotrophoblast
cytotropic
    c. antibody
cytotropism
Cytoxan
Czapek-Dox agar

D

D — deciduous
 density
 deuterium
 deuteron
 dextro
 diopter
 distal
 dorsal
 duration
 vitamin D unit
D_{CO} — diffusing capacity for carbon monoxide
D_L — diffusing capacity of lung
d — day(s)
 diurnal
DA — degenerative arthritis
 developmental age
 direct agglutination
 disaggregated
 dopamine
 ductus arteriosus
DAB — dimethylaminoazobenzene
DAC — digital-to-analog converter
D/A converter
dacryoadenitis
dacryoblennorrhea
dacryocyst
dacryocystitis
dacryocystography
dacryocyte
dactinomycin
dactyl
DADDS — diacetyl diaminodiphenylsulfone
DAGT — direct antiglobulin test
DAH — disordered action of the heart
Dakin's solution
DALA — delta-aminolevulinic acid
dalapon
Dale-Laidlaw's clotting time method
Dalen-Fuchs nodules
dalton
Dalton's law
DAM — degraded amyloid
 diacetyl monoxime
damage
 irradiation d.
 radiation d.
dAMP — deoxyadenosine monophosphate
 deoxyadenosine phosphate
damping
D and C — dilatation and curettage
 dilation and curettage
dandruff
dandy fever
Dandy-Walker syndrome
Dane's
 method
 particle
DANS — 1-dimethylaminonaphthalene-5-sulphonyl chloride
dansyl chloride
danthron
dantrolene sodium
DAO — diamine oxidase

DAP — dihydroxyacetone
  phosphate
  direct agglutination
  pregnancy (test)
dapsone
DAPT — direct agglutination
  pregnancy test
Dapt — Daptazole
Darier's disease
dark
  d. current
  d. reactions
  d. reactivation
darkfield microscope
darkground microscope
Darkshevich's nucleus
Darling's disease
dartos
darwinian
  d. point
  d. tubercle
darwinism
DAT — differential agglutination titer
  diphtheria antitoxin
  direct agglutination test
data
  d. acquisition system
  d. display
  d. processing
  d. reduction
database
daughter
daunomycin
daunorubicin
Davainea
Davaineidae
Davenport graph
Davidsohn differential test
DB — dextran blue
  distobuccal
db — decibel

DBA — dibenzanthracene
DBC — dye-binding capacity
DBCL — dilute blood clot lysis
  (method)
DBI — development-at-birth
  index
DBM — dibromomannitol
DBO — distobucco-occlusal
DBP — diastolic blood pressure
  distobuccopulpal
DC — deoxycholate
  diphenylarsine cyanide
  distocervical
DC, dc — direct current
D & C — dilatation and curettage
  dilation and curettage
DCA — deoxycholate-citrate
  agar
  desoxycorticosterone
  acetate
DCc — double concave
DCF — direct centrifugal flotation
DCG — disodium cromoglycate
DCHFB — dichlorohexafluorobutane
DCI — dichloroisoproterenol
DCLS — deoxycholate citrate
  lactose saccharose
dCMP — deoxycytidine monophosphate
  deoxycytidine phosphate
D colony
DCT — direct Coombs' test
DCTMA — desoxycorticosterone trimethylacetate
DCTPA — desoxycorticosterone triphenylacetate

DCx — double convex
DDAVP — 1-deamino-(8-D-arginine)-vasopressin
DDC — diethyldithiocarbamic acid
DDD — dense deposit disease
dichlorodiphenyldichloroethane
dihydroxydinaphthyl disulfide
DDS — diaminodiphenylsulfone
dystrophy-dystocia syndrome
DDT — chlorophenothane
dichlorodiphenyltrichloroethane
DDVP — dichlorvos
D & E — dilation and evacuation
DEA — dehydroepiandrosterone
diethanolamine
deactivation
deacylase
deacylate
dead time
DEAE — diethylaminoethanol
diethylaminoethyl
diethylaminoethyl-cellulose
DEAE-D — diethylaminoethyl dextran
deafferentation
deafness
  conduction d.
  high frequency d.
  mixed-type d.
  nerve d.
  tone d.
dealcoholization
deallergization

deamidase
deaminase
  adenosine d.
  adenylic acid d.
  cytidine d.
  guanine d.
  guanosine d.
  guanylic acid d.
deamination
deanol acetamidobenzoate
deaquation
death
  brain d.
  cell d.
  crib d.
  fetal d.
  d. fever
  functional d.
  natural d.
DEBA — diethylbarbituric acid
Debaryomyces
  D. hansenii
  D. hominis
  D. neoformans
debrancher deficiency limit dextrinosis
debranching enzyme
debridement
debris
debubbling
debug
debye
decacurie
decagram
decahydronaphthalene
decalcification
decaliter
decameter
decamethonium
  d. bromide
  d. iodide
decanoic acid

decantation
decapeptide
decapitation
decarbazine
decarbonization
decarboxylase
    acetoacetate d.
    acetolactate d.
De Castro's fluid
decavitamin
decay
    beta d.
    d. coefficient
    d. constant
    d. mode
    d. product
    radioactive d.
    d. rate
    d. scheme
deceration
decerebrate
decibel
decidua
    basal d.
    capsular d.
    menstrual d.
    parietal d.
    reflex d.
    d. vera
decidual
    d. alteration
    d. cast
    d. cells
    d. change
    d. membrane
    d. metaplasia
deciduous
decigram
decile
deciliter
decimal
    d. reduction time

decimeter
decision table
decoagulant
decode
decoder
decolorize
decompensation
    cardiac d.
    d. injury
    d. sickness
decomposition
    d. potential
decompression
    d. sickness
decontamination
decortication
decoy cell
decrement
decrementing
    d. response
decubation
decubitus
    dorsal d.
    left lateral d.
    right lateral d.
    d. ulcer
    ventral d.
decussate
decussation
    dorsal tegmental d.
    d. of inferior cerebellar peduncles
    d. of pyramids
    d. of superior cerebellar peduncles
    pons d.
    pyramidal d.
    supramammillary d.
    ventral tegmental d.
dedifferentiation
DEEG — depth electroencephalogram

DEEG (continued)
depth electroencephalography
depth electrography

deep
- d. brachial artery
- d. cervical lymphatics
- d. circumflex iliac vein
- d. infrapatellar bursa
- d. lymphatics
- d. middle cerebral vein
- d. palmar arch
- d. peroneal nerve
- d. plantar branch
- d. sylvian vein
- d. temporal nerve
- d. transverse fibers
- d. volar arch

def — deficiency
defecation
defecography
defect
- acquired d.
- atrial septal d.
- congenital d.
- ectodermal d.
- endocardial cushion d's
- fibrous cortical d.
- neural tube d.
- septal d.
- surgical d.
- ventricular septal d.

defective
- d. insight
- d. judgment
- d. recent memory
- d. remote memory
- d. virus

defenestration
deferoxamine
- d. hydrochloride
- d. mesylate

defervescence
defibrillation
defibrillator
defibrination
- d. syndrome

deficiency
- d. disease
- vitamin d.

deficit
definition
definitive
deflection
- d. signal

deflorescence
defoliant
deformability
deformation
deformity
- acquired d.
- congenital d.
- Klippel-Feil d.
- lobster claw d.
- pigeon breast d.
- valgus d.
- varus d.

deg — degeneration
degree
De Galantha's method for urates
degenerate code
degenerated
- d. intervertebral disc
- d. intervertebral fibrocartilage
- d. meniscus

degenerating
- d. myelin demonstration

degeneration
- albuminous d.
- amyloid d.
- ascending d.
- axonal d.

degeneration *(continued)*
  ballooning d.
  basophilic d.
  calcareous d.
  cellular d.
  cloudy swelling d.
  collagen d.
  colloid d.
  Crooke's hyaline d.
  cystic d.
  cystoid d.
  cytologic d.
  descending d.
  fatty d.
  feathery d.
  fibrinoid d.
  fibrinous d.
  floccular d.
  granular d.
  hepatolenticular d.
  hyaline d.
  hydatid d.
  hydropic d.
  lipid d.
  lipoid d.
  liquefactive d.
  medial d.
  mucinous d.
  mucoid d.
  myelin d.
  myxoid d.
  myxomatous d.
  parenchymatous d.
  pigmentary d.
  pseudomucinous d.
  secondary d.
  subacute combined d.
  trans-synaptic d.
  wallerian d.
  waxy d.
  Zenker's d.

degenerative
  d. arthritis
  d. change
  d. index
deglutition
deglycerolization
degradation
degranulation
degree
  d's of freedom
dehiscence
dehydratase
dehydrate
dehydration
dehydroacetic acid
dehydroascorbic acid
dehydrobilirubin
dehydrocholesterol
  activated 7-d.
dehydrocholic acid
11-dehydrocorticosterone
dehydroepiandrosterone
dehydrogenase
  isocitric d.
  lactate d. (LDH)
dehydrogenate
dehydrogenation
dehydropeptidase
deionization
Deiters' nucleus
Dejerine-Sottas disease
Delaney clause
de Lange's syndrome
delay
  d. circuit
  d. line
delayed
  d. adrenarche
  d. climacteric
  d. hypersensitivity reaction
  d. menopause

delayed *(continued)*
   d. puberty
de-lead
deletion
   chromosomal d.
   d. theory
deliquescence
deliquescent
delirium (deliria)
   d. tremens
delivery
   precipitous d.
Delphian node
delta
   d. band
   d. cell islet
   d. check
   d. ray
delta activity
   intermittent rhythmic d. a.
   polymorphic d. a.
deltoideus muscle
delusion
Dem — Demerol (meperidine)
demarcation
   line of d.
Dematiaceae
dematiacious fungi
Dematium
demecarium bromide
demeclocycline
   d. hydrochloride
dementia
   presenile d.
   senile d.
Demerol (meperidine)
demethylchlortetracycline
demeton
demilune
demineralization
Demodex
   D. folliculorum

demyelinate
demyelinating disease
demyelination
demyelinization
denaturation
   protein d.
dendrite
dendritic
dengue
   hemorrhagic d.
   d. virus, types 1, 2, 3, 4
Dennis technique
dens (dentes)
   d. in dente
dense
   d. body
   d. connective tissue
   d. deposit disease
densimeter
densitometer
densitometry
density
   base d.
   calcific d.
   decreased d.
   d. function
   d. gradient centrifugation
   increased d.
   intermediate d.
   radiographic d.
   water d.
dental
   d. calculus
   d. caries
   d. fluorosis
   d. follicular cyst
   d. granuloma
   d. plaque
   d. radiography
dentate
   d. gyrus
   d. ligament

dentate *(continued)*
   d. nucleus
denticle
denticulated
dentigerous
   d. cyst
   d. mixed tumor
dentin
   d. crystal alteration
   d. dysplasia
   d. formation
dentinal
dentinogenesis imperfecta
dentinoma
   fibroameloblastic d.
dentistry
dentition
Denver classification
deoxyadenosine monophosphate
deoxyadenosine phosphate
deoxyadenylic acid
deoxycholate
   d. citrate lactose saccharose
deoxycholic acid
deoxycholylglycine
11-deoxycorticosterone
11-deoxycortisol
deoxycytidine monophosphate
deoxycytidine phosphate
deoxycytidylic acid
6-deoxygalactose
2-deoxy-D-glucose
deoxyguanosine monophosphate
deoxyguanosine phosphate
deoxyguanylic acid
deoxyhemoglobin
6-deoxy-mannose
deoxyribonuclease
   d. digestion

deoxyribonuclease *(continued)*
   d. (DNase) test
   d. I
   d. II
deoxyribonucleic acid
   d. a. staining
deoxyribonucleoside
deoxyribonucleotide
deoxyribose
deoxysugar
deoxyuridine
   d. monophosphate
   d. phosphate
   d. suppression test
deoxyuridylic acid
deparaffinization
dependence
   drug d.
dependent
   d. variable
dephospho-coenzyme A
   d.-c. A kinase
   d.-c. A pyrophosphorylase
depigmentation
deplasmolysis
depletion
   d. layer
   lipid d.
   plasma d.
depolarization
depolarizer
depolymerization
deposit
deposition
   bilharzial pigment d.
   calcium d.
   cholesterol d.
   fatty d.
   ferrocalcinotic d.
   foreign material d.
   hemosiderin d.

Dermatophagoides pteronyssimus (m.

deposition *(continued)*
- malarial pigment d.
- particulate crystalline material d.
- xanthomatous d.

depressant

depressed
- d. fracture
- d.-type manic-depressive psychosis

depression
- psychoneurotic d.
- reactive d.

deprivation

deproteinization

depth
- d. electroencephalogram
- d. electroencephalography
- d. electrography
- d. of field
- d. of focus

deQuervain's
- disease
- thyroiditis

DeR — reaction of degeneration

der — derivative chromosome

deradelphus

derangement

Dercum's disease

derepression

De Ritis ratio

derivation

derivative
- d. chromosome

derived protein

Dermacentor
- *D. andersoni*
- *D. occidentalis*
- *D. reticulatus*
- *D. variabilis*

Dermacentroxenus
- *D. sibericus*

dermal
- d. eccrine cylindroma
- d. epidermal nevus
- d. nevus
- d. papilla

Dermanyssus
- *D. gallinae*

dermatan sulfate

dermatitis
- actinic d.
- allergic d.
- atopic d.
- d. atrophicans
- d. atrophicans diffusa
- d. atrophicans maculosa
- chronica atrophicans idiopathica d.
- contact d.
- eczematoid d.
- d. escharotica
- exfoliative d.
- factitious d.
- d. gangrenosa infantum
- d. herpetiformis
- lichenoid d.
- d. medicamentosa
- photo contact d.
- phototoxic contact d.
- pigmented purpuric lichenoid d.
- psoriasiform d.
- radiation d.
- d. repens
- seborrheic d.
- stasis d.
- toxic d.
- d. venenata

Dermatobia
- *D. hominis*

dermatofibroma

dermatofibrosarcoma
- d. protuberans

Desulfovibrio desulfuricans

dermatofibrosis
    d. lenticularis disseminata
dermatogen
dermatoglyphics
dermatographism
dermatologic
dermatology
dermatome
dermatomycin
dermatomycosis
dermatomyositis
dermatopathic
    d. lymphadenitis
    d. lymphadenopathy
Dermatophilaceae
dermatophilosis
Dermatophilus
    D. congolensis
    D. penetrans
dermatophyte
dermatophytid
Dermatophytin "O"
dermatophytosis
dermatosis (dermatoses)
    progressive pigmentary d.
dermis
dermographia
dermoid
    d. cyst
dermopathy
derodidymus
DES – diethylstilbestrol
desalt
desaturation
Descemet's
    membrane
    posterior lamina
descending
    d. colon
    d. degeneration
    d. hypoglossal nerve
    d. limb

descending *(continued)*
    d. thoracic aorta
desensitization
desensitize
deserpidine
desferrioxamine
desiccant
desiccate
desiccation
desiccator
desipramine
    d. assays
    d. hydrochloride
deslanoside
desmepithelium
desmoid
desmolase
desmoplasia
desmosine
desmosome
desmosterol
desolvation
11-desoxycorticosterone
11-desoxy,17-OH-corticosterone
despeciate
desquamation
desquamative
    d. interstitial pneumonitis
destructive
desynapsis
desynchronization
desynchronized
    d. sleep
DET – diethyltryptamine
detachment
    retinal d.
detector
    NP d.
    d. transfer function
detergent
determinant

determination
deterministic
detoxification
　　metabolic d.
detritus
detubation
detumescence
deutan
deuteranomaly
deuteranopia
deuterium
deuterohemophilia
Deuteromycetes
deuteron
deuterosome
deuterotoxin
DEV — duck embryo vaccine
develop
development
developmental
　　d. genetics
　　d. jaw cyst
　　d. synchronism
deviation
device
Devic's disease
dew
　　d. point
Dewar flask
dexamethasone
　　d. suppression test
dexbrompheniramine
　　d. maleate
dexchlorpheniramine
　　d. maleate
dextran
dextranase
dextrin
dextrinase
dextrin-1,6-glucosidase
dextroamphetamine
dextrocardia
　　isolated d.
dextromethorphan hydrobromide
dextroposition
dextrorotatory
dextrose
dextrosuria
dextrothyroxine sodium
DF — decapacitation factor
　　deficiency factor
　　desferrioxamine
　　discriminant function
　　disseminated foci
df — degrees of freedom
DFDT — difluorodiphenyltrichloroethane
DFO — deferoxamine
DFP — diisopropylfluorophosphate
DFU — dead fetus in utero
　　dideoxyfluorouridine
DG — deoxyglucose
　　diastolic gallop
　　diglyceride
　　distogingival
dg or dgm — decigram
dGMP — deoxyguanosine monophosphate
　　deoxyguanosine phosphate
dGTP — 2-deoxyguanosine-5'-triphosphate
DH — delayed hypersensitivity
DHA — dehydroepiandrosterone
　　dihydroxyacetone
DHAP — dihydroxyacetone phosphate
DHAS — dehydroepiandrosterone sulfate

DHE — dihydroergotamine
DHEA — dehydroepiandrosterone
DHEAS — dehydroepiandrosterone sulfate
DHFR — dihydrofolate reductase
DHIA — dehydroisoandrosterone
DHL — diffuse histocytic lymphoma
DHMA — dihydroxymandelic acid
dhobie itch
DHT — dihydrotachysterol
    dihydrotestosterone
DI — diabetes insipidus
diabetes
    bronzed d.
    d. insipidus
    juvenile-onset d.
    d. mellitus
diabetic
    d. angiopathy
    d. coma
    d. dermopathy
    d. glomerulosclerosis
    hyperosmolar d. coma
    d. ketoacidosis
    d. lipemia
    d. myelopathy
    d. retinopathy
diacetate
diacetic acid
diacetylaminoazotoluene
diacylglycerol
diag — diagnosis
Diagnex Blue test
diagnosis
    clinical d.
    cytologic d.
    differential d.

diagnosis *(continued)*
    laboratory d.
    pathologic d.
    physical d.
    provocative d.
    roentgen d.
    serum d.
diagram
diakinesis
Dialister
dialkyl
    d. dimethyl ammonium chloride
    d. sodium sulfosuccinate
dial unit
dialysance
dialysate
dialysis
dialyzer
diamagnetic
diameter
    Mantoux d.
diamide
diamine
    diethylene d.
    d. oxidase
diaminoacid aminotransferase
diaminodiphenylsulfone
2,4-diaminophenol hydrochloride
Diamond-Blackfan anemia
diamthazole dihydrochloride
diapedesis
diaphane
diaphanometer
diaphanoscope
diaphoresis
diaphragm
    eventration of the d.
    field d.
    iris d.
    Potter-Bucky d.

DIAPHRAGMA – DICHLORODEPHENYLDICHLOROETHANE

diaphragma
   d. pelvis
   d. sellae
   d. urogenitale
diaphragmatic
   d. hernia
   d. lymph node
   d. pleura
diaphysis (diaphyses)
diapophysis
diapositive
Diaptomus
diarrhea
diarthrosis (diarthroses)
diaschisis
diascope
diastase
diastasis
diastematomyelia
diastereoisomer
diastereoisomerism
diastereomer
diastole
diastolic
   d. hypertension
   d. murmur
   d. pressure
diathermy
diathesis
   hemorrhagic d.
diatom
diatomaceous
diatrizoate
diauxic
diauxie
diaxon
diazepam
   d. assays
diazine
diazinon
diazomethane
   d. generator

diazonium salt
diazo staining method
diazotize
diazoxide
dibasic acid
dibenzanthracene
dibenzepin hydrochloride
diborane
dibothriocephaliasis
Dibothriocephalus
dibromethane
dibromosalicylaldehyde
dibucaine
   d. hydrochloride
   d. number
dibutoline sulfate
dibutyl
   d. adipate
   d. phthalate
   d. succinate
DIC – diffuse intravascular coagulation
   disseminated intravascular coagulation
dic – dicentric
dicarbamylamine
dicarboxylic acid
dicentric
dicephalus
   d. dipus dibrachius
   d. dipus tetrabrachius
   d. dipus tribrachius
   d. dipygus
   d. tripus tribrachius
dicheirus
dichlobenil
dichlorisone
dichlorobenzene
dichloro-chloroaniline-triazine
dichlorodiethyl sulfide
dichlorodiphenyldichloroethane

dichlorodiphenyltrichloroethane
dichloroethane
1,1-dichloroethylene
dichloroethyl ether
dichloromethane
dichloronaphthoquinone
1-1-dichloro-1-nitroethane
dichlorophene
2,4-dichlorophenoxyacetic acid
dichlorophenyl dimethyl urea
dichlorophenyl methyl butyl-
  urea
dichloropropane
1,3-dichloro-2-propanol
dichloropropene
dichloropropionic acid
dichlorphenamide
dichlorvos
dichogeny
dichotomize
dichotomous
  d. variable
dichotomy
dichroism
  circular d.
dichromate
Dick test
dicloxacillin sodium
dicofol
Dicrocoelium
  D. dendriticum
dicrotic notch
dictyokinesis
dictyosome
dictyotene
dicumarol
dicyclomine hydrochloride
dicycloxylamine
Diego antigen
dieldrin

dielectric
  d. constant
  d. strength
diencephalic
  d. periventricular fibers
  d. syndrome
diencephalon
diene
diener
dienestrol
Dientamoeba
  D. fragilis
dietary
Dieterle's method
dietetics
diethanolamine
diethyl
  d. 2-chlorovinyl phosphate
  d. *p*-nitrophenyl phosphate
  d. toluamide
  d. xanthogen disulfide
diethylamine
diethylaminoethylcellulose
diethylcarbamazine citrate
diethyldithiocarbamate
diethylene glycol
diethylenetriaminepentaacetic
  acid
diethyl ether
diethylpropion hydrochloride
diethylstilbestrol
diethyl sulfate
diethyltoluamide
diethyltryptamine
diff — differential
differential
  d. agglutination titer
  d. diagnosis
  d. leukocyte count
  d. leukocyte count automa-
    tion

differential *(continued)*
    d. medium
    d. segments
differentiation
differentiator
diffraction
    d. grating
    x-ray d.
diffusate
diffuse
    d. acute inflammation
    d. acute peritonitis
    d. amyloidosis
    d. bronchopneumonia
    d. chronic inflammation
    d. enlargement
    d. esophageal spasm
    d. fibrosis
    d. hyperplasia
    d. hypertrophy
    d. illumination
    d. interstitial fibrosis
    d. lymphatic tissue
    d. meningiomatosis
    d. necrosis
    d. neuroendocrine system
    d. nontoxic goiter
    d. pneumonia
    d. pyelonephritis
    d. septal cirrhosis
    d. ulceration
diffusible
diffusing
    d. capacity of the lungs
diffusion
    d. coefficient
    d. current
    facilitated d.
    d. method
    d. potential
diffusivity
digalen

digastric
    d. branch
    d. lobe
    d. muscle
digenetic
DiGeorge's syndrome
digestion
    d. vacuole
digestive
    d. disorder
    d. system
digit
digital
    d. cassette recorder
    d. computer
    d. radiography
    d. readout
    d. subtraction angiography
    d.-to-analog converter
    d. voltmeter
digitalis
    d. glycosides
digitalization
digitize
digitizer
digitonin
digitoxin
digitoxose
diglyceride
diglycocoll hydroiodide
digoxin
Digramma brauni
Di Guglielmo's syndrome
dihydric alcohol
dihydrobiopterin
dihydrocodeine
dihydrocoenzyme I
dihydroergotamine mesylate
dihydrofolate
    d. dehydrogenase
    d. reductase
dihydrofolic acid

dihydrofolliculin
dihydromorphinone hydrochloride
dihydro-orotase
dihydropteridine
   d. reductase
dihydropyrimidinase
dihydrorotenone
dihydrosphingosine
dihydrotachysterol
dihydrotestosterone
dihydroubiquinone
dihydro-uracil dehydrogenase
dihydrouridine
dihydroxyacetone
   d. phosphate
dihydroxyacetonetransferase
dihydroxycholecalciferol
4-dihydroxymandelic acid
5-dihydroxyphenylacetic acid
3,4-dihydroxy-L-phenylalanine decarboxylase
diiodohydroxyquin
diiodothyronine
diiodothyrosine
di-isobutyl cresolyl ethoxy ethyl dimethyl benzyl ammonium chloride
di-isobutyl phenoxy ethoxy ethyl dimethyl benzyl ammonium chloride
di-isopropylfluoro-phosphatase
diisopropyl phosphofluoridate
dikaryon
diktyoma
dil — dilute
   dissolve
dilatation
   aneurysmal d.
   poststenotic d.
dilation

DILD — diffuse infiltrative lung disease
diloxanide
diluent
dilut — diluted
dilute
   d. acetic acid
   d. hydrochloric acid
   d. phosphoric acid
dilution
   d. coefficient
   doubling d.
   log d.
   nitrogen d.
   serial d.
   d. test
dilutor
DIM — divalent ion metabolism
Dimastigamoeba
dimefadane
dimefline hydrochloride
dimefox
dimenhydrinate
dimension
dimer
   thymine d.
dimercaprol
dimercaptopropanol
dimerization
dimetan
dimethicone
dimethindene maleate
dimethisoquin hydrochloride
dimethisterone
dimethoate
dimethoxanate hydrochloride
2,5-dimethoxy-4-methylamphetamine
3,4-dimethoxyphenylethylamine
dimethpyrindene

dimethylacetamide
dimethylallyl diphosphate
p-dimethylaminoazobenzene
1-dimethylaminonaphthalene-t-sulphonyl chloride
dimethylbenzanthracene
dimethylcarbamate
O, O-dimethyl *O*,2,2-dichlorovinyl phosphate
dimethyl ether
dimethylformamide
dimethylguanosine
dimethylketone
dimethylnitrosamine
5,5-dimethyl-2,4-oxazolidinedione
dimethylphthalate
dimethyl sulfate
dimethyl sulfoxide
dimethylthetin homocysteine methyltransferase
dimethyltryptamine
diminazene aceturate
dimorphic
   d. pathogenic fungi
dimorphism
dinitroaminophenol
dinitrobenzene
dinitrobutyl phenol
dinitrochlorobenzene
dinitrocresol
dinitro-*o*-cyclohexyl phenol
dinitrofluorobenzene
dinitrogen
   d. monoxide
   d. tetroxide
dinitroorthocresol
dinitrophenol
dinitrophenylhydrazine test
dinitrotoluene
Dinobdella
   D. ferox

dinucleotide
Dioctophyma
   D. renale
dioctyl sodium sulfosuccinate
diode
   varactor d.
   Zener's d.
diopter
dioxane
dioxathion
dioxin
dioxygenase
dioxyline phosphate
DIP — desquamative interstitial pneumonia
   desquamative interstitial pneumonitis
   diisopropyl phosphate
   distal interphalangeal
   dual-in-line package
dipalmitoylphosphatidylcholine
dipeptidase
dipeptide hydrolase
Dipetalonema
   D. perstans
   D. streptocerca
dipetalonemiasis
diphacinone
diphasic
   d. meningoencephalitis virus
   d. milk fever virus
diphemanil methylsulfate
diphenadione
diphenhydramine hydrochloride
diphenidol
p-diphenol oxidase
diphenoxylate hydrochloride
diphenyl
diphenylamine

diphenylchlorarsine
diphenylcyanarsine
diphenylhydantoin
diphenylmethane
diphenylpyraline hydrochloride
2,3-diphosphoglycerate
    d. mutase
    d. phosphatase
diphosphoglyceromutase
diphosphoinositide
diphosphonate
diphosphopyridine nucleotide
diphtheria
    d. antitoxin
    d. bacillus
    d. toxin immunization reaction
diphtheritic
diphtheroid
    aerobic d.
    anaerobic d.
    d. bacilli
diphyllobothriasis
Diphyllobothrium
    D. latum
dipicolinic acid
dipipanone hydrochloride
DIPJ — distal interphalangeal joint
diplegia
diplobacillus
diplobacterium
diploblastic
diplochromosome
Diplococcus
    D. constellatus
    D. magnus
    D. morbillorum
    D. mucosus
    D. paleopneumoniae
    D. plagarumbelli
    D. pneumoniae
diplococcus (diplococci)
    d. of Morax-Axenfeld
    d. of Neisser
    Weichselbaum's d.
diploë
Diplogaster
Diplogonoporus
    D. brauni
    D. grandis
diploic vein
diploid
    d. number
diploidy
Diplomate of the National Board of Medical Examiners
diplonema
diplont
diplopia
diplopod
Diplopoda
diplosome
Diplosporium
diplotene
dipolar structure
dipole
    d. moment
dipropyl isocinchomeronate
dipstick
Diptera
dipterous
dipygus
    d. parasiticus
Dipylidium
    D. caninum
dipyridamole
dipyrone
diquat
    d. assays
direct
    d. access
    d. agglutination test
    d. antiglobulin test

direct *(continued)*
    d. current
    d. hernia
    d. light reflex
    d. memory access
    d. transport
Dirofilaria
    D. conjunctivae
    D. immitis
    D. repens
    D. tenuis
dirofilariasis
disaccharidase
disaccharide
    d. tolerance test
disc, disk
    articular d.
    d. diffusion test
    d. electrophoresis
    embryonic d.
    germ d.
    interpubic d.
    intervertebral d.
    Merkel's tactile d.
discharge
    d. frequency
disclosing solution
discocyte
discography
    cervical d.
    lumbar d.
discoid
    d. lupus erythematosus
discordance
discordant
discrete
discriminator
disease
disfigurative
dish
    Petri d.
    Stender d.
disinfect
disinfectant
disinfection
disintegration
    d. constant
    radioactive d.
disjunction
disk. *See* disc.
diskocyte
diskogram
diskography
    cervical d.
    lumbar d.
dislocation
    closed d.
    complete d.
    compound d.
    congenital d.
    fracture d.
    pathologic d.
dismutase
    superoxide d.
disodium
    d. chromoglycate
    d. 3,6-endoxohexahydrophthalate
    d. ethylene bis-(dithiocarbamate)
disome
disomic
disomy
disorder
    element d.
    functional d.
    intestinal flow d.
    ion d.
    peristalsis d.
    ureteral peristalsis d.
disorganization
disorientation
    spatial d.
dispermy

disperse
    d. phase
dispersion
    colloidal d.
    molecular d.
dispireme
displacement
disposable
disposition
disproportion
    cephalopelvic d.
dissect
dissecting aneurysm
dissection
disseminated
    d. acute lupus erythematosus
    d. inflammation
    d. intravascular coagulation
    d. lupus erythematosus
    d. sclerosis
dissemination
Disse's spaces
dissociation
    albuminocytologic d.
    bacterial d.
    constant d.
    microbic d.
dissolution
dissolve
dissymmetry
distal
    d. anterior closed space
    d. convoluted renal tubule
    d. latency
    d. myopathy
    d. radioulnar joint
    d. tibiofibular joint
    d.-type progressive muscular dystrophy
distance
distension, distention

distill
distillate
distillation
    destructive d.
    fractional d.
    molecular d.
    vacuum d.
Distoma
distome
distomiasis
distortion
distractibility
distribution
    d. coefficient
    d. curve
    dose d.
    d. function
    Poisson d.
    reference d.
    sample d.
disturbance
    consciousness d.
disulfide
    d. bond
disulfiram
    d. assays
disulfoton
disuse atrophy
DIT – diiodotyrosine
dithiazanine iodide
dithionite
dithiothreitol
diuresis (diureses)
diuretic
    cardiac d.
    hemopiesic d.
    loop d.
    mechanical d.
    osmotic d.
    thiazide d.
diurnal
diuron

divergence
diverticular
diverticulitis
   hemorrhagic d.
   obstructive d.
   perforated d.
diverticulosis
diverticulum (diverticula)
   colonic d.
   epiphrenic d.
   false d.
   intestinal d.
   Meckel's d.
   pharyngoesophageal d.
   pressure d.
   pulsion d.
   traction d.
   Zenker's d.
division
   cell d.
   equational d.
   maturation d.
   reduction d.
Dixon's test
dizygotic
dizziness
DJD — degenerative joint disease
DK — decay
   diseased kidney
DL — difference limen
   diffusing capacity of the lung
   distolingual
   Donath-Landsteiner (test)
dl — deciliter
DLA — distolabial
D-L Ab — Donath-Landsteiner antibody
DLAI — distolabioincisal
DLCO — diffusing capacity of the lung for carbon monoxide
DLE — discoid lupus erythematosus
   disseminated lupus erythematosus
DLI — distolinguoincisal
DLO — distolinguo-occlusal
DLP — distolinguopulpal
DM — diabetes mellitus
   diastolic murmur
   dopamine
D.M. — diphenylamine-arsine chloride
dm — decimeter
DMA — dimethyladenosine
   direct memory access
DMAB — dimethylaminobenzaldehyde
DMAC — dimethylacetamide
DMBA — dimethylbenzanthracene
DMCT — demethylchlortetracycline
DMD — Duchenne's muscular dystrophy
DME — dimethyl ether (of D-tubocurarine)
DMF — dimethylformamide
DMM — dimethylmyleran
DMN — dimethylnitrosamine
DMO — dimethyloxazolidinedione
DMPA — depomedroxyprogesterone acetate
DMPE — 3,4-dimethoxyphenylethylamine
DMPP — dimethylphenylpiperazinium
DMS — dimethylsulfoxide

DMSO — dimethylsulfoxide
DMT — dimethyltryptamine
DN — dextrose-nitrogen (ratio)
   dibucaine number
Dn. — dekanem
dn — decinem
DNA — deoxyribonucleic acid
DNA
   complexity
   ligase
   nucleotidylexotransferase
   nucleotidyltransferase
   polymerase
   reassociation
   renaturation
   repair
   synthesis
DNase — deoxyribonuclease
DNase agar
DNB — dinitrobenzene
      Diplomate of the
        National Board of
        Medical Examiners
DNC — dinitrocarbanilide
DNCB — dinitrochlorobenzene
DNFB — dinitrofluorobenzene
DNOC — dinitro-orthocresol
DNP — deoxyribonucleoprotein
   dinitrophenol
DNPH — dinitrophenylhydrazine
DNPM — dinitrophenylmorphine
DO — diamine oxidase
   disto-occlusal
   Doctor of Osteopathy
DOA — dead on arrival
dobutamine
   d. hydrochloride
DOC — deoxycholate
   deoxycorticosterone

DOCA — deoxycorticosterone
   acetate
docimasia
   auricular d.
   hepatic d.
   pulmonary d.
DOCS — deoxycorticoids
Doctor of Osteopathy
document
documentation
dodecylguanidine acetate
Döderlein's bacillus
DOE — dyspnea on exercise
   dyspnea on exertion
Döhle-Heller aortitis
Döhle's inclusion bodies
Dold's
   reaction
   test
dolichol
   d. phosphate
Dolichos
   D. biflorus
dolipore
doll's eye movements
DOM — deaminated-*O*-methyl
   metabolite
   dimethoxymethyl
   amphetamine
   2,5-dimethoxy-4-
   methylamphetamine
DOMA — dihydroxymandelic
   acid
domain
dominant
   d. complementarity
domiphen bromide
DON — diazo-oxonorleucine
Donath-Landsteiner
   antibody
   test

Donnan's potential
Donné's
    bodies
    corpuscles
    test
Donohue's syndrome
donor
    F d.
Donovania
    D. granulomatis
Donovan's bodies
DOPA — dihydroxyphenylalanine
dopa
    d. reaction
DOPAC — dihydroxyphenylacetic acid
dopamine
    d. hydroxylase
    d. monooxygenase
dopaminergic
dopaquinone
Doppler
    echocardiography
    effect
dormancy
dormant
Dorner stain
Dorothy Reed cells
dorsal
    d. accessory olivary nucleus
    d. cutaneous nerve
    d. digital artery
    d. digital vein
    d. displacement
    d. fascia
    d. funiculus
    d. intermediate sulcus
    d. lateral nucleus
    d. lateral sulcus
    d. longitudinal fasciculus
    d. median sulcus

dorsal *(continued)*
    d. mesentery
    d. metacarpal vein
    d. metatarsal artery
    d. metatarsal vein
    d. motor nucleus
    d. nasal artery
    d. nerve
    d. nucleus
    d. paraflocculus
    d. proper fasciculus
    d. root ganglion
    d. spinal nerve root
    d. spinocerebellar tract
    d. spinothalamic tract
    d. subaponeurotic space
    d. tegmental nucleus, pons
    d. thoracic nerve
    d. ventral nucleus
    d. vertebra
dorsalis pedis artery
dorsiflex
dorsiflexion
dorsolateral
dorsomedial nucleus
dorsoplantar
dorsum (dorsa)
    d. sellae
dosage
    d. compensation
dose
    absorbed d.
    d. account
    air d.
    booster d.
    d. calibrator
    depth d.
    divided d.
    effective d.
    epilating d.
    erythema d.
    d. estimate

dose *(continued)*
    exit d.
    genetically significant d.
    integral d.
    lethal d.
    loading d.
    maximal permissible d.
    mean d.
    mean d. per unit cumulated activity
    median effective d.
    median infectious d.
    median lethal d.
    minimal lethal d.
    organ tolerance d.
    radiation d.
    radiation absorbed d.
    d. rate
    sensitizing d.
    skin d.
    threshold d.
    threshold erythema d.
    tissue tolerance d.
    tumor lethal d.
dosimeter
    pencil d.
    pocket d.
    thermoluminescent d.
    ultraviolet fluorescent d.
dosimetry
dot
    Maurer's d's
    Mittendorf's d's
    d. product
    d. scan
    Schüffner's d's
double
    d. albuminemia
    d. aortic arch
    d. artery
    d.-beam photometer
    d.-blind

double *(continued)*
    d. cardiac valve orifice
    d.-contrast study
    d. diffusion test
    d. discharge
    d. ductus arteriosus
    d. helix
    d. kidney
    d. oxalate
    d.-pole double-throw switch
    d.-pole single-throw switch
    d.-precision variable
    d. renal pelvis
    d. ureter
doubling time
Douglas's
    cul-de-sac
    pouch
Dowex
Downey
    cells
    -type lymphocyte
Down's syndrome
downtime
doxepin hydrochloride
    d. h. assays
doxorubicin
    d. hydrochloride
doxycycline
doxylamine succinate
DP — dementia praecox
          diastolic pressure
          distopulpal
DPA — dipropylacetate
DPC — delayed primary closure
DPD — diffuse pulmonary disease
DPDL — diffuse, poorly differentiated lymphoma
dpdt — double-pole double-throw (switch)

DPG — diphosphoglycerate
    displacement placentogram
DPGM — diphosphoglyceromutase
DPGP — diphosphoglycerate phosphatase
DPH — diphenylhydantoin
DPL — distopulpolingual
dpm — disintegrations per minute
DPN — diphosphopyridine nucleotide
DPN synthetase
DPP — dimethoxyphenyl penicillin
DPS — dimethylpolysiloxane
dpst — double-pole single-throw (switch)
DPT — diphtheria, pertussis, and tetanus
    dipropyltryptamine
DPTA — diethylenetriamine pentaacetic acid
DQ — developmental quotient
DR — diabetic retinopathy
    reaction of degeneration
dr — drachm
    dram
Drabkin's reagent
dracontiasis
dracunculiasis
dracunculosis
Dracunculus
    D. medinensis
Dragendorff's
    solution
    test
dragon worm infection
drain
drainage
Drechslera hawaiiensis

drench hose
Drepanidotaenia
    D. lanceolata
drepanocyte
drepanocytemia
drepanocytic
drepanocytosis
Drepanospira
DRF — dose-reduction factor
drift
    antigenic d.
    random genetic d.
Drinker respirator
drip
    intravenous d.
dromostanolone proprionate
drop
    Ir d.
droperidol
droplet
    d. nuclei
dropper
Drosophila
drowning
drowsiness
droxacin sodium
drug
    d. addiction
    d. dependence
    d. desensitization
    d.-induced thrombocytopenia
    d. interference
    d.-resistant
    d. screening assays
drumstick
    d. spore
drunkenness
drusen
dry
    d. catarrh
    d. gangrene

dry *(continued)*
   d. ice
drying agent
DS — defined substrate
   dehydroepiandrosterone sulfate
   dextrose-saline
   Down's syndrome
DSA — digital subtraction angiography
DSAP — disseminated superficial actinic porokeratosis
DSC or DSCG — disodium cromoglycate
DSM — dextrose solution mixture
DST — dexamethasone suppression test
DT — delirium tremens
   duration tetany
   dye test
DTBC — D-tubocurarine
DTBN — di-t-butyl nitroxide
DTC — D-tubocurarine
dTDP — thymidine diphosphate
DTF — detector transfer function
DTIC — dacarbazine
DTM — dermatophyte test medium
DTMP — deoxythymidine monophosphate
dTMP — thymidine phosphate
DTN — diphtheria toxin normal
DTNB — dithiobisnitrobenzoic acid
DTP — diphtheria, tetanus, and pertussis
   distal tingling on percussion
DTPA — diethylenetriaminepentacetic acid
DTR — deep tendon reflex
dTTP — thymidine triphosphate
DTZ — diatrizoate
DU — duodenal ulcer
dU — deoxyuridine
du — dial unit
dual
   d.-contrast study
   d.-in-line package
dualism
Duane-Hunt relation
duazomycin
Dubin-Johnson syndrome
duboisine
Duchenne's
   disease
   -type muscular dystrophy
Ducrey's bacillus
duct
   aberrant d.
   alveolar d.
   d. of Arantius
   Bellini's papillary d.
   bile d.
   cochlear d.
   Cuvier's d.
   cystic d.
   d. ectasia
   ejaculatory d.
   endolymphatic d.
   d. of epididymis
   Gartner's d.
   hepatic d.
   intercalated d.
   interlobular bile d.
   lacrimal d.
   lactiferous d.
   Luschka's d's
   lymphatic d.

duct *(continued)*
- mesonephric d.
- Müller d.
- müllerian d.
- nasolacrimal d.
- omphalomesenteric d.
- pancreatic d.
- paramesonephric d.
- parotid d.
- prostatic d.
- salivary d.
- Santorini's d.
- semicircular d.
- Stensen's d.
- suderiferous d.
- thoracic d.
- thyroglossal d.
- utriculosaccular d.
- vitelline d.
- Wharton's d.
- Wirsung's d.
- wolffian d.

ductal

ductus
- d. arteriosus
- d. deferens
- d. venosus

Duffy antibodies, Fy^a, Fy^b

Duke's
- classification
- method of bleeding time

dullness
- Gerhardt's d.
- shifting d.
- tympanitic d.

Dumdum fever

dummy
- d. variable

dUMP — deoxyuridine monophosphate
deoxyuridine phosphate

dumping syndrome

duod — duodenum

duodenal
- d. lumen
- d. mucous membrane
- d. muscularis propria
- d. serosa
- d. submucosa
- d. subserosa
- d. ulcer

duodenography
- hypotonic d.

duodenojejunal recess

duodenoscopy

duodenum

duovirus

duplication
- caudal d.
- caudal dipygus d.
- congenital d.
- cranial d.
- cranial monocephalus d.
- facial diprosopus d.
- fetal d.
- trunk d.

duplicity theory

Dupuytren's
- contracture
- fibromatosis

dural

dura mater

Dürck's nodes

Durham's tube

dust
- blood d.
- d. cell
- chromatin d.

Duttonella

d. v. — double vibration
DVA — distance visual acuity
DVM — digital voltmeter
DW — distilled water

D5W, D5 & W or D₅W — 5 per cent dextrose in water
D/W — dextrose in water
dwarf
    achondroplastic d.
    constitutional d.
    pituitary d.
    primordial d.
    d. tapeworm
dwarfism
    pituitary d.
DX — dextran
DXM — dexamethasone
DXT — deep x-ray therapy
D-xylose tolerance test
Dy — dysprosium
dyad
dyclonine hydrochloride
dydrogesterone
dye
    acridine d.
    aminoketone d.
    aniline d.
    anthraquinone d.
    azine d.
    azo d.
    azoic d.
    diphenylmethane d.
    d. excretion tests
    hydroxyketone d.
    indamine d.
    indigoid d.
    indophenol d.
    lactone d.
    methine d.
    nitro d.
    nitroso d.
    oxazine d.
    phthalocyanine d.
    polymethine d.
    quinoline d.
    stilbene d.

dye *(continued)*
    sulfur d.
    thiazine d.
    thiazole d.
    triarylmethane d.
    xanthene d.
dyn — dyne
dynamic
dyne
dynein
dyphylline
dysarthria
dysaudia
dysautonomia
    familial d.
dysbarism
dysbasia
dysbetalipoproteinemia
    familial d.
dysbolism
dyschezia
dyschondroplasia
dyscrasia
    blood d.
    lymphatic d.
dysdiadochokinesia
dysdiemorrhysis
dysentery
    amebic d.
    bacillary d.
    balantidial d.
    bilharzial d.
    catarrhal d.
    ciliary d.
    ciliate d.
    epidemic d.
    flagellate d.
    Flexner's d.
    fulminant d.
    giardiasis d.
    malarial d.
    protozoal d.

dysentery *(continued)*
   scorbutic d.
   Sonne d.
   spirillar d.
   sporadic d.
   viral d.
dyserythropoiesis
dyserythropoietic
   d. congenital anemia
dysfibrinogenemia
dysfunction
   constitutional hepatic d.
   uterine d.
   vasomotor d.
dysfunctional
   d. bleeding
dysgammaglobulinemia
dysgenesis
   familial gonadal d.
dysgenetic
dysgerminoma
dysglobulinemia
dysgonic
dyshesion
dyshidrosis
dyshormonogenesis
dyskaryosis
dyskeratosis
   d. congenita
   hereditary benign intra-
     epithelial d.
dyskinesia
   tardive d.
dyslexia
dyslipoproteinemia
dysmenorrhea
dysmentation
dysmorphism
dysmyelopoietic syndrome
dysostosis
   cleidocranialis d.
   Crouzon's craniofacial d.

dyspareunia
dyspepsia
dysphagia
   sideropenic d.
dysphasia
dysphonia
dysphoria
dysplasia
   acquired d.
   chondroectodermal d.
   dentin d.
   fibrous d.
   fibrous familial d.
   fibrous monostotic d.
   fibrous polyostotic d.
   hereditary d., ectodermal
   mammary d.
   polyostotic fibrous d.
   precancerous d.
   thymic d.
   vesical d.
   Zenker's d.
dyspnea
   cardiac d.
   exertional d.
   paroxysmal d.
   paroxysmal nocturnal d.
dyspneic
dyspoiesis
dysprosium
dysproteinemia
dysprothrombinemia
dysrhythmia
dyssynergia
   progressive cerebellar d.
dystaxia
dystocia
dystonia
dystonic
dystrophic
dystrophy
   adiposogenital d.

dystrophy *(continued)*
   Becker's d.
   distal muscular d.
   Duchenne-type muscular d.
   d.-dystocia syndrome
   facioscapulohumeral muscular d.
   Landouzy-Dejerine progressive muscular d.

dystrophy *(continued)*
   limb-girdle muscular d.
   lipoid d.
   myotonic d.
   progressive muscular d.
dysuria
DZ — dizygous

E

E — cortisone (compound E)
   electric charge
   electron
   emmetropia
   energy
   epinephrine
   erythrocyte
   extraction fraction
   eye
E. — *Entamoeba*
   Escherichia
E_1 — estrone
E_2 — estradiol
E_3 — estriol
E_4 — estetrol
EA — early antigen
   ethacrynic acid
EAC — Ehrlich ascites carcinoma
   external auditory canal
EACA — epsilon-aminocaproic acid
Eadie-Hofstee equation
EAE — experimental allergic encephalomyelitis
EAHF — eczema, asthma. hay fever

EAHLG — equine antihuman lymphoblast globulin
EAHLS — equine antihuman lymphoblast serum
EAM — external auditory meatus
EAN — experimental allergic neuritis
E antigen
EAP — epiallopregnanolone
ear
   external e.
   internal e.
   e. lobule
   middle e.
   scroll e.
eastern
   e. equine encephalitis
   e. equine encephalomyelitis virus
Eaton agent
Eaton-Lambert syndrome
EB — epidermolysis bullosa
   Epstein-Barr (virus)
   estradiol benzoate

Eberthella
   E. typhi
EBI — emetine bismuth iodide
EBL — estimated blood loss
EBNA — EBV nuclear antigen
Ebner's gland
Ebola virus
Ebstein's
   anomaly
   malformation
eburnation
EBV — Epstein-Barr virus
EC — electron capture
   enteric-coated
   Escherichia coli
   excitation-contraction
   experimental control
   extracellular
ECA — ethacrynic acid
ECBO virus — enteric cytopathogenic bovine orphan virus
ECBV — effective circulating blood volume
ECC — extracorporeal circulation
ecchondroma
ecchordosis physalifora
ecchymosis
eccrine
   e. gland
   e. poroma
   e. spiradenoma
ECD — electron capture detector
EC detector
ECDO virus — enteric cytopathogenic dog orphan virus
ECF — effective capillary flow
   extracellular fluid
ECF-A — eosinophil chemotactic factor of anaphylaxis
ECFV — extracellular fluid volume
ECG — electrocardiogram
ecgonine
Echinochasmus
   E. perfoliatus
echinococciasis
echinococcosis
Echinococcus
   E. granulosus
   E. multilocularis
echinocyte
echinocytosis
echinoderm
Echinorhynchus
echinosis
Echinostoma
   E. cinetorchis
   E. ilocanum
   E. lindoensis
   E. malayanum
   E. melis
   E. paryphostomum
   E. perfoliatum
   E. revolutum
echinostomiasis
ECHO — enteric cytopathogenic human orphan (virus)
echocardiogram
echocardiography
   contrast e.
   cross-sectional e.
   Doppler e.
echoencephalography
echogenic
echogram
echography
echolucent

echo-ophthalmography
echophonocardiography
echothiophate
ECHO virus — enteric cytopathogenic human orphan virus
ECHO virus
   type 1
   type 12
ECHO 28 virus
ECI — electrocerebral inactivity
ECI or ECIB — extracorporeal irradiation of blood
ECIL — extracorporeal irradiation of lymph
ECL — emitter-coupled logic
eclampsia
   puerperal e.
   uremic e.
eclipse
ECLT — euglobulin clot lysis time
ECM — erythema chronicum migrans
   extracellular material
ECMO virus — enteric cytopathogenic monkey orphan virus
ECoG — electrocorticogram
   electrocorticography
E. coli — *Escherichia coli*
ecology
ecosystem
ECSO virus — enteric cytopathogenic swine orphan virus
ECT — euglobulin clot test
ectasia
   mammary duct e.
ecthyma
   e. gangrenosum
   e. infectiosum
ectoderm
ectodermal dysplasia
ectoparasite
ectopia
ectopic
   e. anus
   e. hormone
   e. pregnancy
   e. tissue
ectoplasm
ectothrix
ectozoon (ectozoa)
ectromelia
ectromelus
ectrometacarpia
ectropion
ectylurea
ECV — extracellular volume
ECW — extracellular water
eczema
   e. herpeticum
   mummular e.
eczematoid dermatitis
ED — effective dose
   Ehlers-Danlos syndrome
   epileptiform discharge
   erythema dose
edathamil calcium-disodium
edema
   angioneurotic e.
   cerebral e.
   peripheral e.
   pulmonary e.
edetate
   calcium disodium e.
   e. disodium
   e. sodium
   e. trisodium
edetic acid

edge
    Compton e.
Edinger-Westphal nucleus
Edman reaction
EDP — end-diastolic pressure
EDR — effective direct radiation
    electrodermal response
edrophonium chloride
EDS — Ehlers-Danlos syndrome
EDTA — edetic acid
    ethylenediaminetetraacetate
EDV — end-diastolic volume
Edwardsiella
    E. tarda
Edwardsielleae
Edwards-Patau syndrome
Edwards' syndrome
EDX — electrodiagnosis
EEA — electroencephalic audiometry
EEC — enteropathogenic *Escherichia coli*
EEE — eastern equine encephalomyelitis
EEE virus — eastern equine encephalomyelitis virus
EEG — electroencephalogram
eelworm
EEME — ethinylestradiol methyl ether
EER — electroencephalic response
EF — ectopic focus
    ejection fraction
    encephalitogenic factor
EFA — essential fatty acids
EFC — endogenous fecal calcium

EFE — endocardial fibroelastosis
effect
    Arias-Stella e.
    Auger e.
    Bohr e.
    Compton e. Somogyi
    Crabtree e.
    Doppler e.
    Faraday e.
    Haldane e.
    Pasteur e.
    Whitten e.
    Wolff-Chaikoff e.
    Zeeman's e.
effective
    e. half-life
    e. renal plasma flow
effector
    allosteric e.
    e. cells
efferent
    e. arteriole
    e. ductule
    e. lymphatics
    e. sacral branch
    e. vagus branch
efficiency
    visual e.
efflorescence
effusion
    chylous e.
    serofibrinous e.
    serosanguineous e.
    serous e.
EFV — extracellular fluid volume
EFVC — expiratory flow-volume curve
EG — esophagogastrectomy
EGG — electrogastrogram

EGL — eosinophilic granuloma
　　　　of the lung
EGM — electrogram
egobronchophony
egophony
EGOT — erythrocyte glutamic
　　　　oxaloacetic trans-
　　　　aminase
EH — essential hypertension
EHBF — estimated hepatic
　　　　blood flow
　　　　exercise hyperemia
　　　　blood flow
EHC — enterohepatic circula-
　　　　tion
　　　　essential hypercholes-
　　　　terolemia
EHDP — ethane hydroxydi-
　　　　phosphate
EHF — exophthalmos-hyper-
　　　　thyroid factor
EHL — endogenous hyper-
　　　　lipidemia
Ehlers-Danlos syndrome
EHO — extrahepatic obstruc-
　　　　tion
EHP — excessive heat produc-
　　　　tion
Ehrlich's
　　diazo reagent
　　postulate
　　reaction
　　test
　　unit
EI — enzyme inhibitor
　　eosinophilic index
E/I — expiration-inspiration
　　　ratio
EIA — enzyme immunoassay
eicosatrienoic acid
EID — electroimmunodiffusion
eighth cranial nerve

Eikenella
　　E. corrodens
einsteinium
Einthoven's
　　law
　　triangle
EIP — extensor indicis proprius
Eisenmenger
　　tetralogy of E.
Eisenmenger's complex
ejaculation
ejaculatory duct
ejection
　　e. fraction
　　e. time
EK — erythrokinase
EKC — epidemic keratocon-
　　　　junctivitis
EKG — electrocardiogram
EKY — electrokymogram
elaidic acid
elastance
elastase
elastic
　　e. connective tissue
　　e. fiber
　　e. lamellae
　　e. lamina
　　e. membrane
　　e. recoil
elastica
elasticity
elastin
elastofibroma
　　e. dorsi
elastosis
　　e. perforans serpiginosa
　　senile e.
elbow
electric
　　e. field vector
　　e. potential difference

electrical
  e. alternans
  e. artifact
electrocardiogram
electrocardiograph
electrocardiography
electrocautery
electrocerebral inactivity
electrochemical cell
electrochemistry
electrocorticogram
electrocorticography
electrode
  Clark's oxygen e.
  Severinghaus e.
electrodiagnosis
electroencephalogram
electroencephalography
electroendosmosis
electroimmunoassay
electroimmunodiffusion
electrolysis
  Faraday's law of e.
electrolyte
  amphoteric e.
  e. balance and homeostasis
  colloidal e.
  e. imbalance
  protein e.
  serum e.
electrolytic cell
electromagnet
electromagnetic
  e. radiation
  e. unit
electrometer
electromotive force
electromyogram
electromyograph
electromyography
  single-fiber e.

electron
  Auger e.
  e. microprobe
  e. microscopy
  e. paramagnetic resonance
  e. spin resonance
  e. transport chain
  e. transport inhibitors
  e. volt
electronegative
electronegativity
electronic
  e. voltmeter
electron microscope
  analytical e. m.
  scanning e. m.
  transmission e. m.
electrooculogram
electroosmosis
electropherogram
electrophile
electrophoresis
  serum protein e.
electrophoretic
  e. mobility
electrophoretogram
electrophysiology
electropositive
electroretinogram
electroretinography
electroscope
electrostatic
  e. unit
electrosurgery
eleidin
Elek test
element(s). *See* Appendix 4,
  Table of Elements.
elementary
  e. body
  e. charge

elementary *(continued)*
   e. particle
elephantiasis
   e. nostras
eleventh cranial nerve
elimination
   immune e.
   e. reaction
ELISA – enzyme-linked immunosorbent assay
elixophyllin
ellipsin
ellipsoid
elliptocyte
elliptocytosis
   hereditary e.
Ellis–van Creveld syndrome
Ellsworth-Howard test
elongation
ELT – euglobulin lysis time
El Tor vibrio
eluate
eluent
elute
elution
elutriation
EM – ejection murmur
       electron microscopy
       erythrocyte mass
Em – emmetropia
emaciation
EMB – eosin-methylene blue
       ethambutol
       ethambutol-myambutol
Embadomonas
EMB agar
Embden-Meyerhof
   cycle
   pathway
embedding
embolectomy
embolic
   e. aneurysm
   e. glomerulonephritis
embolism
   air e.
   amniotic fluid e.
   arterial e.
   bacillary e.
   bone-marrow e.
   capillary e.
   cerebral e.
   coronary e.
   fat e.
   gas e.
   infective e.
   lymph e.
   miliary e.
   paradoxical e.
   plasmodium e.
   pulmonary e.
   pyemic e.
   retinal e.
   saddle e.
   spinal e.
   trichinous e.
   venous e.
embolus (emboli)
   air e.
   amniotic fluid e.
   atheromatous e.
   bland e.
   bone marrow e.
   fat e.
   foreign body e.
   massive e.
   paradoxical e.
   parasitic e.
   recent e.
   septic e.
   tumor e.
   valvular tissue e.

embryo
  cylindrical e.
  nodular e.
  stunted e.
embryocardia
embryology
embryoma
embryonal
  e. adenoma
  e. carcinoma
  e. cell carcinoma
  e. duct cyst
  e. nephroma
  e. rest
  e. rhabdomyosarcoma
  e. teratoma
embryonic
  e. blood vessel
  e. disc
  e. ependymal layer
  e. hemoglobin
  e. mantle layer
  e. marginal layer
  e. structure
embryoniform
embryonization
EMC — electron microscopy
  encephalomyocarditis
EMC virus — encephalomyocarditis virus
emesis
emetine
EMF — electromagnetic flowmeter
  electromotive force
  endomyocardial fibrosis
  erythrocyte maturation factor
EMG — electromyogram
  exophthalmos, macroglossia, gigantism

emigration
  e. of white cells
eminence
  frontal e.
  hypothenar e.
  median e.
  parietal e.
  thenar e.
emissary vein
emission
  e. line
  e. spectroscopy
  e. spectrum
EMIT — enzyme-multiplied immunoassay technique
emitter
  e.-coupled logic
Emmonsia
Emmonsiella
emperipolesis
emphraxis
emphysema
  bullous e.
  centrilobular e.
  compensatory e.
  interstitial e.
  obstructive e.
  panacinar e.
  pulmonary e.
  subcutaneous e.
  vesicular e.
emphysematous
  e. bleb
  e. vaginitis
empty sella syndrome
empyema
  subdural e.
emu — electromagnetic unit
emulsify
emulsion
emylcamate

EN — erythema nodosum
ENA — extractable nuclear antigen
enamel
    e. hypoplasia
    mottled e.
enamelogenesis imperfecta
enantiobiosis
enantiomer
enantiomerism
enantiomorph
enantiomorphism
encapsulated
encephalitis (encephalitides)
    arthropod-borne virus e.
    California e.
    eastern equine e.
    e. herpes simplex
    e. lethargica
    post-infectious allergic e.
    post-vaccination allergic e.
    St. Louis e.
    Venezuelan equine e.
    western equine e.
encephalocystocele
encephalogram
encephalography
encephalomalacia
encephalomeningocele
encephalomyelitis
    autoimmune e.
encephalomyelopathy
encephalomyocarditis
encephalon
encephalopathy
    anoxic e.
    hepatic e.
    hypercapnic e.
    hypertensive e.
    hypoglycemic e.
    lead e.
    uremic e.

encephalopathy *(continued)*
    Wernicke's e.
encephalotrigeminal angiomatosis
enchondroma
enchondrosarcoma
enchondrosis
encode
encoder
end — endoreduplication
Endamoeba
    E. blattae
endarterectomy
endarteritis
    e. obliterans
end bulb
    Krause's e. b.
endemic
    e. goiter
    e. hemoptysis
    e. typhus
endergonic reaction
endoamylase
endobronchial
endocardial
    e. fibroelastosis
    e. sclerosis
endocardiosis
    nonbacterial verrucal e.
endocarditis
    atypical verrucal e.
    bacterial e.
    Libman-Sacks e.
    marantic e.
    nonbacterial thrombotic e.
    rheumatic e.
    vegetative e.
    verrucous e.
endocardium
endocervical
    e. canal
    e. connective tissue

endocervical *(continued)*
   e. epithelium
endocervicitis
endocervix
endochondral
endocrine
   e. adenomatosis
   e. gland
endocrinology
endocrinopathy
endocytosis
endodeoxyribonuclease
endoderm
endodermal
   e. sinus tumor
Endodermophyton
endoenzyme
endogenote
endogenous
   e. antigen-transferred antibody reaction
   e. antigen-transferred cell-bound antibody reaction
   e. hemosiderosis
Endolimax
   E. nana
endolymph
endolymphatic
   e. duct
   e. sac
   e. stromal myosis
endometrial
   e. atrophy
   e. cast
   e. cavity
   e. gestational alteration
   e. gland
   e. hyperplasia
   e. polyp
   e. secretion
   e. stroma
   e. stromal sarcoma

endometrial *(continued)*
   e. stromatosis
   e. zona basalis
   e. zona functionalis
endometrioma
endometriosis
   stromal e.
endometritis
   syncytial e.
endometrium (endometria)
   anovulatory cycle e.
   atrophic e.
   cyclic alteration e.
   estrin-type e.
   inactive e.
   interval e.
   late interval e.
   menopausal e.
   menstrual e.
   postmenopausal e.
   postmenstrual e.
   premenstrual e.
   progestational e.
   proliferative e.
   regenerative e.
   secretory e.
   senile e.
endomitosis
Endomyces
   E. albicans
   E. capsulatus
   E. epidermatidis
   E. epidermidis
endomycosis
endomyocardial
   e. fibrosis
   e. sclerosis
endomysium
endoneurium
endonuclease
endoparasite
endopeduncular nucleus

endopeptidase
endophlebitis
endophthalmitis
endoplasm
endoplasmic reticulum
endopolyploidy
endoreduplication
endoribonuclease
endorphin
endoscopic
    e. retrograde cholangio-
      pancreatography
endoscopy
endosmosis
endospore
endosteum
endosulfan
endothelial
    e. metaplasia
    e. sarcoma
endotheliocyte
endothelioma
endothelium (endothelia)
    continuous e.
    discontinuous e.
    fenestrated e.
endothermic
endothrix
endotoxemia
endotoxic shock
endotoxin
end-plate
    e. potential
endrin
energy
    binding e.
    bond e.
    free e.
    kinetic e.
    potential e.
    e. resolution

enflagellation
enflurane
ENG — electronystagmograph
engulfment
    cytologic e.
enhancement
    immunologic e.
enkephalin
ENL — erythema nodosum
    leproticum
enlargement
    nuclear e.
enol
enolase
enostosis
enoyl–coenzyme A hydratase
entamebiasis
Entamoeba
    E. buccalis
    E. buetschlii
    E. coli
    E. gingivalis
    E. hartmanni
    E. histolytica
    E. nana
    E. nipponica
    E. polecki
    E. tetragena
    E. tropicalis
enteric
    e. cytopathogenic human
      orphan virus
Enteritidis
    E. salmonella
enteritis
    regional e.
    staphylococcal e.
Enterobacter
    E. aerogenes
    E. agglomerans
    E. alvei

Enterobacter (continued)
   E. cloacae
   E. gergoviae
   E. hafniae
   E. liquefaciens
   E. sakazakii
   E. subgroup C.
Enterobacteriaceae
enterobiasis
Enterobius
   E. vermicularis
enterocele
enterochromaffin
   e. cells
   e. staining
enterococcus (enterococci)
enterocolitis
   acute necrotizing e.
   cicatrizing e.
   pseudomembranous e.
   regional e.
enterocolostomy
enteroenterostomy
enterogastrone
enteroglucagon
enterokinase
enterolith
Enteromonas
   E. hominis
enteropathy
   gluten-sensitive e.
   protein-losing e.
enteropeptidase
enterostomy
enterotoxigenic
enterotoxin
enterovirus
enterozoon (enterozoa)
enthalpy
Entner-Doudoroff pathway
entoderm
Entoloma lividum

Entomophthora
   E. coronata
entomophthoromycosis
entopic
entropion
entropy
enucleate
enucleation
enuresis
envelope
   nuclear e.
envenomation
environment
environmental stress
enz. — enzymatic
enzootic
enzymatic
enzyme
   activating e.
   allosteric e.
   amylolytic e.
   autolytic e.
   catheptic e.
   coagulating e.
   constitutive e.
   converting e.
   glycolytic e.
   hydrolytic e.
   e. immunoassay
   inducible e.
   inhibitory e.
   inverting e.
   e.-linked antibody test
   e.-linked immunosorbent
      assay
   lipolytic e.
   microsomal e.
   e.-multiplied immunoassay
      technique
   proteolytic e.
   serum e.
   steatolytic e.

enzymic fat necrosis
EO — eosinophils
 ethylene oxide
EOG — electrooculogram
EOM — extraocular movement
eos — eosinophil
eosin
 e.-methylene blue
eosinopenia
eosinophil
 e. adenoma
 e. chemotactic factor of anaphylaxis
 e. leukocytic infiltrate
 polymorphonuclear e.
 e. stimulation promoter
eosinophilia
eosinophilic
 e. fasciitis
 e. granuloma
 e. hyperplasia
 e. index
 e. leukemia
 e. leukocyte
 e. metamyelocyte
 e. myelocyte
 e. promyelocyte
eosinotactic
EOT — effective oxygen transport
EP — ectopic pregnancy
 electrophoresis
 erythrocyte protoporphyrin
EPC — epilepsia partialis continua
EPEC — enteropathogenic *Escherichia coli*
ependyma
ependymal
 e. cells
 e. layer
ependymitis
ependymoblastoma
ependymoma
 epithelial e.
 Grade I e.
 Grades II – IV e.
 malignant e.
 myxopapillary e.
 papillary e.
EPF — exophthalmos-producing factor
ephedrine
ephelis
Epi — epinephrine
epicanthus
epicarcinogen
epicardium
epichlorohydrin
epicondyle
epicondylitis
epicranial aponeurosis
epicranius muscle
epidemic
 hemorrhagic fever e.
 parotitis virus e.
 typhus e.
epidemiology
epidermal
 e. cyst
 e. dermal nevus
 e. inclusion cyst
epidermidization
 e. of cervix
epidermis (epidermides)
epidermodysplasia
 e. verruciformis
epidermoid
 e. carcinoma
 e. carcinoma-in-situ
 e. cyst
 e. inclusion cyst
 e. metaplasia

epidermolysis
   e. bullosa
epidermophytid
Epidermophyton
   E. floccosum
   E. inguinale
   E. rubrum
epidermophytosis
epididymal
   e. fluid
   e. lumen
epididymis (epididymides)
epididymitis
epididymography
epididymovesiculography
epidural
   e. hematoma
   e. space
epigastric
   e. artery
   e. lymph node
epigastrius parasiticus
epigenesis
epigenetics
epigenotype
epiglottic
   e. cartilage
   e. mucus
epiglottis
epignathus
epilepsy
   familial myoclonic e.
   focal e.
   focal cortical e.
   grand mal e.
   jacksonian e.
   minor e.
   myoclonic e.
   petit mal e.
   post-traumatic e.
   psychomotor e.
   rolandic e.

epilepsy *(continued)*
   temporal lobe e.
   uncinate e.
epileptiform
epiloia
epimer
epimerase
epimerization
epimysium
epinephrine
epineurium
epiphenotype
epiphyseal
   e. giant cell tumor
   e. plate
epiphysis
epiphyte
episcleritis
   rheumatoid e.
episode
episomal
episome
epispadias
epistasis
epistaxis
epitestosterone
epith — epithelium
epithalamus
epithelial
   e. cyst
   e. ependymoma
   e. hyperplasia
   e. inclusion cyst
   e. neoplasm
   e. rest
   e. tumor
epithelialization
epithelioceptor
epithelioid
   e. cell melanoma
   e. cell nevus
   e. sarcoma

epithelioma
    e. adenoides cysticum
    basal cell e.
    benign e.
    Borst-Jadassohn intraepidermal basal cell e.
    Malherbe's calcifying e.
epitheliosis
epithelium (epithelia)
    Barrett's e.
    ciliated e.
    endocervical e.
    exocervical e.
    germinal e.
    tubal e.
epitope
epitrochlear lymph node
epizootic
eponychium
eponym(s). *See* Appendix 2, Eponymic Diseases and Syndromes.
epoophoron
epoxide
epoxy
EPP — end-plate potential
    equal pressure point
    erythropoietic protoporphyria
EPR — electron paramagnetic resonance
    electrophrenic respiration
    estradiol production rate
EPS — exophthalmos-producing substance
Epstein-Barr virus
epulis (epulides)
eq — equivalent
equal pressure point

equation
    Bohr e.
    Eadie-Hofstee e.
    Hanes e.
    Henderson-Hasselbalch e.
    Hill e.
    Lineweaver-Burke e.
    Michaelis-Menten e.
    Nernst e.
    Scatchard e.
    van der Waals e.
equilibration
equilibrium
    chemical e.
    dynamic e.
    physiologic e.
    radioactive e.
    secular e.
    thermal e.
    thermodynamic e.
    transient e.
equine encephalitis
    eastern e. e.
    Venezuelan e. e.
    western e. e.
equipotential
equivalence
equivalent
ER — ejection rate
    endoplasmic reticulum
    estrogen receptors
Er — erbium
ERA — evoked response audiometry
ERBF — effective renal blood flow
erbium
Erb's
    palsy
    point
    waves

ERC — erythropoietin-responsive cell
ERCP — endoscopic retrograde cholangiopancreatography
Erdheim rest
erector muscle of spine
ERG — electroretinogram
erg
ergastoplasm
ergastoplasmic
ergocalciferol
ergoloid mesylates
ergometer
ergonovine
   e. maleate
ergosterol
ergot
ergotamine
   e. tartrate
ergothioneine
ergotism
ergotoxine
Erlenmeyer flask
erosion
erosive
   e. aneurysm
   e. esophagitis
   e. gastritis
   e. inflammation
ERP — effective refractory period
      equine rhinopneumonitis
ERPF — effective renal plasma flow
eructation
eruption
   bullous e.
   Kaposi's varicelliform e.
   macular e.
   maculopapular e.

eruption *(continued)*
   polymorphic light e.
   polymorphous e.
ERV — expiratory reserve volume
Erwinia
   E. amylovora
   E. herbicola
Erwinieae
erysipelas
erysipeloid
Erysipelothrix
   E. insidiosa
   E. rhusiopathiae
erythema
   e. ab igne
   e. annulare centrifugum
   e. chronicum migrans
   e. elevatum diutinum
   e. figuratum
   e. induratum
   e. infectiosum
   e. marginatum rheumaticum
   e. multiforme
   e. multiforme exudativum
   e. neonatorum
   e. nodosum
   Osler's e.
   palmar e.
   e. pernio
   e. perstans
   toxic e.
erythrasma
erythremia
erythremic myelosis
erythritol
erythrityl tetranitrate
Erythrobacillus
erythroblast
erythroblastic
erythroblastoma

erythroblastomatosis
erythroblastosis
   e. fetalis
   e. neonatorum
erythrocuprein
erythrocytapheresis
erythrocyte
   e. sedimentation rate
erythrocythemia
erythrocytic
erythrocytophagy
erythrocytosis
   leukemic e.
   e. megalosplenica
erythroderma
erythrodextrin
erythrodontia
erythrogenesis
erythrogenic
erythroid
   e. aplasia
   e. hyperplasia
   e. hypoplasia
erythrokinetics
erythroleukemia
erythromycin
erythromyeloblastic leukemia
erythron
erythroneocytosis
erythropenia
erythrophagocytosis
erythroplasia
   Queyrat's e.
erythropoiesis
   extramedullary e.
   megaloblastic e.
erythropoietic
   e. porphyria
   e. protoporphyria
   e. tissue
erythropoietin
   e.-responsive cell

erythrose isomerase
ES — emission spectrometry
Es — einsteinium
ESB — electrical stimulation to brain
escape
   e. beats
   nodal e.
   vagal e.
   ventricular e.
Esch. — *Escherichia*
Escherichia
   E. aerogenes
   E. alkalescens
   E. aurescens
   E. coli
   E. dispar
   E. dispar var. *ceylonensis*
   E. dispar var. *madampensis*
   E. freundii
   E. intermedia
Escherichieae
Escherich's bacillus
ESF — erythropoietic-stimulating factor
ESL — end-systolic length
ESM — ejection systolic murmur
eso — esophagoscopy
   esophagus
esophageal
   e. achalasia
   e. adventitia
   e. artery
   e. branch
   e. contraction ring
   e. gland
   e. lumen
   e. manometry
   e. mucous membrane
   e. mucus
   e. muscularis propria

esophageal *(continued)*
- e. plexus
- e. sphincter
- e. submucosa
- e. varices
- e. vein

esophagitis
- corrosive e.
- erosive e.
- infectious e.
- monilial e.
- peptic e.
- reflux e.

esophagoduodenostomy
esophagogastroduodenoscopy
esophagogastroscopy
esophagogastrostomy
esophagography
esophagojejunostomy
esophagomalacia
esophagoscopy
esophagostomy
esophagotracheal
esophagus
- Barrett's e.

ESP — end-systolic pressure
  eosinophil stimulation promoter
ESR — erythrocyte sedimentation rate
esr — electron spin resonance
ESS — erythrocyte-sensitizing substance

essential
- e. atrophy
- e. hypercholesterolemia
- e. hyperlipemia
- e. hypertension
- e. pentosuria

ester
esterase
esterification
estetrol
esthesioneuroblastoma
esthesioneurocytoma
esthiomene
estradiol
estramustine
Estren-Dameshek anemia
estrin-type endometrium
estriol
- conjugated e.
- free e.
- serum e.
- total e.
- unconjugated e.
- urinary e.

estrogen
- e. receptor

estrogenic
estrone
estrous
- e. cycle

ESU — electrostatic unit
ESV — end-systolic volume
ET — effective temperature
  endotracheal
  etiology
  eustachian tube
Et — ethyl
ETA — ethionamide
ETF — eustachian tube function
ETH — elixir terpin hydrate
ethacrynic acid
ethambutol
ethamivan
ethane
ethanedial
ethanoic acid
ethanol
ethanolamine
ethanolaminephosphate cytidylyltransferase

ethanolaminephosphotransferase
ETH/C — elixir of terpin hydrate with codeine
ethchlorvynol
ethene
ether
    alkyl phenol polyglycol e.
    dichloroethyl e.
    ethyl e.
    propylene glycol monomethyl e.
    vinyl e.
ethinamate
ethinyl estradiol
ethionamide
ethionine
ethisterone
ethmoid
    e. antrum
    e. bone
    e. sinus
ethmoidal
    e. artery
    e. bulla
ethmoidomaxillary suture
ethoheptazine
ethohexadiol
ethopropazine
ethosuximide
ethotoin
ethoxzolamide
ethyl
    e. acetate
    e. alcohol
    e. aminobenzoate
    e. benzene
    e. biscoumacetate
    e. bromide
    e. butyl propanediol
    e. carbamate

ethyl *(continued)*
    e. chloride
    e. di-(*p*-chlorophenyl) glycollate
    e. dipropylthiocarbamate
    e. ether
    e. formate
    e. hexanediol
    e. iodide
    e. iodophenylundecylate
    e. mercaptan
    e. mercaptoethyl diethyl thiophosphate
    e. mercury chloride
    e. mercury phosphate
    e. nitrate
    e. nitrophenyl benzene thiophosphate
    e. nitrophenyl thiobenzene
    e. phosphate
ethylamine
ethylene
    e. chlorobromide
    e. chlorohydrin
    e. dibromide
    e. dichloride
    e. glycol
    e. oxide
ethylenediamine
ethylenediaminetetraacetate
ethylenediaminetetraacetic acid
ethylidene dichloride
N-(ethylmercuri)-*p*-toluenesulfonanilide
ethylmorphine hydrochloride
ethyne
etiocholanolone
etiocobalamine
etiol — etiology
etiology
    genetic e.

etiology *(continued)*
   unknown e.
ETKM — every test known to mankind
ETM — erythromycin
ETOH — ethyl alcohol
etoprine
ETOX — ethylene oxide
ETP — eustachian tube pressure
ETT — extrathyroidal thyroxine
EU — Ehrlich unit
   enzyme unit
Eu — europium
EUA — examination under anesthesia
eubacteria
Eubacteriales
Eubacterium
   E. aerofaciens
   E. alactolyticum
   E. contortum
   E. endocarditis
   E. lentum
   E. limosum
   E. parvum
   E. rectale
   E. ventriosum
eucalyptol
eucalyptus oil
eucaryote
eucatropine
   e. hydrochloride
euchromatin
eudermol
eugenol
Euglena
   E. gracilis
euglenoid
euglobulin
   e. clot test
eugonic

eukaryon
eukaryosis
eukaryote
eukaryotic
Eulenburg's disease
eumelanin
Eumycetes
eumycotic
eunuchoidism
euploid
euploidy
Euproctis
   E. chrysorrhoea
European
   blastomycosis
   hookworm
   rat flea
europium
Eurotium
   E. malignum
eurythermal
Eusimulium
eustachianography
eustachian tube
Eustrongylus
euthyroid
euthyroidism
Eutriatoma
Eutrombicula
   E. alfreddugesi
eutrophic
EV — extravascular
ev — electron volt
evaporation
eventration
eversion
evisceration
EVM — electronic voltmeter
evoked potential
   brain stem auditory e. p.
   scalp-recorded somatosensory e. p.

evoked potential *(continued)*
   somatosensory e. p.
   spinal somatosensory e. p.
   visual e. p.
evolution
E wave
EWB — estrogen withdrawal bleeding
Ewing's
   sarcoma
   tumor
EWL — egg-white lysozyme
ex — excision
   exophthalmos
examination
   double-contrast e.
exanthem
   Boston e.
   e. subitum
exanthematous
EXBF — exercise hyperemia blood flow
exc — excision
excessive
   e. cornification
   e. fatigue
   e. lacrimation
   e. sweating
   e. tearing
   e. weakness
   e. weeping
   e. weight gain
   e. weight loss
excipient
excision
excoriation
excretion
   pseudouridine e.
excretory
exenteration
exergonic reaction
exertional dyspnea

exfoliation
exfoliative
   e. cytologic alteration
   e. dermatitis
   e. psoriasis
exhalation
exhaustion
   e. atrophy
   heat e.
exocellular
exocelomic
   e. cavity
   e. membrane
exocervical
   e. connective tissue
   e. epithelium
exocervix
exocrine
exocytosis
exoenzyme
exogenote
exogenous
   e. antigen cell-bound antibody reaction
   e. antigen-circulating antibody reaction
   e. hemosiderosis
exonuclease
exopeptidase
Exophiala
   E. jeanselmei
   E. mycetoma
   E. werneckii
exophthalmos
exophytic
exoribonuclease
exosmosis
exostosis
   cartilaginous e.
   osteocartilaginous e.
exothermic
exotoxin

expectancy wave
experiment
experimental
expiration
expiratory
    e. reserve volume
explosion
explosive
exponent
exponential
exposure
exsanguination
exsiccant
exsiccate
exsiccation
exstrophy
ext — exterior
    external
    extract
Extended Binary Coded Decimal Interchange Code
extension
extensor
extensor carpi radialis brevis muscle
extensor carpi radialis longus muscle
extensor carpi ulnaris muscle
extensor digiti minimi muscle
extensor digitorum muscle
extensor hallucis brevis muscle
extensor hallucis longus muscle
extensor plantar reflex
extensor pollicis brevis muscle
extensor pollicis longus muscle
external
    e. arcuate fibers
    e. auditory canal
    e. auditory meatus
    e. capsule
    e. carotid artery
    e. carotid nerve

external *(continued)*
    e. ear
    e. endometriosis
    e. hemorrhoids
    e. hydrocephalus
    e. iliac artery
    e. iliac vein
    e. inguinal ring
    e. jugular vein
    e. limiting membrane
    e. maxillary artery
    e. medullary lamina
    e. nasal branch
    e. os
    e. pudendal artery
    e. pudendal vein
externalia
exteroceptor
exterofection
exterofective
exterogestate
extracellular
    e. alteration
    e. background material alteration
    e. fiber
    e. fluid
    e. granule
    e. ground substance
    e. lipid aggregate
    e. macromolecule aggregate
    e. matrix
    e. plasma
    e. sap
    e. space
    e. structural alteration
    e. vacuole
extracerebral
extracorpuscular
extract
extractable nuclear antigen
extraembryonic mesoblast

extrafusal fibers
extrahepatic bile duct
extrahypothalamic
extramammary Paget's disease
extramedullary
    e. erythropoiesis
    e. hematopoiesis
    e. megakaryocytopoiesis
    e. myelopoiesis
extrapancreatic
extrapyramidal tract
extraskeletal
extrasystole
extrauterine pregnancy
extravasation
extravascular
extreme capsule
extremital
extremity
extrinsic
    e. ocular muscle
    e. tongue muscle
extrude
exudate
    acute inflammatory e.

exudate *(continued)*
    inflammatory e.
    mucopurulent e.
exudation
exudative
    e. glomerulonephritis
    e. inflammation
eye
    e. appendages
eyeball
    tunica fibrosa of the e.
    tunica interna of the e.
    tunica vasculosa of the e.
eyebrow
eyelash
eyelid
    third e.
eyepiece
    comparison e.
    compensated e.
    high eyepoint e.
    huygenian e.
    Ramsden's e.
    widefield e.
eyeworm

F

F — Fahrenheit
    farad
    feces
    female
    field of vision
    fluorine
    foramen
    force
    formula
    French (catheter size)
    gilbert (unit of magnetomotive force)

F *(continued)*
    hydrocortisone (compound F)
F_1 — first filial generation
F_2 — second filial generation
F. — *Filaria*
    Fusiformis
FA — fatty acid
    femoral artery
    fluorescent antibody
    free acid

FAB — formalin ammonium
    bromide
Fabricius
    bursa of F.
Fabry's disease
face
    adenoid f.
    cleft f.
    hippocratic f.
    f. presentation
facial
    f. artery
    f. bones
    f. diprosopus duplication
    f. lymph node
    f. muscle
    f. myiasis
    f. nerve
    f. palsy
    f. vein
facies
    adenoid f.
    cushingoid f.
    f. hepatica
    hippocratic f.
    leonine f.
    leprechaun f.
    Parkinson's f.
    scaphoid f.
facilitated diffusion
facioscapulohumeral-type progressive muscular dystrophy
factitious
    f. dermatitis
    f. urticaria
factor
    Christmas f.
    coagulation f's I, II, III, IV, V, VII, VIII, IX, X, XI, XII, XIII
    deficiency f's I, II, V, VII, VIII, IX, X, XI

factor *(continued)*
    F f.
    fibrin-stabilizing f.
    Fitzgerald f.
    Fletcher f.
    G f.
    Hageman f.
    Laki-Lorand f.
    Passovoy f.
    Prower f.
    Stuart f.
    von Willebrand's f.
factorial
facultative
FAD — flavin adenine dinucleotide
FADF — fluorescent antibody darkfield
Fahr — Fahrenheit
Fahrenheit
    temperature scale
    thermometer
failure
    circulatory f.
    heart f.
fainting
faintness
falciform
fallopian tube
    f. t. ampulla
    f. t. fimbria
    f. t. infundibulum
    f. t. isthmus
    f. t. lumen
    f. t. lymphatics
    f. t. secretion
Fallopius' aqueduct
Fallot
    tetralogy of F.
false
    f. aneurysm
    f. diverticulum

false *(continued)*
- f. knot, umbilical cord
- f. negative
- f. positive

falx (falces)
- f. cerebelli
- f. cerebri
- f. inguinalis

familial
- f. benign pemphigus
- f. cardiomyopathy
- f. cerebellar ataxia
- f. erythrophagocytic lymphohistiocytosis
- f. fibrous dysplasia
- f. gonadal dysgenesis
- f. hemolytic anemia
- f. hypercholesterolemia
- f. Mediterranean fever
- f. myoclonic epilepsy
- f. nephritis
- f. nephronophthisis
- f. nonhemolytic jaundice
- f. periodic paralysis
- f. polyposis
- f. primary systemic amyloidosis

family

FAN — fuchsin, amido black, and naphthol yellow

FANA — fluorescent antinuclear antibody

Fanconi's
- anemia
- syndrome

Fanconi-Zinssen syndrome

F and R — force and rhythm (of pulse)

Fannia
- *F. canicularis*
- *F. scalaris*

farad

faraday

Faraday's
- constant
- effect
- law of electrolysis

Farber's
- disease
- lipogranulomatosis

farcy

farmer's lung

farnesyl-pyrophosphate synthetase

Farrant's medium

fascia (fasciae)
- antebrachial f.
- axillary f.
- brachial f.
- cervical f.
- clavipectoral f.
- clitoridal f.
- cremasteric f.
- crural f.
- dorsal f.
- f. lata
- masseter f.
- nuchal f.
- f. occludens
- orbit f.
- parotid f.
- pectoral f.
- pelvic f.
- penile f.
- perirenal f.
- renal f.
- superficial f.
- temporal f.
- thoracolumbar f.
- transversalis f.
- urogenital diaphragmatic f.

fascial
- f. fibrosarcoma
- f. space

fascicle
fascicular
fasciculation
   f. potential
fasciculus (fasciculi)
   f. arcuate
   f. cingulate
   f. comma
   f. cuneatus
   dorsal proper f.
   frontotemporal f.
   f. gracilis
   inferior fronto-occipital f.
   inferior longitudinal f.
   f. interfascicularis
   lateral proper f.
   lenticular f.
   longitudinal f.
   medial longitudinal f.
   perpendicular f.
   subthalamic f.
   sulcomarginal f.
   superior fronto-occipital f.
   superior longitudinal f.
   temporo-occipital f.
   thalamic f.
   uncinate f.
   ventral proper f.
   vertical occipital f.
fasciitis
   eosinophilic f.
   infiltrative f.
   necrotizing f.
   nodular f.
   pseudosarcomatous f.
Fasciola
   F. gigantica
   F. hepatica
fasciolar gyrus
fascioliasis
fasciolopsiasis

Fasciolopsis
   F. buski
FASEB — Federation of American Societies for Experimental Biology
fast
   f. green
   f. hemoglobin
fastigiobulbar projection
fasting blood sugar
FAT — fluorescent antibody test
fat
   f. absorption test
   f. cells
   f. embolism
   f. embolus
   f. necrosis
   subcutaneous f.
fatigue
fatty
   f. atrophy
   f. change
   f. degeneration
   f. deposition
   f. infiltration
   f. metamorphosis
   f. nutritional cirrhosis
   f. phanerosis
   f. tissue
fatty acid
   essential f. a.
   free f. a.
   nonesterified f. a.
   f. a. oxidation
   f. a. profile
   f. a. synthesis
   unesterified f. a.
fauces
faucial

FAV — feline ataxia virus
favism
favus
FB — foreign body
FBE — full blood examination
F body
FBP — femoral blood pressure
   fibrinogen breakdown products
FBS — fasting blood sugar
   fetal bovine serum
FCA — ferritin-conjugated antibodies
FCC — follicular center cells
FD — fatal dose
   focal distance
   forceps delivery
FD_{50} — median fatal dose
FDA — Food and Drug Administration
   frontodextra anterior
FDNB — fluorodinitrobenzene
F donor
FDP — fibrin degradation product
   flexor digitorum profundus
   frontodextra posterior
   fructose 1,6-diphosphate
FDS — flexor digitorum superficialis
FDT — frontodextra transversa
Fe — iron
febrile
   f. agglutination test
FEC — free erythrocyte coproporphyrin
fecal
   f. impaction
   f. incontinence
   f. vomitus
fecalith
feces
   extravasation f.
   impacted f.
FECG — fetal electrocardiogram
FECP — free erythrocyte coproporphyria
FECV — functional extracellular fluid volume
Federation of American Societies for Experimental Biology
feedback
FEF — forced expiratory flow
Fehleisen's streptococcus
Fehling's
   solution
   test
FEKG — fetal electrocardiogram
FEL — familial erythrophagocytic lymphohistiocytosis
Felton phenomenon
Felty's syndrome
female
   f. breast
   f. carrier
   f. genital fluids
   f. genital spaces
   f. genitalia
   f. hormones
   f. pseudohermaphroditism
   f. sex chromatin pattern
   f. urethra
feminization
   f. syndrome, adrenal
   testicular f.
feminizing tumor
femoral
   f. artery

femoral *(continued)*
   f. canal
   f. circumflex vein
   f. cutaneous vein
   f. lymph node
   f. nerve
   f. vein
femorocele
femtoliter
femtometer
femtomole
femur (femora)
fenestra (fenestrae)
   f. cochleae
   f. vestibuli
fenestrated
fenestration
   atrophic f.
fenfluramine
fennel oil
fenoprofen calcium
fentanyl citrate
FEP or FEPP — free erythrocyte protoporphyrin
ferment
fermentation
   mannitol f.
   mixed acid f.
fermium
ferning
Ferrata's cell
ferredoxin
Ferribacterium
ferric
   f. chloride
   f. chloride test
   f. ferricyanide reduction test
   f. ferrocyanide
   f. oxide
ferrihemoglobin
ferrimagnetic
ferrite
ferritin
   f.-coupled antibody
ferrocalcinosis
ferrocalcinotic deposition
ferrochelatase
ferrocyanide
ferroflocculation
ferrohemoglobin
ferrokinetic
ferromagnetic
ferrous
   f. carbonate
   f. chloride
   f. citrate
   f. ferricyanide
   f. fumarate
   f. gluconate
   f. sulfate
ferroxidase
ferruginous
   f. micelles
fertile
fertility
fertilization
FES — flame emission spectroscopy
      forced expiratory spirogram
festinating gait
FET — forced expiratory time
fetal
   f. abnormality
   f. adenoma
   f. adrenal cortex
   f. antigen
   f. duplication
   f. fat cell lipoma
   f. fluids
   f. hemoglobin
   f. implantation site

fetal *(continued)*
    f. lipoma
    f. lobulation
    f. membrane
    f. pupillary membrane
    f. spaces
    f. surface
fetid rhinitis
fetoglobulin
fetography
fetoplacental
fetoprotein
fetor
    f. hepaticus
    f. oris
fetoscopy
FETS — forced expiratory time, in seconds
fetus
    f. acardiacus
    f. amorphus
    f. compressus
    f. in fetu
    macerated f.
    f. papyraceus
    parasitic f.
    stunted f.
Feulgen's
    reaction
    stain
    test
FEV — forced expiratory volume
fever
    Bullis f.
    Bwamba f.
    chikungunya f.
    Colorado tick f.
    Dumdum f.
    familial Mediterranean f.
    Haverhill f.
    Malta f.

fever *(continued)*
    Mediterranean f.
    Omsk hemorrhagic f.
    O'nyong-nyong f.
    Oroya f.
    pappataci f.
    Pel-Ebstein f.
    Pontiac f.
    Q. f.
    Rocky Mountain spotted f.
    San Joaquin f.
    undulant f.
    West Nile f.
FF — fat free
    fecal frequency
    filtration fraction
FFA — free fatty acids
F factor
FFDW — fat-free dry weight
FFM — fat-free mass
FFP — fresh frozen plasma
FFWW — fat-free wet weight
FG — fibrinogen
FGD — fatal granulomatous disease
FHR — fetal heart rate
FHS — fetal heart sound
FHT — fetal heart
    fetal heart tones
FI — fever caused by infection
    fibrinogen
    forced inspiration
FIA — fluorescent immunoassay
fib — fibrillation
    fibrinogen
fiber
    Purkinje's f's
    Reissner's f.
    Sharpey's f's
    Tomes' f's
fiberoptic

fibril
- collagen f's
- fibroglia nerve f.
- muscular f.

fibrillar

fibrillary
- f. astrocyte
- f. astrocytoma

fibrillated

fibrillation
- atrial f.
- auricular f.
- cardiac f.
- muscular f.
- ventricular f.

fibrin
- f. degradation product
- gluten f.
- f. monomer
- myosin f.
- f. stabilizing factor
- stroma f.
- f. titer test

fibrinogen
- f. deficiency

fibrinogenase

fibrinogenopenia

fibrinogenous

fibrinoid
- f. necrosis
- f. necrotizing inflammation

fibrinokinase

fibrinolysin
- seminal f.

fibrinolysis

fibrinolytic purpura

fibrinopenia

fibrinopeptide

fibrinopurulent

fibrinous
- f. acute lobar pneumonia
- f. acute pleuritis

fibrinous *(continued)*
- f. adhesion
- f. exudation
- f. inflammation
- f. peritonitis
- f. pleurisy
- f. pleuritis

fibroadenoma
- giant f.
- intracanalicular f.
- juvenile f.
- pericanalicular f.

fibroadenosis

fibroameloblastic
- f. dentinoma
- f. odontoma

fibroblast

fibroblastic meningioma

fibroblastoma
- perineural f.

fibrocalcific

fibrocartilage
- intervertebral f.
- f. matrix alteration

fibrocartilaginous annulus

fibrocaseous

fibrocongestive
- f. hypertrophy
- f. splenomegaly

fibrocystic
- f. disease, breast
- f. mastitis
- f. mastopathy

fibroelastic
- f. cartilage
- f. membrane

fibroelastosis
- endocardial f.

fibroepithelial
- f. papilloma
- f. polyp

fibroepithelioma

fibrogenesis
    f. imperfecta ossium
fibroid
    f. uterus
fibrolipoma
fibroliposarcoma
fibroma
    ameloblastic f.
    cementifying f.
    chondromyxoid f.
    myxoid f.
    nonossifying f.
    odontogenic f.
    ossifying f.
    periosteal f.
    peripheral odontogenic f.
fibromatosis
    f. colli
    Dupuytren's f.
    palmar f.
    plantar f.
fibromuscular
fibromyoma
fibromyositis
fibromyxoid
fibromyxolipoma
fibromyxoma
fibromyxosarcoma
fibronectin
fibroplasia
    retrolental f.
fibrosarcoma
    fascial f.
    medullary f.
    odontogenic f.
    periosteal f.
fibrosiderotic nodule
fibrosing
    f. adenomatosis
    f. adenosis
    f. alveolitis
fibrosis
    condensation f.
    cystic f.
    diffuse f.
    endomyocardial f.
    focal f.
    hepatic f.
    inflammation with f.
    interstitial f.
    mediastinal f.
    multifocal f.
    nodular f.
    pulmonary f.
    retroperitoneal f.
    septal f., liver
    subepidermal f.
fibrotic
fibrous
    f. adhesion
    f. ankylosis
    f. astrocyte
    f. astrocytoma
    f. body
    f. cortical defect
    f. dysplasia
    f. histiocytoma
    f. hypertrophic pachymeningitis
    f. layer
    f. mesothelioma
    f. nodule
    f. obliteration
    f. osteoma
    f. repair
    f. replacement
    f. tendon sheath
    f. thyroiditis
    f. tissue
    f. tubercle
    f. union
fibroxanthoma

fibula
fibular
ficin
Fick's
   bacillus
   law
   principle
Ficoll-Hypaque technique
FID — flame ionization detector
Fiedler's myocarditis
field
   low-power f.
   f. of microscope
   f. of view
FIF — forced inspiratory flow
fifth
   f. cranial nerve
   f. disease virus
   f. metacarpal
   f. metatarsal
FIGLU — formiminoglutamic acid
FIGO — International Federation of Gynecology and Obstetrics
FIGO classification of staging
filament
filamentous
Filaria
   F. bancrofti
   F. conjunctivae
   F. demarquayi
   F. hominis oris
   F. juncea
   F. labialis
   F. lentis
   F. loa
   F. lymphatica
   F. medinensis
   F. ozzardi
   F. palpebralis

Filaria (continued)
   F. philippinensis
   F. sanguinis
   F. tucumana
   F. volvulus
filaria (filariae)
filariasis
   Bancroft's f.
   Malayan f.
filaricide
Filarioidea
filiform
   f. hyperkeratosis
   f. papillae
filix
   f. mas
filling
   f. defect
   f. gallop
   f. rumble
film
   fixed blood f.
   gelatin f.
   spot f.
   sulfa f.
   x-ray f.
Filobasidiella
   F. bacillisporus
   F. neoformans
filter
   bacterial f.
   barrier f.
   Berkefeld f.
   blocking f.
   Chamberland f.
   collodion f.
   exciter f.
   gelatin f.
   Gelman f.
   inherent f.
   interference f.
   membrane f.

filter *(continued)*
    microaggregate f.
    Seitz f.
    Selas f.
filterable
filtrate
filtration
filum terminale (fila terminalia)
    f. t. externum
    f. t. internum
fimbria
fimbriated
fimbriodentate sulcus
finder
fine structure
finger
    clubbed f.
    hippocratic f's
    mallet f.
    rudimentary f.
finite
firmware
first
    f. branchial arch
    f. cranial nerve
    f. division, fifth cranial nerve
    f. division, trigeminal nerve
    f. metacarpal
    f. metatarsal
    f. pharyngeal pouch
    f. trimester pregnancy
first degree
    f. d. burn
    f. d. frostbite
    f. d. heart block
    f. d. radiation injury
Fischer projection
Fishberg's concentration test
fission
fissural

fissure
    f. in ano
    ansaparamedian f.
    calcarine f.
    centrolingual f.
    cerebellar f.
    hippocampal f.
    horizontal f.
    inferior orbital f.
    interhemispheric f.
    intrabiventral f.
    intraculminate f.
    intrapyramidal f.
    lateral cerebral f.
    longitudinal cerebral f.
    parietooccipital f.
    postcentral f.
    posterolateral f.
    postlingual f.
    postlunate f.
    postnodular f.
    prebiventral f.
    precentral f.
    preculminate f.
    prepyramidal f.
    primary f.
    Rolando's f.
    secondary f.
    superior posterior f.
    f. of Sylvius
    ventral medial f.
    ventral median f.
fissured nucleus
fist — fistula
fistula
    f. in ano
    arteriovenous f.
    biliary f.
    branchial f.
    inflammatory f.
    thyroglossal f.

fistulous
FITC — fluorescein isothiocyanate
Fite's method
Fitzgerald factor
fixation
   f. artifact
   autotrophic f.
   complement f.
   nitrogen f.
   secondary f.
fixative
   Brasil's f.
   Carnoy's f.
   Heidenhain's Susa f.
   Saccomanno's f.
   Zenker's f.
fixed-point variable
FJN — familial juvenile nephrophthisis
fl — femtoliter
   fluid
FLA — left frontoanterior (*frontolaeva anterior*)
flaccid
flaccidity
flagellar
Flagellata
flagellate
flagellin
flagellum (flagella)
flame
   capillary f's
   f. cell
   f. ionization detector
   manometric f.
   f. photometry
flammable
flank
flashcard
flash-point temperature
flask
   Dewar f.
   Erlenmeyer f.
   Florence f.
flatulence
flatworm
flavin
   f.-adenine dinucleotide
   f. mononucleotide
flavivirus
Flavobacterium
   F. meningosepticum
flavoenzyme
flavoprotein
fld — fluid
fl dr — fluid dram
flea
   American rat f.
   dog f.
   European rat f.
   human f.
   Indian rat f.
Flechsig's tract
fleckmilz
Fletcher factor
flexion
Flexner's
   bacillus
   dysentery
Flexner-Strong bacillus
flexor
flexor carpi radialis muscle
flexor carpi ulnaris muscle
flexor digiti minimi brevis muscle
flexor digitorum longus muscle
flexor digitorum muscle
flexor dititorum pedis longus muscle
flexor hallucis brevis muscle
flexor hallucis longus muscle

flexor plantar reflex
flexor pollicis brevis muscle
flexor pollicis longus muscle
flexure
   hepatic f.
   left colic f.
   right colic f.
   splenic f.
floating-point variable
floccose
floccular degeneration
flocculation
   cephalin f.
   Ramon f.
   f. test
floccule
   toxoid-antitoxin f.
flocculonodular lobe
flocculoreaction
flocculus (flocculi)
floppy valve syndrome
flora
florantyrone
Florence flask
Florentine iris
flotation
flow
   abnormal f.
   f. chart
   f. cytometry
   f.-volume curve
flowmeter
floxuridine
fl oz — fluid ounce
FLP — left frontoposterior (*frontolaeva posterior*)
FLS — fibrous long-spacing (collagen)
FLSA — follicular lymphosarcoma
FLT — left frontotransverse (*frontolaeva transversa*)
flu — influenza
fluctuation
flucytosine
fludrocortisone
fluid
   f. alteration
   amniotic f.
   f. balance
   Bensley's osmic dichromate f.
   Bouin's f.
   cerebrospinal f.
   Ciaccio's f.
   Clarke's f.
   cutaneous f.
   De Castro's f.
   epididymal f.
   female genital f.
   fetal f.
   Gendre's f.
   Helly's f.
   left pleural f.
   male genital f.
   mammary f.
   menstrual f.
   pancreatic f.
   pericardial f.
   peritoneal f.
   placental f.
   pleural f.
   f. retention
   seminal f.
   seminal vesicle f.
   synovial f.
   urinary tract f.
fluke
   blood f.
   cat liver f.

fluke *(continued)*
    Chinese liver f.
    giant intestinal f.
    giant liver f.
    liver f.
    oriental lung f.
    sheep liver f.
    Yokogawa's f.
flumethiazide
fluocinolone
fluor. – fluorometry
fluoracetate
fluorescein
    f. isothiocyanate
    f. mercuric acetate
    f. sodium
fluorescence
fluorescent
    f. antibody technique
    f. immunoassay
    f. treponemal antibody absorption test
fluoride
fluorine
fluoroacetamide
fluoroacetate
fluoroacetic acid
fluorocarbon
fluorochrome
5-fluorocytosine
fluorodinitrobenzene
fluorometer
fluorometholone
fluorometry
fluoroscope
fluoroscopy
fluorosis
    dental f.
    endemic f.
fluorouracil
fluosilicate salt
fluoxymesterone

fluphenazine
    f. enanthate
    f. hydrochloride
fluprednisolone
flurandrenolone
flurazepam hydrochloride
flutamide
flutter
    atrial f.
    ventricular f.
flux
fly
    black f.
    bot f.
    deer f.
    horse f.
    house f.
    larva f.
    stable f.
    tsetse f.
    warble f.
FM – flowmeter
Fm – fermium
fm – femtometer
FMF – familial Mediterranean fever
FMN – flavin mononucleotide
fmol – femtomole
FMS – fat-mobilizing substance
FN – false-negative
FO – foramen ovale
       fronto-occipital
foam
    f. cell
    f. stability test
FOAVF – failure of all vital forces
focal
    f. distance
    f. epilepsy
    f.-film distance
    f. length

focal *(continued)*
    f. plane
    f. plane tomography
    f. segmental glomerulo-
      sclerosis
    f. zone
focus (foci)
    conjugate f.
    principal f.
fog
folacin
folate
    f. deficiency anemia
    f. reductase
fold
    aryepiglottic f.
    circular f. of intestine
    epicanthic f.
    ileocecal f.
folded
    f. cell
    f. nucleus
foliate papillae
folic acid
Folin-Ciocalteu reagent
folinic acid
folium, cerebellar
follicle
    atretic f.
    cyst f.
    cystic ovarian f.
    graafian f.
    hair f.
    lymphatic f.
    malpighian f.
    mature ovarian f.
    nabothian f.
    ovarian f.
    splenic lymphatic f.
    f.-stimulating hormone
    thyroid f.

follicular
    f. adenocarcinoma
    f. adenoma
    f. carcinoma
    f. center cells
    f. conjunctivitis
    f. cyst
    f. dermatitis
    f. inflammation
    f. inverted keratosis
    f. lymphoma
    f. and papillary adenocar-
      cinoma
    f. salpingitis
    f. urethritis
folliculitis
    f. decalvans
    f. keloidalis
    f. ulerythematosa reticulata
fomite
Fonsecaea
    F. compactum
    F. dermatitidis
    F. jeanselmei
    F. pedrosoi
Fontana-Masson staining
    method
Fontana's spaces
fontanelle
food
    f. deprivation
    f. intolerance
    f. poisoning
Food and Drug Administration
foodball
foot
    Madura f.
foot-and-mouth disease
foot-and-mouth disease virus,
    types A, B, C
Foot's reticulin method

foramen (foramina)
- Bochdalek's f.
- cecum f.
- interventricular f.
- jugular f.
- f. lacerum
- Luschka's f.
- Magendie's f.
- f. magnum
- Monro's f.
- obturator f.
- optic f.
- f. ovale
- primary interventricular f.
- f. primum
- f. rotundum
- f. spinosum
- stylomastoid f.
- f. venae cavae
- Winslow's epiploic f.
- zygomaticofacial f.
- zygomaticotemporal f.

foramen ovale
- anatomically patent f. o.
- functionally patent f. o.
- incompetent valve f. o.
- patent f. o.
- prematurely closed f. o.
- probe patent f. o.

Forbes' disease

force
- van der Waals f's

forced
- f. expiratory flow
- f. expiratory volume
- f. vital capacity

forceps

Fordyce's disease

forearm

forefinger

foregut

forehead

foreign
- f. body
- f. material deposition

Forel's commissure

forensic medicine

foreskin

forespore

formaldehyde
- f. dehydrogenase
- f.-induced fluorescence method

formalin
- alcoholic f.
- f. ammonium bromide buffered neutral f.
- f.-ether sedimentation method
- f. pigment

formamidase

formamide

formate dehydrogenase

forme
- f. fruste
- f. tardive

formic acid

formication

formiminoglutamic acid

formiminotetrahydrofolate cyclodeaminase

formula (formulae, formulas)
- Arneth's f.
- Haworth f.

formulary

formyltetrahydrofolate
- f. deformylase
- f. synthetase

formyltransferase

fornix (fornices)
- f. of cerebrum
- conjunctival f.

FORTRAN — formula translation

fosfomycin
fossa (fossae)
    anterior f.
    cranial f.
    cubital f.
    ischiorectal f.
    middle f.
    oval f. of heart
    pituitary f.
    posterior f.
    pterygoid f.
    pyriform f.
    rhomboid f.
    Rosenmüller's f.
    subhepatic f.
    subphrenic f.
    temporal f.
    tonsillar f.
    Treitz's f.
fourchette
Fourier analysis
fourth
    f. branchial arch
    f. cranial nerve
    f. cranial nerve nucleus
    f. metacarpal
    f. metatarsal
    f. metatarsophalangeal joint
    f. pharyngeal pouch
    f. ventricle
fourth degree
    f. d. burn
    f. d. frostbite
    f. d. radiation injury
fovea centralis
foveate
foveola (foveolae)
Fowler's solution
Fox-Fordyce disease
FP — false-positive
    freezing point

FP *(continued)*
    frontoparietal
    frozen plasma
FPA — fluorophenylalanine
FPC — fish protein concentrate
F pilus (pili)
FPM — filter paper microscopic (test)
FR — Fisher-Race (notation)
    flocculation reaction
    flow rate
Fr — francium
    French (catheter gauge)
fract — fracture
fraction
fractionation
fracture
    chip f.
    closed f.
    comminuted f.
    compound f.
    compressed f.
    depressed f.
    f. dislocation
    greenstick f.
    healed f.
    impacted f.
    incomplete f.
    linear f.
    nonunion f.
    oblique f.
    pathologic f.
    simple f.
    spiral f.
    stellate f.
    transverse f.
    ununited f.
frag — fragility
fragilitas ossium
fragility
    capillary f.
    erythrocyte f.

fragility *(continued)*
   mechanical f.
   osmotic f.
   red cell f.
fragillograph
fragment
   Klenow f.
fragmentation
   f. of myocardium
frambesia
frame
framework
   scleral f.
   uveal f.
Francis' skin test
Francisella
   F. tularensis
francium
Franklin's disease
Frank-Starling mechanism
fraternal twins
FRC — frozen red cells
        functional reserve
          capacity
        functional residual
          capacity
freckle
   Hutchinson's melanotic f.
free
   f. electron
   f. energy
   f. erythrocyte protoporphyrin
   f. fatty acids
   f. radical
   f. thyroxine index
   f. triiodothyronine index
freeze
   f.-clamp
   f.-cleave method
   f.-etch method
   f.-fracture-etch method

freeze *(continued)*
   f.-substitution
freezing
   f. injury
   f. point
   f. point depression osmometer
Frei test
frenulum
   f. clitoridis
   f. labii inferioris
   f. labii superioris
   f. linguae
frequency
   angular f.
   f. distribution
   f. polygon
   urinary f.
Fresnel zone plate
Freund's adjuvant
friable
frict — friction
friction rub
   pericardial f. r.
   pleural f. r.
Friedländer's
   bacillus
   pneumobacillus
   pneumonia
Friedman's test
Friedreich's ataxia
frigidity
Fröhlich's syndrome
Frommel-Chiari syndrome
frons
   f. cranii
frontal
   f. bone
   f. gyrus
   f. horn, lateral ventricle
   f. lobe
   f. nerve

frontal *(continued)*
    f. pole
    f. process
    f. region, subdural space
    f. sinus
    f. sulcus
    f. suture
frontomarginal sulcus
frontoparietal operculum
frontopolar
frontopontine
frontotemporal fasciculus
frostbite
frozen
    f. red blood cells
    f. section method
FRP — functional refractory period
FRS — furosemide
fructofuranose
beta-fructofuranosidase
fructokinase
fructopyranose
fructose
    f. biphosphate
    f. diphosphate
    ferric f.
fructosemia
fructosuria
fructosyl
FS — full scale (IQ)
    function study
FSD — focal skin distance
FSF — fibrin-stabilizing factor
FSH — follicle-stimulating hormone
FSP — fibrinogen split products
    fibrinolytic split products
FSR — fusiform skin revision
FT — false transmitter
    fibrous tissue

FT_4 — free thyroxine
FT_3I — free triiodothyronine index
FTA — fluorescent treponemal antibody
FTA-AB or FTA-ABS — fluorescent treponemal antibody absorption test
FTI — free thyroxine index
FU — fecal urobilinogen
    fluorouracil
fuchsin
    acid f.
    basic f.
    carbol f.
fucosidase
fucosidosis
FUDR — fluorodeoxyuridine
fugacity
Fujiwara reaction
full-width half-maximum
fumagillin
fumarase
fumarate hydratase
fumarylacetoacetase
fumigation
function
    Boolean f.
    liver f.
functional
    f. residual capacity
functionally patent foramen ovale
fundal
fundus (fundi)
fungal
fungicidal
fungicide
fungiform papillae
Fungi Imperfecti
fungus (fungi)
    ascospore-forming f.

212 FUNGUS (FUNGI) – FZ

fungus (fungi) *(continued)*
    cutaneous f.
    fission f.
    mosaic f.
    mycelial f.
    yeast f.
funnel chest
FUO – fever of undetermined origin
       fever of unknown origin
FUR – fluorouracil riboside
furan
furanose
furanoside
furazolidone
furfural
furfuraldehyde
furosemide
furuncle
furunculosis
fusariomycosis
Fusarium   epicoccum (per AHH)
    F. javanicum
    F. moniliforme
    F. oxysporum
    F. roseum
    F. solanae
    F. sporotrichoides
fuseau (fuseaux)
Fusidium terricola
fusiform
    f. aneurysm
    f. bronchiectasis
    f. cell

fusiform *(continued)*
    f. gyrus
Fusiformis
    F. necrophorus
fusion
    splenogonadal f.
Fusobacterium
    F. aquatile
    F. fusiforme
    F. glutinosum
    F. gonidiaformans
    F. mortiferum
    F. naviforme
    F. necrophorum
    F. nucleatum
    F. plautivincenti
    F. prausnitzii
    F. symbiosum
    F. varium
fusocellular
fusospirillary
fusospirillosis
fusospirochetal
fusospirochetosis
fusostreptococcicosis
FV – fluid volume
FVC – forced vital capacity
FVL – femoral vein ligation
FW – Felix-Weil (reaction)
       Folin and Wu's (method)
F wave
FWHM – full width half-maximum
FWR – Felix-Weil reaction
FZ – focal zone

G

G — an immunoglobulin
    giga
    gingival
    glucose
    gonidial (colony)
    gravida
    gravitational constant
    Greek
g — force (the pull of gravity)
    gram
GA — gastric analysis
    general anesthesia
    gestational age
    gingivoaxial
    glucuronic acid
    gut-associated
Ga — gallium
GABA — gamma-aminobutyric acid
GAD — glutamic acid decarboxylase
gadfly
gadolinium
Gaffkya
    G. tetragena
gag
    g. reflex
gain
    antigen g.
Gaisböck's disease
gait
    athetotic g.
    choreic g.
    g. disturbance
    dystonic g.
    festinating g.
    reeling g.
    shuffling g.

gait *(continued)*
    spastic g.
    staggering g.
    steppage g.
    g. unsteadiness
    waddling g.
gal — gallon
galactan
galactic
galactin
galactitol
galactocele
galactocerebroside
    g. galactosidase
galactography
galactokinase
galactolipid
galactolipin
galactonolactone dehydrogenase
galactorrhea
galactosamine
galactose
    g. assay
    g. dehydrogenase
    g.-1-phosphate uridylyltransferase
    g. tolerance test
galactosemia
alpha-galactosidase
beta-galactosidase
galactoside
galactosuria
galactosylceramidase
galactosylceramide
    g. galactosyl-hydrolase
galactowaldenase
galacturia

gale
galea
    g. aponeurotica
galenic
Galen's
    great cerebral vein
    ventricle
Galerina
    G. autumnalis
    G. marginata
    G. venerata
gall
gallamine triethiodide
gallbladder
Gall body
gallium
    g. citrate
    g. scan
gallocyanin
Gallogen
gallop
    filling g.
    presystolic g.
    protodiastolic g.
    rhythm g.
gallstone
gal-1-P — galactose-1-phosphate
GALT — gut-associated lymphoid tissue
GaLV — gibbon ape lymphosarcoma virus
Galv — galvanic
galvanic
    g. cell
galvanism
galvanization
galvanochemical
galvanometer
Gambian trypanosomiasis
gamboge
gamete
gametocide
gametocyte
gametocytemia
gametogenesis
gamma
    g. amino butyric acid
    g. benzene hexachloride
    g. camera
    g. globulin
    g.-glutamyl-cysteine synthetase
    g. glutamyl transferase
    g. heavy chain disease
    g.-lactone
    g.-pipradol
    g. radiation
    g. ray
    g.-ray spectrum
    g. spectrometer
    g. spectrometry
    g. streptococcus
    g.-well counter
gammaglobulinopathy
gammagram
gammagraphic
gammopathy
    monoclonal g.
    polyclonal g.
Gamna-Gandy nodules
ganglioglioma
ganglion (ganglia)
    accessory g.
    aorticorenal g.
    autonomic g.
    basal g.
    g. blocker
    cardiac g.
    celiac g.
    cell g.
    cell layer g.
    ciliary g.
    Corti's g.
    g. cyst

ganglion (ganglia) *(continued)*
    dorsal root g.
    gasserian g.
    geniculate g.
    inferior cervical g.
    inferior, glossopharyngeal nerve g.
    inferior mesenteric g.
    inferior ninth cranial nerve g.
    inferior vagus nerve g.
    jugular glossopharyngeal nerve g.
    jugular tenth cranial nerve g.
    jugular vagus nerve g.
    mesenteric g., superior
    middle cervical g.
    nodose tenth cranial nerve g.
    nodose vagus nerve g.
    otic g.
    petrous glossopharyngeal nerve g.
    pterygopalatine g.
    Scarpa's g.
    semilunar g.
    sphenopalatine g.
    spinal g.
    spiral g.
    stellate g.
    submaxillary g.
    superior cervical g.
    superior glossopharyngeal nerve g.
    superior ninth cranial nerve g.
    superior vagus nerve g.
    g. of sympathetic trunk
    thoracic sympathetic g.
    trigeminal g.
    trigeminal motor root g.

ganglion (ganglia) *(continued)*
    trigeminal sensory root g.
    vestibular g.
ganglioneuroblastoma
ganglioneuroma
ganglionic
ganglioside
    g. GM_1
    g. GM_2
gangliosidosis (gangliosidoses)
    generalized g.
    GM_1 g.
    GM_2 g.
gangosa
gangrene
    dry g.
    gas g.
    progressive bacterial synergistic g.
    static g.
    trophic g.
    venous g.
gangrenous
    g. appendicitis
    g. inflammation
    g. necrosis
Ganser's syndrome
gap
    auscultatory g.
    chromatid g.
    isochromatid g.
    g. junction
GAPD or GAPDH — glyceraldehyde phosphate dehydrogenase
Gardner's syndrome
gargoylism
Garré's sclerosing osteomyelitis
Gärtner's
    bacillus
    duct
    duct cyst

gas
- g. amplification
- g. chromatograph
- g. chromatography
- g. constant
- g. embolism
- extravasation g.
- g. gangrene
- g. law
- g.-liquid chromatography
- g. retention
- g.-solid chromatography
- g. sterilizer
- g. storage limits

gaseous
gasometry
gasping
gaster
Gasteromycetes
Gasterophilus
gastric
- g. argentaffin cell
- g. artery
- g. atrophy
- g. branch, vagus nerve
- g. cardia
- g. cardiac gland
- g. corpus
- g. foveolae
- g. function tests
- g. fundal gland
- g. fundus
- g. inhibitory polypeptide
- g. lavage
- g. lumen
- g. lymph node
- g. mucosa
- g. mucous membrane
- g. muscularis
- g. myiasis
- g. parietal cell
- g. parietography

gastric *(continued)*
- g. pyloric gland
- g. residue examination
- g. rugae
- g. serosa
- g. submucosa
- g. subserosa
- g. ulcer, perforated
- g. vein
- g. vomitus
- g. zymogenic cell

gastrin
- g. assay
- g.-calcium infusion stimulation test
- g.-protein meal stimulation test
- g.-secretin stimulation test

gastrinoma
gastritis
- acute g.
- antral g.
- atrophic g.
- chronic atrophic g.
- chronic hypertrophic g.
- erosive g.
- giant hypertrophic g.
- hemorrhagic g.
- hypertrophic g.
- phlegmonous g.

gastrocele
gastrocnemius muscle
gastrocolic
gastrodisciasis
Gastrodiscoides
- *G. hominis*

Gastrodiscus
- *G. hominis*

gastroduodenal
gastroduodenoscopy
gastroenteric
gastroenteritis

gastroenterologist
gastroenterology
gastroenteropancreatic endo-
　crine system
gastroenteropathy
gastroenteroptosis
gastroenterostomy
gastroepiploic
gastroesophageal
gastrofiberscope
gastrogavage
gastrograph
gastrohepatic
gastrointestinal
　g. blood loss test
　g. contents
　g. fistula
　g. fluids
　g. motility study
　g. protein loss test
　g. series
　g. spaces
　g. tract
gastrojejunal
　g. fistula
gastromalacia
gastroparesis
gastrophrenic
gastrophthisis
gastroscope
　fiberoptic g.
gastroscopic
gastroscopy
gastrosia
　g. fungosa
gastrula
gastrulation
gating
Gaucher's
　cell
　disease
　type of histiocyte

gauge
gauss
gaussian
　g. curve
　g. distribution
gavage
Gay-Lussac's law
GB — gallbladder
　　　Guillain-Barré syndrome
GBA — ganglionic-blocking
　　　　agent
　　　gingivobuccoaxial
G-banding
GBH — graphite–benzalkoni-
　　　　um-heparin
GBIA — Guthrie bacterial in-
　　　　hibition assay
GBM — glomerular basement
　　　　membrane
GC — ganglion cells
　　　gas chromatography
　　　glucocorticoid
　　　gonococcus
　　　gonorrhea
　　　granular casts
　　　guanine cytosine
g-cal — gram-calorie
g-cm — gram-centimeter
GC-MS — gas chromatography–
　　　　　mass spectrometry
Gd — gadolinium
GDA — germine diacetate
GDH — glutamic acid dehydro-
　　　　genase
　　　glycerophosphate de-
　　　　hydrogenase
GDP — guanosine diphosphate
GE — gastroenterostomy
G/E — granulocyte-erythroid
　　　　ratio
Ge — germanium
Gee-Herter-Heubner disease

Gee-Thaysen disease
Geiger counter
Geiger-Müller counter
gel
    g.-filtration chromatography
    g.-permeation chromatography
gelatin
    g. slide adhesive
gelatinous
    g. acute inflammation
    g. acute pneumonia
    g. adenocarcinoma
    g. atrophy
    g. carcinoma
    g. inflammation
Gelman filter
gelsemine
gemellus muscle
geminal
geminate
gemistocyte
gemistocytic
    g. astrocytoma
    g. tumor
gemma
gemmation
gemmule
Gendre's fluid
gene
    allelic g's
    g. cloning
    complementary g's
    derepressed g.
    dominant g.
    g. dosage
    g. flow
    g. frequency
    H g.
    histocompatibility g.
    holandric g's

gene *(continued)*
    hologynic g's
    immune response g's
    Ir g's
    Is g's
    g. library
    major g.
    g. mapping
    modifying g's
    mutant g.
    nonstructural g's
    operator g.
    g. pool
    recessive g.
    regulator g.
    repressor g.
    sex-linked g.
    g. splicing
    structural g.
    supplementary g's
    X-linked g.
general
    g. radiation
generalization
generation
    spontaneous g.
    g. time
generative
generator
generic
    g. name
genesis
genesistasis
genestatic
genetic
    g. code
    g. counseling
    g. drift
    g. engineering
    g. map
    g. mapping
    g. marker

genetic *(continued)*
    g. regulation
    g. screening
genetics
    bacterial g.
    bacteriophage g.
    behavior g.
    biochemical g.
    clinical g.
    developmental g.
    immunogenetic g.
    mathematical g.
    medical g.
    mendelian g.
    molecular g.
    population g.
    somatic cell g.
genicular
geniculate
    g. bodies
    g. ganglion
geniculocalcarine tract
geniculotemporal tract
geniculum (genicula)
genin
genioglossus muscle
geniohyoid
genital
    g. disorder
    g. fluids
    g. spaces
    g. tubercle
genitalia
genitocrural
genitofemoral
    g. nerve
genitography
genitourinary
    g. myiasis
    g. tract
Gennari's line
genoblast

genocopy
genome
genotype
genotypic
gentamicin
    g. sulfate
gentian
    g. violet
gentiobiase
gentisate oxygenase
genu (genua)
    g. corpus callosum
    g. internal capsule
    g. recurvatum
    g. valgum
    g. varum
genus (genera)
Geodermatophilus
geographic
    g. pathology
    g. tongue
geometric
    g. efficiency
    g. isomerism
    g. mean
geophagia
geophilic
geotrichosis
Geotrichum
    G. candidum
    G. immite
geotropism
GEP — gastroenteropancreatic
            endocrine system
geranyl
    g. diphosphate
Gerhardt's
    dullness
    test
geriatric
geriatrician
geriatrics

germ
   g. cell
   g. cell tumor
   g. layers
   g. tube
germanium
German measles virus
germicide
germinal
   g. center
   g. epithelial inclusion cyst
   g. epithelium
   g. inclusion cyst
   g. vesicle
germinoblast
germinoma
   pineal g.
geroderma
   g. osteodysplastica
gerontologist
gerontology
gerüstmark
gestagen
gestation
gestational
   g. alteration
   g. trophoblastic disease
gestosis
GET — gastric emptying time
GET½ — gastric emptying half-time
GeV — giga electron volt
GF — gastric fluid
   germ-free
   gluten-free
G factor
GFR — glomerular filtration rate
GG — gamma globulin
GG or S — glands, goiter or stiffness (the neck)
GGA — general gonadotropic activity
GGG — gummi guttae gambiae (gamboge)
GGT — gamma-glutamyl transferase
   glutamyltransferase
GGTP — gamma-glutamyl transpeptidase
GH — growth hormone
GHD — growth hormone deficiency
Ghon's
   complex
   tubercle
Ghon-Sachs bacillus
ghost
   blood g.
   g. cell
GH-RF — growth hormone–releasing factor
GH-RH — growth hormone–releasing hormone
GH-RIH — growth hormone release-inhibiting hormone
GHz — gigahertz
GI — gastrointestinal
   globin insulin
giant
   g. blue nevus
   g. fibroadenoma
   g. follicle lymphoma
   g. hairy nevus
   g. intestinal fluke
   g. intracanalicular fibroadenoma
   g. liver fluke
   g. neutrophilia
   g. osteoid osteoma
   g. platelets
   g. rugal hypertrophy

giant *(continued)*
   g. urticaria
giant cell
   g. c. arteritis
   g. c. carcinoma
   foreign body g. c's
   g. c. granuloma
   g. c. hepatitis
   Langhans' g. c's
   multinucleated g. c's
   g. c. myocarditis
   g. c. pneumonia
   g. c. sarcoma
   g. c. thyroiditis
   Touton g. c's
   g. c. tumor
   Warthin-Finkeldey g. c's
giantism
Giardia
   G. intestinalis
   G. lamblia
giardiasis
Gibberella fujikuroi
gibbon ape lymphosarcoma virus
Giemsa stain
Gierke's disease
giga
   g. electron volt
gigahertz
gigantism
gigantomastia
GIGO – garbage in, garbage out
gigohm
GIK – glucose, insulin and potassium
Gilbert's syndrome
Gilchrist's disease
gill-arch skeleton
Gilles de la Tourette's syndrome

GIM – gonadotropin-inhibitory material
Gimenez stain
gingiva
gingival
   g. epithelial attachment
   g. hyperplasia
   g. lamina propria
   g. mucous membrane
gingivitis
   diphenylhydantoin g.
   hypertrophic g.
   scorbutic g.
gingivosis
gingivostomatitis
   herpetic g.
   necrotizing ulcerative g.
GIP – gastric inhibitory polypeptide
girdle
GIS – gastrointestinal system
GI series – gastrointestinal series
GIT – gastrointestinal tract
gitalin
gitaloxin
gitoxin
GITT – glucose-insulin tolerance test
gitter cell
GK – glycerol kinase
GL – greatest length
Gl – glucinium
gl – gill
   gland
GL 54 – athomin
GLA – gingivolinguoaxial
glabella
glabelloalveolar line
glabellomeatal line
glabrous

glacial
    g. acetic acid
gland
    adrenal g.
    apocrine g.
    Bartholin's g.
    Bowman's g's
    Brunner's g's
    buccal g's
    bulbourethral g.
    ceruminous g's
    cervical g's
    Cowper's g.
    Ebner's g.
    endocrine g's
    esophageal g's
    gastric g's
    interscapular g.
    jugular g.
    lacrimal g.
    lingual g's
    lymph g's
    mammary g.
    mesenteric g's
    Moll's g.
    mucous g's
    parathyroid g.
    pituitary g.
    salivary g.
    Skene's g.
    sublingual g.
    suprarenal g.
    thyroid g.
    vaginal g.
glanders
glandular
    g. epithelium
    g. metaplasia
glans (glandes)
    g. clitoridis
    g. penis

Glanzmann-Naegeli thrombasthenia
Glanzmann's thrombasthenia
glass
    g.-bead retention method
    borosilicate g.
    cover g.
    g. fiber filter
    heat-resistant g.
    low-actinic g.
    optical g.
glassy
    g. cell carcinoma
    g. membrane
glaucarubin
glaucoma
    angle closure g.
    congenital g.
    infantile g.
    open angle g.
    primary g.
    secondary g.
GLC — gas-liquid chromatography
glenoid cavity
Glenospora
    G. graphii
Glenosporella
    G. loboi
glia
    ameboid g.
    fibrillary g.
    plasmic g.
gliadin
glial
glioblast
glioblastoma
    g. multiforme
Gliocladium
glioma
    malignant g.

glioma *(continued)*
    mixed g.
    nasal g.
    subependymal g.
gliomatosis
gliosarcoma
gliosis
gliosome
gliotoxin
Glisson's capsule
Gln — glutamine
glob — globulin
globin
globoid
    g. leukodystrophy
globose
globoside
globular
    g. protein
globule
globulin
    A-1 g's
    A-2 g's
    alpha g's
    antidiphtheritic g.
    antihemophilic g.
    antilymphocytic g.
    beta g's
    gamma g's
    immune serum g.
    rabies immune g.
    thyroxine-binding g.
    g. X
    zoster immune g.
globulinuria
globulomaxillary
    g. cyst
globus (globi)
    g. hystericus
    g. pallidus
glomangioma
glomera aortica

glomerular
    g. basal lamina
    g. capillary basement membrane
    g. capillary endothelium
    g. crescents
    g. filtration
    g. filtration rate
    g. mesangium
    g. urinary pole
    g. vascular pole
glomerulitis
glomerulonephritis
    acute g.
    acute exudative g.
    acute hemorrhagic g.
    antibasement membrane g.
    chronic g.
    diffuse g.
    embolic g.
    exudative g.
    focal g.
    healed g.
    hemorrhagic g.
    induced g.
    lobular g.
    membranous g.
    membranous-proliferative g.
    mesangial proliferative g.
    necrotizing g.
    postinfectious g.
    proliferative g.
    rapidly progressive g.
    subacute g.
glomerulopathy
glomerulosclerosis
    cirrhotic g.
    diabetic g.
    intercapillary g.
    nodular g.
glomerulus (glomeruli)

glomus (glomera)
    g. caroticum
    g. coccygeum
    g. intravagale
    g. jugulare
    g. tumor
glossal
Glossina
glossitis
    Hunter's g.
    median rhomboid g.
glossopalatine arch
glossopharyngeal
    g. nerve
    g. neuralgia
    g. nucleus
glottal
glottis (glottides)
glow modular tube
Glu — glutamic acid
    glutamine
glu or gluc — glucose
glucagon
glucagonoma
glucan
    g. branching enzyme
    g.-branching glycosyltransferase
alpha-glucan
glucaric acid
glucatonia
glucide
glucitol
glucoamylase
glucocerebrosidase
glucocerebroside
glucocorticoid
glucocorticosteroid
glucofuranose
glucogenesis
glucogenic
glucokinase

gluconate
    g. dehydrogenase
    ferrous g.
gluconeogenesis
gluconeogenetic
gluconolactonase
glucoproteinase
glucopyranose
glucosamine
    acetyl g.
glucosan transglucosylase
glucosazone
glucose
    g. assays
    g. dehydrogenase
    g. metabolism
    g. monophosphate synthetase
    g. oxidase
    g.-1-phosphatase
    g.-6-phosphatase
    g.-1-phosphate
    g.-6-phosphate
    g.-6-phosphate dehydrogenase
    g.-6-phosphate dehydrogenase test
    g. phosphomutase
    renal threshold for g.
    g. tolerance test
    g. transport system
    UDP-g.
    UDP-g.-glycogen glucosyltransferase
glucosephosphate isomerase
    g. i. assays
    g. i. deficiency
glucose-1-phosphate phosphodismutase
glucose-1-phosphate uridylyltransferase
alpha-glucosidase

alpha-1,3-glucosidase
beta-glucosidase
glucoside
glucosulfone sodium
glucosuria
glucosyl
glucosylceramidase
   g. assays
glucosyltransferase
glucurolactone
glucuronate reductase
glucuronic acid
glucuronidase
beta-glucuronidase
glucuronide
glucuronolactone reductase
glucuronyl-transferase
glutamate
   g. decarboxylase
   g. dehydrogenase
   g. formiminotransferase
   g.-pyruvate transaminase
   g. semialdehyde
glutamic acid
   g. a. decarboxylase
glutamic-oxaloacetic transaminase
glutamic-pyruvic transaminase
glutaminase
glutamine
   g.-fructose-6-phosphate aminotransferase
   g.-ketoacid aminotransferase
   g. phenylacetyltransferase
   g. synthetase
glutaminyl
   g.-peptide-glutamyltransferase
glutamyl
   gamma-g. cysteine synthetase

glutamyl *(continued)*
   gamma-g. transferase
   g. transfer cycle
   g. transpeptidase
glutaraldehyde
glutaric acid
glutaryl-coenzyme A synthetase
glutathione
   g.-homocystine transhydrogenase
   oxidized g.
   g. peroxidase
   g. reductase
   g. stability test
   g. synthetase
   g. thiolesterase
glutathionemia
glutathionuria
gluteal
   g. artery
   g. nerve
   g. region
   g. sulcus
   g. vein
gluten
   g.-sensitive enteropathy
glutenin
glutethimide
   g. assays
gluteus maximus muscle
gluteus medius muscle
gluteus minimus muscle
gluteus muscle
glutin
glutinous
Gly — glycine
glycan
glyceraldehyde
   g. phosphate
   g.-phosphate dehydrogenase

glycerate
- g. dehydrogenase
- g. kinase
- g. phosphomutase

glyceric acid
glyceride
glycerin
glycerite
glycerol
- g. dehydrogenase
- g. gelatin medium
- g. kinase

glycerolization
glycerolize
glycerophosphatase
glycerophosphate
glycerophosphatide
glycerophosphorylcholine diesterase
glyceryl
- g. ether lipids
- g. guaiacolate
- g. monostearate
- g. triacetate
- g. trinitrate

glycine
- g. acyltransferase
- g. amidinotransferase
- g. formiminotransferase

glycinemia
glycinuria
Glyciphagus
- *G. buski*
- *G. domesticus*

glycobiarsol
glycocalyx
glycochenodeoxycholate
glycochenodeoxycholic acid
glycocholate
glycocholic acid
glycodeoxycholic acid

glycogen
- g. branching enzyme
- g. digestion
- hepatic g.
- g. phosphorylase
- g. staining
- g. storage disease
- g. (starch) synthase
- g. synthesis
- tissue g.

glycogenase
glycogenesis
glycogenic
glycogenolysis
glycogenolytic
glycogenosis (glycogenoses)
- hepatophosphorylase deficiency g.
- hepato-renal, glucose-6-phosphatase deficiency g.
- idiopathic generalized g.
- myophosphorylase deficiency g.

glycol
- g. methacrylate

glycolaldehydetransferase
glycolic acid
glycolipid
- g. staining

glycolithocholic acid
glycollate oxidase
glycolysis
glycolytic
glycone
glyconeogenesis
glycopeptide
glycophorin
glycoprotein
- g. hormone
- g. staining

glycopyrrolate

glycopyrronium bromide
glycosaminoglycan
glycosaminolipid
glycosidase
glycoside
    cardiac g.
    cyanophoric g.
    g. hydrolase
    sterol g.
glycosphingolipid
glycosulfatase
glycosuria
    pathologic g.
    renal g.
    toxic g.
glycosuric
    g. melituria
glycosyl
    g. ceramide
glycosylated
    g. hemoglobin
glycosyltransferase
    α-glucan-branching g.
glycyl-glycine dipeptidase
glycyl-leucine dipeptidase
Glycyphagus
    G. domesticus
glyodin
glyoxalase
glyoxylate reductase
GM — gastric mucosa
    geometric mean
    grand multiparity
Gm — gamma
Gm (gamma)
    Gm allotype
    Gm marker
gm — gram
g-m — gram-meter
GMA — glyceryl methacrylate
GMP — guanosine monophosphate

GMP *(continued)*
    guanosine phosphate
GMT — geometric mean titer
GMW — gram-molecular weight
GN — glomerulonephritis
    glucose nitrogen (ratio)
    gram-negative
Gnathostoma
    G. hispidum
    G. spinigerum
gnathostomiasis
GNID — gram-negative intracellular diplococci
gnotobiota
gnotobiote
gnotobiotic
gnotobiotics
gnotophoresis
GnRH — gonadotropin-releasing hormone
goblet cell
GOE — gas, oxygen and ether
goiter
    adenomatous g.
    colloid g.
    congenital g.
    diffuse g.
    dyshormonogenic g.
    endemic g.
    exophthalmic g.
    hyperplastic g.
    lymphadenoid g.
    multinodular g.
    nodular g.
    parenchymatous g.
    simple g.
    sporadic diffuse g.
    sporadic nodular g.
    substernal g.
    toxic g.
gold
    g. assays

gold *(continued)*
    g. chloride
    g. chloride reagent
    g. sodium thiomalate
    g. thioglucose
    g. toning
Goldblatt's
    hypertension
    kidney
Goldflam's disease
Golgi-Mazzoni corpuscle
Golgi's
    alteration
    cavity alteration
    complex
    corpuscle
    cycle
    membrane alteration
    neuron
    organ
    vacuole alteration
    vesicle alteration
Goll's tract
Gomori's
    method for chromaffin
    trichrome stain
gonad
gonadal
    g. dysgenesis
    g. endocrine disorder
    g. stromal tumor
gonadoblastoma
gonadotrope
gonadotropic
gonadotropin
    chorionic g.
    human chorionic g.
    g.-releasing hormone
Gongylonema
    G. pulchrum
gongylonemiasis
gonion (gonia)
gonococcal arthritis-dermatitis syndrome
gonococcus (gonococci)
gonorrhea
gonorrheal
Goodell's sign
Goodpasture's
    stain
    syndrome
Good's syndrome
Gordius
    G. aquaticus
    G. robustus
Gordon's
    agent
    body
    test
Gorham's disease
GOT — glutamic-oxaloacetic transaminase
gout
gouty
Gowers' tract
GP — general paresis
    glycoprotein
    gutta-percha
G6P — glucose-6-phosphate
GPAIS — guinea pig anti-insulin serum
GPC — gastric parietal cell
GPD or GPDH — glucose phosphate dehydrogenase
G6PD or G6PDH — glucose-6-phosphate dehydrogenase
G6PDA — glucose-6-phosphate dehydrogenase enzyme variant A
GPI — glucosephosphate isomerase
GPIMH — guinea pig intestinal mucosal homogenate

GPIPID — guinea pig intraperitoneal infectious dose
GPK — guinea pig kidney (antigen)
GPKA — guinea pig kidney absorption (test)
GPS — guinea pig serum
GPT — glutamic-pyruvic transaminase
GPUT — galactose phosphate uridyl transferase
GR — gastric resection
    glutathione reductase
gr — grain
GRA — gonadotropin-releasing agent
graafian follicle
gracilis muscle
gradient
graduated
    g. cylinder
graft
    allogenic g.
    autologous g.
    heterologous g.
    isogenic g.
    material g.
    g. rejection
    g.-versus-host reaction
Graham-Cole test
Graham's law
grain
    g. count halving time
    g. itch
    g. itch mite
graininess
gram
    g. negative
    g. positive
gramicidin

gram-negative
    bacilli
    bacteria
    cocci
gram-positive
    bacilli
    bacteria
    cocci
Gram's stain
Gram-Weigert stain
grand mal
Granger method
granular
    g. atrophy
    g. cell myoblastoma
    g. cell tumor
    g. degeneration
    g. endoplasmic reticulum
    g. layer
    g. leukocyte
    g. pneumocyte
    g. urethritis
granulation
    arachnoid g.
    pacchionian g.
    g. tissue
granule
    Babès-Ernst g's
    g's of developing neutrophils
    Langerhans' g's
    sand g's
granuloblastosis
granulocyte
    band-form g.
    g. concentrate
    segmented g.
granulocytic
    g. aplasia
    g. cells
    g. hyperplasia

granulocytic *(continued)*
    g. hypoplasia
    g. leukemia
    g. series
granulocytopenia
granulocytopoiesis
granulocytopoietic
granulocytosis
granulogenesis
granuloma
    g. annulare
    apical g.
    beryllium g.
    calcified g.
    caseating g.
    dental g.
    eosinophilic g.
    g. faciale
    foreign body g.
    giant cell reparative g.
    histiocytic g.
    Hodgkin's g.
    g. inguinale
    lethal midline g.
    lipoid g.
    Majocchi's g.
    mineral oil g.
    multifocal eosinophilic g.
    non-necrotizing g.
    plasma cell g.
    pyogenic g.
    reticulohistiocytic g.
    sarcoid g.
    spermatogenic g.
    suture g.
    swimming pool g.
    tuberculoid g.
    unifocal eosinophilic g.
granulomatosis
    allergic g.
    angiitic g.

granulomatosis *(continued)*
    Wegener's g.
granulomatous
    g. colitis
    g. inflammation
    g. polyp
    g. thyroiditis
granulopenia
granulophthisis
granulopoiesis
granulopoietic
granulopoietin
granulosa cell
    g. c. carcinoma
    g. c. theca cell tumor
    g. c. tumor
graph
    Davenport g.
    g. tablet
graphic
    g. analysis
    g. terminal
Graphium
grating
    replica g.
grav I — pregnancy one
    primigravida
Graves' disease
gravid
gravida
gravimetric
Gravindex test
gravitation
gravity
    specific g.
Gravlee jet wash
Grawitz's tumor
gray
    g. commissures
    g.-patch ringworm
    g. platelet syndrome

gray *(continued)*
- g. ramus
- g. scale

gray matter
- cerebral g. m.
- cervical spinal cord g. m.
- frontal lobe g. m.
- insula g. m.
- lumbosacral spinal cord g. m.
- occipital lobe g. m.
- paramammillary g. m.
- parietal lobe g. m.
- periventricular g. m.
- spinal cord g. m.
- temporal lobe g. m.
- thoracic spinal cord g. m.

greater
- g. alar cartilage
- g. auricular nerve
- g. occipital nerve
- g. omentum
- g. splanchnic nerve
- g. superficial petrosal nerve

greenstick
- g. compound fracture
- g. fracture

grenz rays

GRF — gonadotropin-releasing factor
- growth hormone–releasing factor

GRH — growth hormone–releasing hormone

grid
- aligned g.
- Bucky g.
- crossed g.
- focused g.
- g. index
- g. lines
- parallel g.

grid *(continued)*
- Potter-Bucky g.
- g. ratio

Gridley stain

Grimelius argyrophil method

grip
- devil's g.

grippe

griseofulvin

Grocott-Gomori methenamine-silver method

groin

gross

ground
- g. glass
- g.-glass hepatocyte
- g. state
- g. substance

groundnut oil

group
- azo g.
- blood g.
- coli-aerogenes g.
- peptide g.
- proteus g.
- salmonella g.

grouping
- antigenic structural g.
- blood g.
- haptenic g.

growth
- g. acceleration
- g. alteration
- g. arrest
- g. disorder
- g. fraction
- g. hormone
- g. hormone release–inhibiting hormone
- g. hormone–releasing factor
- g. retardation

Gruber-Widal reaction

G/S — glucose and saline
GSA — Gross virus antigen
    guanidinosuccinic acid
GSC — gas-solid chromatography
    gravity-settling culture
GSD — genetically significant dose
    glycogen storage disease
GSE — gluten-sensitive enteropathy
GSH — reduced glutathione
GSR — galvanic skin response
    generalized Shwartzman reaction
GSSG — oxidized glutathione
GSSR — generalized Sanarelli-Shwartzman reaction
GT — generation time
    glucose tolerance
    glutamyl transpeptidase
GTD — gestational trophoblastic disease
GTH — gonadotropic hormone
GTN — glyceryl trinitrate
GTP — glutamyl transpeptidase
    guanosine triphosphate
GTT — glucose tolerance test
GU — gastric ulcer
    genitourinary
    gonococcal urethritis
guaiac
guaiacol
Guama virus
guanase
guanethidine
    g. monosulfate
    g. sulfate
guanidinemia
guanidinoacetate
    g. kinase

guanidinoacetate *(continued)*
    g. methyl-transferase
guanidino-aminovaleric acid
guanine
    g. deaminase
    g. nucleotide
guanosine
    g. cyclic phosphate
    g. diphosphate
    g. monophosphate
    g. phosphate
    g. triphosphate
guanylate cyclase
guanylic acid
guanylyl
guarding
Guarnieri's bodies
Guaroa virus
gubernaculum
    chorda g.
    g. testis
Guillain-Barré syndrome
guinea pig
    g. p. intestinal mucosal homogenate
    g. p. intraperitoneal infectious dose
    g. p. kidney (antigen)
    g. p. kidney absorption (test)
    g. p. serum
Gull's disease
L-gulonate dehydrogenase
gum
    g. arabic
    g. karaya
gumma (gummas, gummata)
gummatous
GUS — genitourinary system
gustin
gut-associated lymphoid tissue
Guthion

Guthrie's
　　bacterial inhibition assay
　　　test
Gutman unit
GV – gentian violet
GVH – graft versus host
GVHR – graft-versus-host
　　　reaction
GXT – graded exercise test
Gy – gray
Gymnoascus
gymnobacterium
GYN – gynecology
gynandroblastoma
gynandromorphism
gynecogen
gynecoid
gynecologic
gynecologist
gynecology
gynecomastia
gynogenesis
gyrate
gyrus (gyri)
　　angular g.
　　g. breves insulae
　　callosal g.
　　callosomarginal g.
　　cingulate g.
　　dentate g.
　　fasciolar g.

gyrus (gyri) *(continued)*
　　g. fornicatus
　　fusiform g.
　　hippocampal g.
　　inferior frontal g.
　　inferior occipital g.
　　inferior temporal g.
　　intralimbic g.
　　lateral occipital g.
　　lateral olfactory g.
　　lingual g.
　　g. longus
　　marginal g.
　　medial olfactory g.
　　middle frontal g.
　　middle temporal g.
　　occipitotemporal g.
　　orbital g.
　　postcentral g.
　　posterior parietal g.
　　precentral g.
　　g. rectus
　　subcallosal g.
　　superior frontal g.
　　superior occipital g.
　　superior temporal g.
　　supracallosal g.
　　supramarginal g.
GZ – Guilford-Zimmerman
　　　personality test

H

H – henry
　　Holzknecht unit
　　horizontal
　　hormone
　　Hounsfield unit
　　hydrogen
　　hypermetropia

H – Hauch (motile micro-
　　　organism)
H. – *Hemophilus*
^1H – protium
^2H – deuterium
^3H – tritium
H^+ – hydrogen ion

H-2^b mouse cells
h — hour(s)
    Planck's constant
HA — headache
    height age
    hemadsorbent
    hemagglutinating antibody
    hemagglutination
    hemolytic anemia
    hydroxyapatite
Ha — hahnium
HAA — hepatitis-associated antigen
HABA — hydroxybenzeneazobenzoic acid
habenula (habenulae)
habenular commissure
habenulopeduncular tract
    nucleus
habitual
habituation
habitus
    asthenic h.
    hypersthenic h.
    hyposthenic h.
    sthenic h.
HAD — hemadsorption
Haemagogus
Haemaphysalis
    H. concinna
    H. leporispalustris
    H. spinigera
Haemonchus
    H. contortus
    H. placei
Haemophilus. See *Hemophilus.*
Haemosporidia
Hafnia
    H. alvei
hafnium
Hageman factor

H agglutination
H agglutinin
HAHTG — horse antihuman thymus globulin
HAI — hemagglutination inhibition
    hemagglutinin inhibition
Hailey-Hailey disease
hair
    beaded h.
    h. follicle
    ingrown h.
    lanugo h.
    telogen h.
hairball
hal — halothane
halazone
Haldane effect
half-life
    biologic h. l.
    physical h. l.
half-value layer
halide
Hallervorden-Spatz disease
Hall's method
hallucination
hallucinatory
hallucinogen
hallux (halluces)
    h. valgus
    h. varus
halogen
halogenated
halogenation
haloperidol
halophile
haloprogin
halothane
hamartia
hamartoma
hamate

hamartoma

hamatum
Hamman-Rich syndrome
Hamman's disease
hammer toe
hamster
Ham test
hamstring
hamular
hamulus (hamuli)
H and D curve
H and E — hematoxylin and eosin
H and E staining
Hand-Schüller-Christian
   disease
   type of histiocyte
H and V — hemigastrectomy and vagotomy
Hanes equation
Hanger's test
hangnail
Hanker-Yates reagent
Hansen's
   bacillus
   disease
Hansenula
H antigen
HAP — heredopathia atactica polyneuritiformis
      histamine phosphate acid
HAPA — hemagglutinating anti-penicillin antibody
hapalonychia
haploid
haploidy
haplophase
haplosomic
haplotype
hapten
   group A h.

haptoglobin, Hp^1 and Hp^2
haptophore
Harada's syndrome
Hardy-Weinberg law
harelip
Hargraves' cell
Harris' alum hematoxylin
Harrison's test
Hartmanella
   H. hyalina
Hartnup disease
HASHD — hypertensive arteriosclerotic heart disease
Hashimoto's
   disease
   struma
   thyroiditis
Hassall's corpuscle
haustrum (haustra)
HAV — hepatitis A virus
Haverhill fever
Haverhillia
   H. moniliformis
   H. multiformis
haversian
   h. canal
   h. glands
   h. lamella
   h. system
Haworth formula
hay fever
Haygarth's nodes
HB — heart block
      hepatitis B
Hb — hemoglobin
HBABA — hydroxybenzeneazobenzoic acid
HB_cAg — hepatitis B core antigen
HB_sAg — hepatitis B surface antigen

H band
HBB — hydroxybenzyl benzimidazole
Hb Barts — Bart's hemoglobin
Hb CO — carboxyhemoglobin
HBD or HBDH — hydroxybutyrate dehydrogenase
HBF — hepatic blood flow
HbF — fetal hemoglobin
HBI — high serum-bound iron
HBO — hyperbaric oxygen
HBP — high blood pressure
HBr — hydrobromic acid
HBV — hepatitis B virus
HBW — high birth weight
HC — hair cell
    head compression
    hepatic catalase
    Huntington's chorea
    hyaline casts
    hydroxycorticoid
HCC — hydroxycholecalciferol
hCG — human chorionic gonadotropin
HCH — hexachlorocyclohexane
HCHO — formaldehyde
HCl — hydrochloric acid
HCN — hydrocyanic acid
HCO$_3$ — bicarbonate
H colony
HCP — hepatocatalase peroxidase
    hereditary coproporphyria
hCS or hCSM — human chorionic somatomammotropin
HCT — hematocrit
    homocytotrophic
    hydrochlorothiazide
HCU — homocystinuria
HCVD — hypertensive cardiovascular disease
HD — heart disease
    high dosage
    Hodgkin's disease
    hydatid disease
HDBH. *See* HBDH.
HDC — histidine decarboxylase
HDH — heart disease history
HDL or HDLP — high-density lipoprotein
HDN — hemolytic disease of the newborn
HDP — hydroxydimethylpyrimidine
HDS — herniated disk syndrome
HE — hereditary elliptocytosis
    human enteric
He — helium
head
    angular h.
    articular h.
    coronoid h.
    humeral h.
    infraorbital h.
    lateral h.
    mandibular h.
    medial h.
    oblique h.
    plantar h.
    quadrate h.
    radial h.
    scapular h.
    transverse h.
    ulnar h.
    zygomatic h.
headache
heart
    abdominal h.
    h. block
    cervical h.
    h. disease
    extracorporeal h.

heart *(continued)*
   h. failure
   hypoplastic h.
   intracorporeal h.
   h.-lung machine
   h. sound
   trilocular h.
heartburn
heartworm
HEAT — human erythrocyte agglutination test
heat
   h. capacity
   h. of combustion
   h. exhaustion
   h. of formation
   h. of fusion
   h. intolerance
   latent h.
   molar h. capacity
   h. precipitation test
   h. prostration
   h. of reaction
   h. of solution
   specific h.
   h. stroke
   h. unit
   h. of vaporization
heavy
   h. chain disease
   h. metals
   h. particle therapy
hebephrenic schizophrenia
Heberden's node
HEC — hydroxyergocalciferol
hectogram
hectometer
HED — unit of roentgen-ray dosage (*Haut-Einheits-Dosis*)
Heerfordt's disease
Hegar's sign

Heidenhain's
   azan stain
   iron hematoxylin stain
   Susa fixative
Heinz body (bodies)
   H. b. hemolytic anemia
   H. b. test
Heinz-Ehrlich bodies
Heister's valve
HEK — human embryo kidney human embryonic kidney
Hektoen agar
HEL — human embryo lung
HeLa cells
Held's space
Heleidae
helenine
helical *[Heliobacter pylori]*
helicotrema
helium
   h. isotope
helix
hellebore
Helly's fluid
helmet cell
helminth
helminthiasis
helminthic
helminthism
helminthology
Helminthosporium
Helophilus
Helvella
   H. esculenta
hemacytometer
hemadsorption
hemagglutination
   h. inhibition
hemagglutinin
   autologous h.
   cold h.

hemagglutinin *(continued)*
    heterologous h.
    homologous h.
    warm h.
hemal
hemalum
hemangioblastoma
hemangioendothelial sarcoma
hemangioendothelioma
hemangiolipoma
hemangioma
    ameloblastic h.
    capillary h.
    cavernous h.
    infantile h.
    sclerosing h.
hemangiomatosis
hemangiopericytoma
hemangiosarcoma
hemapheresis
hemarthrosis
hematein
hematemesis
hematencephalon
hematidrosis
hematin
hematocele
hematochezia
hematoclasis
hematoclastic
hematocrit
    large vessel h.
    mean circulatory h.
    total body h.
hematocrystallin
hematogen
hematogenesis
hematogenous
hematohyaloid
hematoidin
hematologist
hematology
hematolysis
hematoma
    epidural h.
    subdural h.
hematometra
hematopoiesis
    extramedullary h.
hematopoietic
    h. aplasia
    h. cell cytoplasmic alteration
    h. hyperplasia
    h. hypoplasia
    h. maturation
    h. system
    h. tissue
hematopoietin
hematosalpinx
hematoside
hematoxylin
    h. body
    Carazzi's h.
    Clara's h.
    Cole's h.
    h. and eosin staining
    Harris' alum h.
    Heidenhain's iron h. stain
    Lillie's h.
    Mayer's h.
    Weigert's iron h. stain
hematuria
heme
hemiacardius
hemiacetal
hemianalgesia
hemianesthesia
hemianopia
hemianopsia
    binasal h.
    bitemporal h.
    homonymous h.
hemiatrophy

hemiazygos vein
hemiballismus
hemiblock
hemic
hemidesmosome
hemiglobin
hemimelia
hemin
hemiparesis
hemiplegia
Hemiptera
hemispheral
    h. lobule
    h. sublobule
hemisphere
    cerebral h.
Hemispora stellata
hemizygosity
hemoagglutination
hemochromatosis
hemochromogen
hemochromometry
hemocystinuria
hemocyt. — hemocytometer
hemocytoblast
hemocytometer
hemodialysis
hemofiltration
hemoflagellate
hemofuscin
hemoglobin
    h. A
    Bart's h.
    h. carbamate
    deoxygenated h.
    h. F
    fetal h.
    glycosylated h.
    h. H
    mean corpuscular h.
    oxygenated h.
    h. pigmentation

hemoglobin *(continued)*
    reduced h.
    unstable h.
hemoglobinated
hemoglobinemia
hemoglobinometry
hemoglobinopathy
    heterozygous h.
    homozygous h.
    mixed h.
hemoglobinorrhea
hemoglobinuria
    bacillary h.
    epidemic h.
    malarial h.
    march h.
    paroxysmal cold h.
    paroxysmal nocturnal h.
    toxic h.
hemoglobinuric
    h. nephrosis
hemogram
hemohistioblast
hemokinesis
hemolymph
    h. heteroagglutinin
    h. node
hemolysate
hemolysin
hemolysis
    alpha h.
    beta h.
    colloid osmotic h.
    extravascular h.
    extrinsic h.
    gamma h.
    immune h.
    intramedullary h.
    intravascular h.
    osmotic h.
    passive h.
    traumatic h.

hemolytic
- h. anemia
- h. disease of the newborn
- h. jaundice

hemolyze
hemopericardium
hemoperitoneum
hemopexin
hemophil
hemophilia
- h. A
- h. B
- h. C
- vascular h.

hemophiliac
hemophilic
Hemophilus
- *H. aegyptius*
- *H. aphrophilus*
- *H. bovis*
- *H. bronchisepticus*
- *H. conjunctivitidis*
- *H. ducreyi*
- *H. duplex*
- *H. hemoglobinophilus*
- *H. hemolyticus*
- *H. influenzae*
- *H. parahemolyticus*
- *H. parainfluenzae*
- *H. parapertussis*
- *H. paraphrohemolyticus*
- *H. paraphrophilus*
- *H. pertussis*
- *H. suis*
- *H. vaginalis*

hemophilus
- h. of Koch-Weeks
- h. of Morax-Axenfeld

hemophthalmia
hemopneumopericardium
hemopneumothorax
hemopoietic
hemoprotein
hemoptysis
- cardiac h.
- oriental h.
- parasitic h.
- vicarious h.

hemorrhage
- petechial h.

hemorrhagic
- acute h. bronchopneumonia
- acute h. cholecystitis
- acute h. cystitis
- acute h. glomerulonephritis
- acute h. inflammation
- acute h. ulcer
- acute h. ulceration
- h. ascites
- h. bronchopneumonia
- h. cyst
- h. cystitis
- h. disease of the newborn
- h. diverticulitis
- h. fever
- h. gastritis
- h. glomerulonephritis
- h. infarct
- h. inflammation
- h. lobar pneumonia
- h. pneumonia
- h. shock
- h. thrombocythemia
- h. ulcer

hemorrhoid
- thrombosed h.

hemorrhoidal
- h. artery
- h. nerve
- h. vein
- h. zone

hemosiderin
hemosiderinuria

hemosiderosis
    endogenous h.
    exogenous h.
    idiopathic pulmonary h.
hemostasis
hemostat
hemostatic
hemotherapy
hemothorax
hemozoin
HEMPAS — hereditary erythrocytic multinuclearity with positive acidified serum
Henderson-Hasselbalch equation
Henle's loop
Henoch-Schönlein syndrome
Henoch's purpura
henry
Henry's law
Hensen's node
HEPA — high-efficiency particulate air (filter)
heparan sulfate
heparin
heparinase
heparinate
heparinize
heparitin sulfate lyase
hepatic
    h. artery
    h. branch, vagus nerve
    h. capsule
    h. cords
    h. duct
    h. encephalopathy
    h. failure
    h. flexure
    h. lobule
    h. lymph node
    h. porphyria
    h. sinusoid

hepatic *(continued)*
    h. vein
hepatitis (hepatitides)
    acute focal h.
    h. antibody
    h. antigen
    A virus h.
    B virus h.
    giant cell h.
    infectious h.
    serum h.
    viral h.
hepatization
hepatoadrenal
hepatoblastoma
hepatocele
hepatocellular
    h. carcinoma
    h. jaundice
hepatocholangitis
hepatocuprein
hepatocyte
hepatoduodenal ligament
hepatogram
hepatolenticular
    h. degeneration
hepatoma
hepatomegaly
hepatopancreatic
hepatophosphorylase deficiency
hepatorenal
    h. glycogenosis
    h. ligament
    h. syndrome
hepatosplenomegaly
hepatotoxicity
heptabarbital
heptachlor
heptachloro-camphene
heptachlorocyclopentadiene
heptane

hereditary
   h. erythroblastic multinuclearity
   h. fructose intolerance
   h. persistence of fetal hemoglobin
   h. plasmathromboplastin component
   h. spherocytosis
heredity
   autosomal h.
   sex-linked h.
   X-linked h.
Herellea
   H. vaginicola
Hering-Breuer reflex
Hering's
   canal
   nerve
Hermansky-Pudlak syndrome
hermaphrodism
hermaphroditism
Hermetia illucens
hermetic
hernia
   diaphragmatic h.
   epigastric h.
   esophageal h.
   femoral h.
   hiatal h.
   incarcerated h.
   inguinal h.
   irreducible h.
   Morgagni's h.
   peritoneal h.
   retrocolic h.
   retrosternal h.
   Richter's h.
   strangulated h.
   umbilical h.
hernial

herniated
   h. nucleus pulposus
hernioplasty
herniorrhaphy
heroin
herpangina
herpes
   h. corneae
   h. febrilis
   h. genitalis
   h. gestationis
   h. simplex
   h. simplex virus, I, II
   h. zoster
   h. zoster virus
herpesvirus
Herpetomonas
Herring bodies
Hers' disease
hertz
Herxheimer's spiral
HES — hydroxyethyl starch
HET — helium equilibration time
hetastarch
heterauxesis
heterecious
heteroagglutination
heteroagglutinin
heteroallele
heteroantibody
heteroantigen
heteroatom
Heterobilharzia
heteroblastic
heterobrachial inversion
heterochromatin
   constitutive h.
   facultative h.
heterochromatinization
heterochthonous

heterocycle
heterocytotropic
Heterodera
   H. marioni
   H. radicicola
heterodyne
heterofermentation
heterogametic
heterogeneous
   h. nuclear RNA
   h. nucleation
heterogenic
heterogenote
heterogenous
heterogony
heterograft
heterokaryon
heterolactic
heterologous
heterolysosome
heterolytic
heteromorphic
   h. bivalent
   h. chromosomes
heterophagic
   h. vacuole
heterophagosome
heterophagy
heterophil
   h. antibody
heterophilic
   h. leukocyte
Heterophyes
   H. heterophyes
   H. katsuradai
Heterophyes/Metagonimus
heterophyiasis
heteroploid
heteroploidy
heteropolymer
heteropolysaccharide
heteropyknotic
heterosis
heterosomal
   h. aberration
heterosome
heterothallism
heterotopia
heterotopic
heterotroph
heterotrophic
heterozygote
heterozygous
   h. hemoglobinopathy
   h. thalassemia
   h. type of hemoglobin disorder
HETP — hexaethyltetraphosphate
heuristic
hexachloroacetone
hexachlorobenzene
hexachlorocyclohexane
hexachloroethane
hexachlorophene
hexadecimal
hexaethyl tetraphosphate
hexafluorenium bromide
hexamer
hexamethonium
   h. bromide
hexamethylenetetramine
hexamethylpararosanilin
hexane
hexanoic acid
hexapradol
hexavalent
hexestrol
hexetidine
hexobarbital
hexocyclium
hexokinase

hexosamine
hexosaminidase
hexose
  h. diphosphate
  h. monophosphate
hexosediphosphatase
hexosephosphate
  h. aminotransferase
  h. dehydrogenase
  h. isomerase
hexose-1-phosphate uridylyl-transferase
hexosephosphoric
hexosyltransferase
hexuronate
hexuronic acid
hexylcaine
hexylresorcinol
HF — Hageman factor
  hay fever
  heart failure
  hemorrhagic fever
  high flow
  high frequency
Hf — hafnium
HFI — hereditary fructose intolerance
HFP — hexafluoropropylene
Hfr — high-frequency recombination
Hg — mercury (*hydrargyrum*)
Hg or Hgb — hemoglobin
HGA — homogentisic acid
H gene
HGF — hyperglycemic-glycogenolytic factor
hGG — human gammaglobulin
hGH — human growth hormone
HGPRT — hypoxanthine guanine phosphoribosyl transferase
HH — hydroxyhexamide
HHA — hereditary hemolytic anemia
HHb — un-ionized hemoglobin
HHD — hypertensive heart disease
H and Hm — compound hypermetropic astigmatism
HHT — hereditary hemorrhagic telangiectasia
HI — hemagglutination inhibition
  hydroxyindole
HIA — hemagglutination-inhibition antibody
5-HIAA — 5-hydroxyindoleacetic acid
hiatus
  h. aorticus
  h. esophageus
  h. hernia
hibernoma
Hicks-Pitney thromboplastin generation test
hidradenitis suppurativa
hidradenoma
  clear cell h.
  nodular h.
  papillary h.
hidrocystoma
high
  h.-energy phosphate
  h.-frequency deafness
  h.-frequency recombination mutant
  h. pressure
high-density
  h.-d. lipoproteins
Highman's
  Congo red technique

Highman's *(continued)*
    method for amyloid
high molecular weight kininogen
high-pressure liquid chromatography
high-voltage transformer
hilar
    h. cell
    h. cell tumor
    h. lymph node
Hill equation
hilum (hila)
hilus (hili)
hindgut
Hine-Duley phantom
Hinton test
HIOMT — hydroxyindole-*O*-methyl transferase
Hippelates
Hippel-Lindau disease
Hippel's disease
hippocampal
    h. commissure
    h. fimbria
    h. fissure
    h. gyrus
    h. pressure groove
hippocampus
hippocratic facies
hippuria
hippuric acid
Hirschsprung's disease
hirsutism
Hirudinea
hirudiniasis
Hirudo (hirudines)
    H. aegyptiaca
    H. medicinalis
His's
    bundle
    space

Histalog test
histaminase
histamine
    h. phosphate
histidase
histidinase
histidine
    h. alpha-deaminase
    h. ammonia-lyase
    h. deaminase
    h. decarboxylase
histidinemia
histidinol dehydrogenase
histidinuria
histiocyte
    gargoylism type of h.
    Gaucher's type of h.
    Hand-Schüller-Christian type of h.
    Niemann-Pick type of h.
histiocytic
    h. granuloma
    h. leukemia
    h. lymphoma
    h. reticulosis, medullary
histiocytoma
histiocytosis
    kerasin-type h.
    lipid h.
    nonlipid h.
    phosphatid-type h.
    h. X
histochemistry
histocompatibility
    h. antigen
    h. complex
histocyte
histodifferentiation
histogenesis
histogram
histologic
histology

histolysis
histolytic
histone
histopathology
Histoplasma
   H. capsulatum
   H. duboisii
   H. farciminosus
histoplasmin
histoplasmosis
historadiography
HIT — hemagglutination-inhibition test
   hypertrophic infiltrative tendinitis
HJ — Howell-Jolly (bodies)
HK — heat-killed
   hexokinase
HKLM — heat-killed *Listeria monocytogenes*
HL — hearing level
   hearing loss
   histiocytic lymphoma
   histocompatibility locus
   hypermetropia, latent
H & L — heart and lungs
HLA — human leukocyte antigen
   human lymphocyte antigen
HLA
  antigens
  complex
HLDH — heat-stable lactic dehydrogenase
hLH — human luteinizing hormone
hLT — human lymphocyte transformation
HLV — herpes-like virus
HM — hydatidiform mole
Hm — manifest hyperopia
hm — hectometer
HMD — hyaline membrane disease
HMF — hydroxymethylfurfural
HMG — human menopausal gonadotropin
   hydroxymethylglutaryl
HML — human milk lysozyme
HMM — hexamethylolmelamine
HMO — health maintenance organization
H-2^b mouse cells
HMP — hexose monophosphate
   hexose monophosphate pathway
HMPG — 4-hydroxy-3-methoxy-phenyl-ethylene glycol
HMPS — hexose monophosphate shunt
HMSAS — hypertrophic muscular subaortic stenosis
HMW — high molecular weight
HN — hereditary nephritis
   hilar node
HN_2 — nitrogen mustard, mechlorethamine
HNP — herniated nucleus pulposus
hnRNA — heterogeneous nuclear RNA
HNSHA — hereditary non-spherocytic hemolytic anemia
HO — high oxygen
   hyperbaric oxygen
H_2O — water
Ho — holmium
HOC — hydroxycorticoid

HOCM — hypertrophic obstructive cardiomyopathy
Hodgkin cycle
Hodgkin's
   disease
   granuloma
   paragranuloma
   sarcoma
hof
Hofbauer cells
Hoffmann's reflex
Hofmann's bacillus
Hogben test
holandric
Hollander test
Hollenhorst plaques
Hollerith code
Holmes'
   alkaline buffer
   method
holmium
holoacardius
   h. acephalus
   h. acormus
   h. amorphus
holocrine
holoenzyme
Holophyra coli
holotype
Holzer's method
Holzknecht unit
Homalomyia
homatropine
   h. hydrobromide
   h. methylbromide
homeostasis
   immunologic h.
homeostatic
homoallele
homobiotin
homobrachial inversion

homocarnosine
homocinchonine
homocitrulline
homocyclic
homocysteine
   h. desulfhydrase
homocystine
homocystinuria
homocytotropic antibody
homodesmotic
homofermentation
homogametic
homogenate
homogeneity
homogeneous
homogenize
homogenous
homogentisate
   h. dioxygenase
   h. oxidase
   h. oxygenase
homogentisic acid
homogentisuria
homograft
homologous
   h. chromosomes
   h. graft
homologue
homology
homolytic
homonymous
   h. hemianopsia
homopolymer
homorphic
homoserine
   h. dehydratase
   h. dehydrogenase
   h. kinase
homosexuality
homosomal
homothallism
homovanillic acid

homozygote
homozygous
    h. hemoglobinopathy
    h. thalassemia
    h.-type hemoglobin disorder
homunculus
hone
honeycomb lung
HOOD — hereditary osteoonycho dysplasia
Hooke's law
hookworm
    American h.
    European h.
    New World h.
    Old World h.
HOP — high oxygen pressure
hordeolum
horizontal
Hormodendrum
    H. algeriensis
    H. carrionii
    H. compactum
    H. dermatitidis
    H. japonicum
    H. pedrosoi
    H. rossicum
hormonal
hormone
    adaptive h.
    adenohypophyseal h.
    adipokinetic h.
    adrenocortical h.
    adrenocorticotropic h.
    adrenomedullary h.
    androgenic h.
    anterior pituitary h.
    antidiuretic h.
    Aschheim-Zondek h.
    chondrotropic h.
    chromaffin h.

hormone *(continued)*
    chromatophorotropic h.
    corpus luteum h.
    cortical h.
    diabetogenic h.
    estrogenic h.
    fat-mobilizing h.
    follicle h.
    follicle-stimulating h.
    galactopoietic h.
    gastrointestinal h.
    gonadotropic h.
    gonadotropin-releasing h.
    growth h.
    hypophysiotropic h.
    inhibiting h's
    inhibitory h.
    interstitial cell–stimulating h.
    juvenile h.
    ketogenic h.
    lactogenic h.
    langerhansian h.
    lipolytic h.
    luteal h.
    luteinizing h.
    luteotropic h.
    mammotropic h.
    melanocyte-stimulating h.
    neurohypophyseal h.
    orchidic h.
    ovarian h.
    parathyroid h.
    placental h.
    posterior pituitary h.
    progestational h.
    proparathyroid h.
    prothoracicotropic h.
    releasing h.
    sex h.
    somatotropic h.
    steroid h.

hormone *(continued)*
   testicular h.
   thyroid-stimulating h.
   thyrotropic h.
   thyrotropin-releasing h.

horn
   Ammon's h.
   anterior h.
   cutaneous h.
   lateral h.
   posterior h.
   ventral h.

Horner's syndrome
horror autotoxicus
horseshoe kidney
Horsley-Clarke apparatus
Horton's syndrome
hospital
   teaching h.

host
   accidental h.
   alternate h.
   definitive h.
   intermediate h.
   h.-parasite relationship
   paratenic h.
   h. of predilection
   reservoir h.
   h. response
   transfer h.

hostility
Hotchkiss-McManus PAS technique
Hounsfield unit
hourglass
   h. gallbladder
   h. stomach

Houssay's syndrome
Howard test
Howell-Jolly bodies
Howell's b's
Howship's lacuna

HP – high protein
     human pituitary
hp – haptoglobin
HPA – hypothalamic-pituitary-adrenal
HPAA – hydroxyphenylacetic acid
HPF – heparin-precipitable fraction
hpf – high power field
HPFH – hereditary persistence of fetal hemoglobin
hPFSH – human pituitary follicle-stimulating hormone
hPG – human pituitary gonadotropin
hPL – human placental lactogen
HPLA – hydroxyphenyllactic acid
HPLC – high-pressure liquid chromatography
HPO – high-pressure oxygen
HPP – hydroxypyrazolopyrimidine
HPPA – hydroxyphenylpyruvic acid
HPPH – hydroxyphenylphenylhydantoin
HPS – hematoxylin-phloxine-saffron
     hypertrophic pyloric stenosis
HPT – hyperparathyroidism
HPV – *Hemophilus pertussis* vaccine
HPVD – hypertensive pulmonary vascular disease
HPVG – hepatic portal venous gas
HR – heart rate

H & R — hysterectomy and
    radiation
Hr — blood type factor
HRBC — horse red blood cells
H reflex
HRIG — human rabies immune
    globulin
HRS — Hamilton Rating Scale
HRT — heart rate
HS — heat-stable
    heme synthetase
    hereditary spherocytosis
    herpes simplex
    horse serum
    Hurler's syndrome
HSA — human serum albumin
HSG — hysterosalpingogram
H spike
H substance
HSV — herpes simplex virus
HSV I — herpes simplex virus I
HSV II — herpes simplex virus II
HT — hemagglutination titer
    histologic technician
    hydroxytryptamine
    hypermetropia, total
    hypertension
    hypodermic tablet
Ht — total hyperopia
ht — heart
    height
HTA — hydroxytryptamine
HTHD — hypertensive heart
    disease
HTLV — human T cell leu-
    kemia-lymphoma
    virus
HTP — hydroxytryptophan
HTV — herpes-type virus
HU — heat unit
    hemagglutinating unit

HU *(continued)*
    hydroxyurea
    hyperemia unit
Hucker-Conn crystal violet
    solution
Huebener-Thomsen-Frieden-
    reich phenomenon
Huebner's recurrent artery
human
    h. chorionic gonadotropin
    h. chorionic somatomam-
        motropin
    h. lymphocyte antigen
    h. pituitary gonadotropin
    h. placental lactogen
    h. T cell leukemia-
        lymphoma virus
humectant
humeral
humeroradial
humeroscapular
humerus (humeri)
humor (humors, humores)
    aqueous h.
    plasmoid h.
    vitreous h.
humoral
Hunner's
    cystitis
    ulcer
Hunter's
    canal
    glossitis
    syndrome
Hunter-Schreger lines
Huntington's chorea
Hurler's syndrome
Hürthle cell
    adenocarcinoma
    adenoma
    carcinoma
    metaplasia

HUS — hemolytic-uremic syndrome
    hyaluronidase unit for semen
Hutchinson-Gilford syndrome
Hutchinson's
    melanotic freckle
    triad
HUTHAS — human thymus antiserum
HV — hepatic vein
    herpesvirus
HVA — homovanillic acid
HVD — hypertensive vascular disease
HVE — high-voltage electrophoresis
HVH — herpesvirus hominis
H-V interval
HVL — half-value layer
HVSD — hydrogen-detected ventricular septal defect
H wave
Hy — hypermetropia
hyalin
    alcoholic h.
    hematogenous h.
hyaline
    h. arteriolosclerosis
    h. cartilage
    h. degeneration
    h. membrane
    h. membrane disease
    h. perisplenitis
    h. thickening
hyalinization
hyaloid
    h. artery
    h. canal
hyalomere

Hyalomma
    H. aegyptium
hyaloplasm
hyaloplasmic
hyaluronate
hyaluronic acid
hyaluronidase
hyaluronoglucosaminidase
hyaluronoglucuronidase
H-Y antigen
hybrid
hybridization
    cellular h.
    cross h.
    DNA-DNA h.
    DNA-RNA h.
    RNA-RNA h.
    saturation h.
hybridoma
hydantoin
hydatid
    alveolar h's
    h. degeneration
    h. mole
    h. of Morgagni
    sessile h.
    unilocular h.
    Virchow's h.
hydatidiform mole
hydatidosis
hydatiduria
Hydatigera
    H. infantis
hydralazine hydrochloride
hydrargyromania
hydrarthrosis
hydrastine
hydratase
hydrate
hydration
hydrazine

hydrazone
hydremia
hydrencephalocele
hydrencephalomeningocele
hydride
hydriodic acid
hydroa
    h. aestivale
hydrobromic acid
hydrocarbon
    alicyclic h.
    aliphatic h.
    aromatic h.
    carcinogenic h.
    cyclic h.
    saturated h.
    unsaturated h.
hydrocele
    h. sac
hydrocephalus
    communicating h.
    noncommunicating h.
hydrochloric acid
hydrochloride
hydrochlorothiazide
hydrocortamate
hydrocortisone
hydrocyanic acid
hydrocytosis
hydroflumethiazide
hydrofluoric acid
hydrogen
    h. chloride
    h. cyanide
    h. fluoride
    h. ion concentration
    h. peroxide
    h. sulfide
    h. sulfide acetyl-transferase
hydrogenase
hydrogenate
hydrogenation

hydrogenlyase
hydrohepatosis
hydrolase
    acetoacetylglutathione h.
    acetyl-CoA h.
    acid h's
    formyl-CoA h.
    guanosine h.
    hydroxyacylglutathione h.
    3-hydroxyisobutyryl-CoA h.
    hydroxymethylglutaryl-CoA h.
    palmitoyl-CoA h.
    succinyl-CoA h.
hydrolysis
hydrolytic
hydrolyze
hydromeningocele
hydrometer
hydromorphone hydrochloride
hydromyelia
hydronephrosis
hydronium
hydropericardium
hydroperitoneum
hydroperoxidase
hydroperoxide
hydrophilic
hydrophobia
hydrophthalmos
hydropic
hydropneumatosis
hydropneumopericardium
hydropneumoperitoneum
hydropneumothorax
hydrops
    h. abdominis
    h. amnii
    h. articuli
    cochlear h.
    endolymphatic h.

hydrops *(continued)*
  h. fetalis
  h. folliculi
  gallbladder h.
  labyrinthine h.
  h. tubae profluens
hydroquinone
hydrosalpinx
hydrostatic
Hydrotaea
hydrothorax
hydrotympanum
hydroureter
hydroxide
hydroxocobalamin
D-2-hydroxyacid dehydrogenase
3-hydroxyacyl-coenzyme A dehydrogenase
hydroxyacylglutathione hydrolase
hydroxyamphetamine hydrobromide
11β-hydroxyandrosterone
hydroxyapatite
hydroxybenzene
p-hydroxybenzoate esters
hydroxybenzoic acid
3-hydroxybutyrate dehydrogenase
hydroxybutyric acid
3-hydroxybutyryl-coenzyme A epimerase
2-hydroxy-2,2-*bis*-(4-chlorophenyl) ethyl acetate
hydroxychloroquine sulfate
alpha-hydroxycholanate dehydrogenase
17-hydroxycorticosteroid
17-hydroxycorticosterone
hydroxydione
β-hydroxydopamine
hydroxyethyl starch
11β-hydroxyetiocholanolone
2-hydroxyglutarate dehydrogenase
hydroxyhexamide
5-hydroxyindoleacetic acid
3-hydroxyisobutyrate dehydrogenase
3-hydroxyisobutyryl-coenzyme A hydrolase
hydroxyketone dye
hydroxyl
hydroxylamine
hydroxylase
hydroxylation
hydroxy-mercurichlorophenol
hydroxy-mercuricresol
hydroxy-mercurinitrophenol
tris-(hydroxymethyl) aminomethane
hydroxymethylglutaryl-coenzyme A
  h.-c. A hydrolase
  h.-c. A lyase
  h.-c. A reductase
  h.-c. A synthase
hydroxymethyltetrahydrofolate dehydrogenase
hydroxyphenamate
hydroxyphenylacetic acid
hydroxyphenyllactic acid
hydroxyphenyl mercurichloride
p-hydroxyphenylpyruvate
  h. dioxygenase
  h. hydroxylase
  h. oxidase
17-hydroxypregnenolone
17-hydroxyprogesterone
hydroxyproline
  h. oxidase
hydroxyprolinuria

8-hydroxyquinolate
8-hydroxyquinoline
17-hydroxysteroid
3-alpha-hydroxysteroid dehydrogenase
beta-hydroxysteroid dehydrogenase
hydroxysteroid oxidoreductase
3-beta-hydroxysteroid sulfotransferase
hydroxystilbamidine isethionate
5-hydroxytryptamine
hydroxytryptophan decarboxylase
hydroxyurea
hydroxyvaline
hydroxyzine
hygroma (hygromas, hygromata)
   cystic h.
   subdural h.
hygrometer
hygrophilous
hygroscopic
Hylemyia
hymen
hymenal tag
hymenolepiasis
Hymenolepididae
Hymenolepis
   H. diminuta
   H. murina
   H. nana
Hymenomycetes
Hymenoptera
hyoid
   h. arch
   h. bone
hyoscine
hyoscyamine
   h. hydrobromide

HYP — hydroxyproline
hypalgesia
hyperacidity
hyperactive
hyperactivity
   motor h.
hyperadrenalism
hyperadrenocorticism
hyperalbuminemia
hyperaldosteronemia
hyperaldosteronism
hyperalgesia
hyperalphaglobulinemia
hyperaminoacidemia
hyperaminoaciduria
hyperammonemia
hyperamylasemia
hyperamylasuria
hyperbaric
   h. chamber
   h. oxygenation
hyperbetaglobulinemia
hyperbetalipoproteinemia
hyperbilirubinemia
   constitutional h.
hyperbilirubinuria
   obstructive h.
hyperbradykinism
hypercalcemia
   familial hypocalciuric h.
   idiopathic h.
hypercalcitoninemia
hypercalcitoninism
hypercalciuria
hypercapnia
hypercapnic
   h. acidosis
hypercarbia
hypercellular
hyperchloremia
hyperchloremic
hyperchlorhydria

hypercholesterinemia
hypercholesterolemia
  essential h.
hyperchromasia
hyperchromatism
hyperchromemia
hyperchromia
hyperchromic
hypercoagulability
hypercoagulable
hypercorticism
hypercorticosolism
hypercortisolism
hypercupremia
hypercupruria
hyperdiploid
hyperdiuresis
hyperechoic
hyperelastosis cutis
hyperemesis
  h. gravidarum
hyperemia
hypereosinophilia
hyperesthesia
hyperestrogenism
hyperfibrinogenemia
hyperflexion
hypergammaglobulinemia
  monoclonal h.
  polyclonal h.
hypergastrinemia
hyperglobulinemia
hyperglycemia
hyperglycemic
  h. glycogenolytic factor
hyperglycinemia
  ketotic h.
  nonketotic h.
hyperglycinuria
hypergonadism
hypergonadotropic
hyperheparinemia

hypericin
hyperimmunity
hyperimmunization
hyperimmunoglobulinemia
hyperinsulinemia
hyperinsulinism
hyperirritability
hyperkalemia
hyperkaluria
hyperkeratosis
  h. eccentrica
  epidermolytic h.
  h. filiform
hyperkeratotic papilloma
hyperkinesis
hyperlipemia
  essential h.
hyperlipidemia
  carbohydrate-induced h.
  fat-induced h.
hyperlipoproteinemia
hyperlucency
hyperlysinemia
hypermagnesemia
hypermelanosis
hypermenorrhea
hypermetropia
hypermobility
hypernatremia
hypernephroma
hyperopia
hyperosmolality
hyperosmolarity
hyperosmotic
hyperostosis
  h. corticalis deformans juvenilis
  h. corticalis generalisata
  h. frontalis interna
hyperoxaluria
hyperparakeratosis
hyperparathyroidism

hyperperistalsis
  ureteral h.
hyperphenylalaninemia
hyperphosphatasia
hyperphosphatemia
hyperphosphaturia
hyperpigmentation
hyperpituitarism
  postpubertal h.
  prepubertal h.
hyperplasia
  adenomatous h.
  atypical h.
  basal cell h.
  basophilic h.
  benign prostatic h.
  cystic endometrial h.
  diffuse h.
  endometrial h.
  eosinophilic h.
  erythroid h.
  focal h.
  granulocytic h.
  hematopoietic h.
  intracystic h.
  intraductal h.
  Leydig cell h.
  lipomelanotic reticulo-
    endothelial cell h.
  lymphoid h.
  mast cell h.
  megakaryocytic h.
  myeloid h.
  neutrophilic h.
  nodular mesothelial h.
  papillary h.
  plasma cell h.
  polypoid h.
  primary h.
  pseudoepitheliomatous h.
  reserve cell h.
  reticuloendothelial cell h.

hyperplasia *(continued)*
  reticulum cell h.
  secondary h.
  stromal h.
  Swiss cheese h.
  wasserhelle h.
hyperplastic
  h. bone marrow
  h. nodular goiter
hyperploid
hyperploidy
hyperpnea
hyperpneic
hyperpolarization
hyperpotassemia
hyperprolactinemia
hyperprolinemia
hyperproteinemia
hyperpyrexia
hyperreflexia
hypersecretion
hypersegmentation
  hereditary h. of neutrophils
  leukocytic h.
hypersensitivity
hypersomia
hypersomnia
hypersplenism
hypersplenosis
hypertelorism
hypertension
  diastolic h.
  essential h.
  Goldblatt's h.
  idiopathic h.
  malignant h.
  mineralocorticoid h.
  orthostatic h.
  paroxysmal h.
  portal h.
  pulmonary h.
  renal h.

hypertension *(continued)*
    renovascular h.
    systolic h.
hypertensive
    h. cardiovascular disease
    h. heart disease
hyperthecosis
hyperthelia
hyperthermia
hyperthyroidism
hyperthyroiditis
hyperthyroxinemia
hypertonia
hypertonicity
hypertonus
hypertrichosis
hypertriglyceridemia
hypertrophic
    h. amphophil cell
    h. arthritis
    h. chronic vulvitis
    h. fibrous pachymeningitis
    h. gastritis
    g. gingivitis
    h. lichen planus
    h. osteoarthropathy
    h. polyneuritic-type muscular atrophy
    h. pulmonary osteoarthropathy
    h. pyloric stenosis
hypertrophy
    benign prostatic h.
    compensatory h.
    diffuse h.
    fibrocongestive h.
    focal h.
    giant rugal h.
    ventricular h.
hypertyrosinemia
hyperuremia
hyperuricemia
hyperuricosuria
hyperuricuria
hyperurobilinogenemia
hypervalinemia
hyperventilation
hyperviscosity
hypervitaminosis
hypervolemia
hypesthesia
    tactile h.
    thermal h.
hypha (hyphae)
Hyphomyces destruens
hypnagogic
    h. hypersynchrony
hypoacidity
hypoadrenalism
hypoadrenocorticism
hypoalbuminemia
hypoaldosteronism
hypoalphaglobulinemia
hypobaric
hypobetaglobulinemia
hypobetalipoproteinemia
hypocalcemia
hypocalciuria
hypocapnia
hypocarbia
hypocellular
hypochloremia
hypochlorhydria
hypochlorite
hypochlorous acid
hypocholesterolemia
hypochondriac region
hypochondriasis
hypochondrium (hypochondria)
hypochromasia
hypochromatism
hypochromemia
    idiopathic h.

hypochromia
hypochromic
  h. anemia
  h. microcytic anemia
hypochrosis
hypocomplementemia
Hypoderma
  H. bovis
hypodermic
hypodiploid
hypoechoic
hypofibrinogenemia
hypogammaglobulinemia
  Swiss-type h.
  X-linked h.
hypoganglionosis
hypogastric
  h. artery
  h. lymph node
  h. plexus
  h. region
  h. vein
hypogastrium
hypoglobulinemia
hypoglossal
  h. muscle
  h. nerve
hypoglycemia
hypoglycin, hypoglycine
hypogonadism
hypogonadotropic
hypoinsulinism
hypokalemia
hypokalemic
  h. nephropathy
  h. nephrosis
hypokaluria
hypoleydigism
hypolipoproteinemia
hypomagnesemia
hypomania

hypomanic
  h. personality
  h.-type manic-depressive psychosis
hypomenorrhea
hyponatremia
hyponatruria
hyponychium
hypoparathyroidism
hypopharynx
hypophosphatasia
hypophosphatemia
  X-linked familial h.
hypophosphaturia
hypophyseal
hypophysiotropic
hypophysis
  h. cerebri
  pharyngeal h.
  h. sicca
hypopigmentation
hypopituitarism
hypoplasia
  erythroid h.
  granulocytic h.
  hematopoietic h.
  lymphoid h.
  megakaryocytic h.
hypoplastic
  h. anemia
  h. bone marrow
hypoploid
hypoploidy
hypopotassemia
hypoproaccelerinemia
hypoproconvertinemia
hypoproteinemia
  prehepatic h.
hypoprothrombinemia
hypopyon
hyporeflexia

hyposecretion
hyposegmentation
   leukocytic nuclear h.
hyposensitization
hypospadias
hyposplenism
hypostatic pneumonia
hyposthenuria
hyposulfite salt
hypotension
   orthostatic h.
hypothalamic
hypothalamicohypophyseal
hypothalamicothalamic
hypothalamic sulcus
hypothalamohypophyseal
hypothalamopituitary
hypothalamus
   caudal area of h.
   dorsal nucleus of h.
   dorsomedial nucleus of h.
   infundibulum of h.
   medial nucleus of h.
   nucleus intercalatus of h.
   periventricular gray matter of h.
   supraoptic region of h.
   tuberal nucleus of h.
   ventromedial nucleus of h.
hypothenar
hypothermia
hypothesis
   Benditt h.
   biogenic amine h.
   cardionector h.
   Lyon h.
   unitarian h.

hypothyroid
hypothyroidism
hypotonia
   vasomotor h.
hypotonic
hypotonicity
hypotonus
hypotransferrinemia
hypotriploid
hypoventilation
hypovitaminosis
hypovolemia
hypovolemic
hypoxanthine
   h. guanine phosphoribosyltransferase
   h. phosphoribosyltransferase
hypoxemia
hypoxia
   anemic h.
   histotoxic h.
   hypoxic h.
   ischemic h.
   stagnant h.
hypoxic
hypsarrhythmia
hypsochrome
hypsochromic
hysterectomy
hysteresis
hysteria
   conversion h.
hysterosalpingography
Hz — hertz

I

I — intensity of magnetism
   iodine
   permanent incisor
^{131}I, ^{132}I — radioactive isotope of iodine
i — deciduous incisor
   optically inactive
IA — impedance angle
   internal auditory
   intra-aortic
   intra-arterial
Ia antigen
IABP — intra-aortic balloon pump
IAC — internal auditory canal
IADH — inappropriate antidiuretic hormone
IADHS — inappropriate antidiuretic hormone syndrome
IAEA — International Atomic Energy Agency
IAGP — International Association of Geographic Pathology
IAM — internal auditory meatus
IAP — International Academy of Pathology
IAS — interatrial septum
   intra-amniotic saline infusion
IASD — interatrial septal defect
IAT — invasive activity test
   iodine-azide test
iatrogenic
   i. agent
   i. anemia
iatrotherapy
IB — inclusion body
I band
IBB — intestinal brush border
IBC — iron-binding capacity
IBF — immunoglobulin-binding factor
IBR — infectious bovine rhinotracheitis
IBU — international benzoate unit
ibuprofen
IBW — ideal body weight
IC — inspiratory capacity
   integrated circuit
   intercostal
   intermittent claudication
   intracavitary
   intracellular
   intracerebral
   intracranial
   intracutaneous
   irritable colon
   isovolumic contraction
ICA — internal carotid artery
   intracranial aneurysm
ICAO — internal carotid artery occlusion
ICC — immunocompetent cells
   Indian childhood cirrhosis
ICD — International Classification of Diseases
   intrauterine contraceptive device
   isocitric dehydrogenase
ice
   dry i.
   i. point
ICF — intracellular fluid

ICG – indocyanine green
ichoroid
ichorrhea
ichthammol
ichthyoacanthotoxism
ichthyohemotoxism
ichthyosarcotoxism
ichthyosis
    i. congenita
    i. hystrix
    i. linguae
    i. uteri
ICM – intercostal margin
ICNND – Interdepartmental Committee on Nutrition in National Defense
icosahedral symmetry
ICS – intercostal space
ICSH – International Committee for Standardization in Hematology
    interstitial cell-stimulating hormone
ICSP – International Council of Societies of Pathology
ICT – indirect Coombs' test
    inflammation of connective tissue
    insulin coma therapy
    isovolumic contraction time
ictal
icteric
icterogenic
    i. spirochetosis
Icterohemorrhagiae
    I. leptospirosis
icterus
    congenital familial i.
    i. gravis

icterus *(continued)*
    i. interference
    i. neonatorum
ict ind – icterus index
ictus (ictus)
ICU – intensive care unit
ICW – intracellular water
ID – identification
    immunodiffusion
    infective dose
    inside diameter
    intradermal
I & D – incision and drainage
id
IDA – image display and analysis
    iron deficiency anemia
IDDM – insulin-dependent diabetes mellitus
Ide test
IDI – induction-delivery interval
idiocy
    amaurotic familial i.
    juvenile amaurotic familial i.
    mongolian i.
idiogram
idioheteroagglutinin
idiopathic
    i. etiology
    i. generalized glycogenosis
    i. hemosiderosis
    i. hypertrophic subaortic stenosis
idiopathy
    toxic i.
idiosyncrasy
idiosyncratic
idiot
    mongolian i.

idiotope
idiotoxin
idiotype
idioventricular
   i. rhythm
iditol
   i. dehydrogenase
   i. dehydrogenase assay
IDL – intermediate-density lipoprotein
IDMS – isotope dilution–mass spectrometry
idoxuridine
IDP – inosine diphosphate
IDR – intradermal reaction
IDS – immunity deficiency state
IDU – idoxuridine
       iododeoxyuridine
iduronic
   i. acid
   i. sulfatase
iduronidase
IDVC – indwelling venous catheter
IE – immunizing unit (*immunitäts Einheit*)
     immunoelectrophoresis
I/E – inspiratory-expiratory ratio
IEMG – integrated electromyogram
IEOP – immunoelectro-osmophoresis
IEP – immunoelectrophoresis
IF – immunofluorescence
    interstitial fluid
    intrinsic factor
IFA – indirect fluorescent antibody
IFC – intrinsic factor concentrate
IFCC – International Federation of Clinical Chemistry
IFR – inspiratory flow rate
IFRA – indirect fluorescent rabies antibody (test)
IFV – intracellular fluid volume
IG – immune globulin
    intragastric
Ig – immunoglobulin
IgA – gamma A immunoglobulin
IgA immunodeficiency nephropathy
IgD – gamma D immunoglobulin
IgE – gamma E immunoglobulin
IgG – gamma G immunoglobulin
IgM – gamma M immunoglobulin
ignition point
IGV – intrathoracic gas volume
IH – infectious hepatitis
IHA – indirect hemagglutination
IHBTD – incompatible hemolytic blood transfusion disease
IHC – idiopathic hypercalciuria
IHD – ischemic heart disease
IHO – idiopathic hypertrophic osteoarthropathy
IHR – intrinsic heart rate
IHSA – iodinated human serum albumin
IHSS – idiopathic hypertrophic subaortic stenosis

IIF − indirect immunofluorescent
IJP − internal jugular pressure
Il − illinium
ILA − insulin-like activity
ILD − ischemic leg disease
   ischemic limb disease
Ile − isoleucine
ileal
   i. artery
   i. lumen
   i. mesentery
   i. mucous membrane
   i. submucosa
ileitis
   distal i.
   regional i.
   terminal i.
ileocecal
ileocolic
   i. artery
   i. lymph node
ileocolitis
   i. ulcerosa chronica
ileum
   duplex i.
ileus
   adynamic i.
   dynamic i.
   gallstone i.
   mechanical i.
   meconium i.
   paralytic i.
   spastic i.
   i. subparta
   ureteral i.
Ilheus virus
iliac
   i. artery
   i. bursa
   i. lymph node
   i. region

iliac *(continued)*
   i. vein
iliocostalis muscle
iliohypogastric
ilioinguinal
iliolumbar
iliopsoas muscle
ilium (ilia)
ill-defined
illuminance
illumination
illusion
IM − infectious mononucleosis
   intramedullary
   intramuscular
im- − (indicates presence of) NH group
IMA − internal mammary artery
IMAA − iodinated macroaggregated albumin
image
   i. intensification
imaging
   electrostatic i.
IMB − intermenstrual bleeding
imbalance
   autonomic i.
   electrolyte i.
   sympathetic i.
   vasomotor i.
IMBC − indirect maximum breathing capacity
imbibition
IMH − idiopathic myocardial hypertrophy
IMHP − 1-iodomercuri-2-hydroxypropane
IMI − intramuscular injection
imidazole
imidazolepyruvic acid
imidazolylethylamine

imide
imidodipeptidase
imine
imino acid
iminoacidopathies
iminodipeptidase
iminoglycinuria
imipramine hydrochloride
immature
immediate hypersensitivity
immersion
    i. blast
    i. foot
    homogenous i.
    oil i.
    i. syndrome
    water i.
immersion-submersion
immiscible
immobility
immobilization
immobilized enzyme
immotile cilia syndrome
immune
    i. adherence
    i. complex
    i. complex diseases
    i. complex glomerulopathy
    i. complex nephropathy
    i. elimination
    i. response
    i. response genes
    i. surveillance
    i. system
immunity
immunization
immunize
immunoadsorbent
immunoassay
    nonradioisotopic i.
    radioisotopic i.
immunobiology
immunoblast
immunocatalysis
immunochemistry
immunochemotherapy
immunocompetence
immunocompromised
immunoconglutinin
immunocyte
immunocytoadherence
immunodeficiency
immunodepression
immunodiagnosis
immunodiffusion
    Ouchterlony i.
    Oudin i.
immunodominance
immunoelectrophoresis
    counter i.
    radio-i.
    reverse i.
    rocket i.
    two-dimensional i.
immunoferritin
immunofiltration
    analytical i.
    preparative i.
immunofixation
    i. electrophoresis
immunofluorescence
immunogen
immunogenetics
immunogenic
    i. determinant
immunogenicity
immunoglobulin
    i.-binding factor
    i. class
    gamma A i. (IgA)
    gamma D i. (IgD)
    gamma E i. (IgE)
    gamma G i. (IgG)
    gamma M i. (IgM)

immunoglobulin *(continued)*
   i. subclass
immunoglobulinopathy
immunohematology
immunohistochemical
immunohistofluorescence
immunoincompetent
immunologic
   i. enhancement
   i. memory
   i. paralysis
   i. tolerance
   i. unresponsiveness
immunologically competent cell
immunologist
immunology
immunomodulation
immunoparalysis
immunopathogenesis
immunopathology
immunoperoxidase
immunopotency
immunopotentiation
immunoprecipitation
immunoproliferative
   i. small intestinal disease
immunoprophylaxis
immunoradiometric
immunoradiometry
immunoreactivity
immunoregulation
immunoselection
immunosenescence
immunosorbent
immunostimulant
immunostimulation
immunosuppression
immunosuppressive
immunosurveillance
immunotherapy
IMP — inosine-5'-phosphate

impacted
   i. feces
   i. fracture
   i. tooth
impaction
   fecal i.
impaired clot retraction
impalpable
impedance
   electrode i.
imperforate
   i. anus
   i. hymen
impermeable
impetigo
   bullous i.
   i. contagiosa
implantation
   circumferential i.
   hypodermic i.
   interstitial i.
   periosteal i.
   i. site
   superficial i.
impotence
   sexual i.
imprecision
impregnation
impulse
   i. sealing
impurity
IMR — infant mortality rate
IMViC tests — indole, methyl red, Voges-Proskauer, and citrate tests
IN — intranasal
In — indium
inactivation
INAD — infantile neuroaxonal dystrophy
INAH — isonicotinic acid hydrazide

inanition
inborn
    i. error of metabolism
inbreeding
    i. coefficient
incarcerated
    i. hernia
incidence
incineration
incised
incision
incisor
    deciduous i.
    mandibular i.
    maxillary i.
incl. — including
inclusion
    blenorrhea i.
    i. body
    i. conjunctivitis
    i. conjunctivitis virus
    i. cyst, epidermal
    i. cyst, epidermoid
    i. cyst, epithelial
    i. cyst, germinal
    i. cyst, germinal epithelial
    cytoplasmic i.
    Döhle's i. bodies
inclusive
incoherent
incompatibility
    ABO i.
    chemical i.
    physiologic i.
incompetence
    valvular i.
incompetency and stenosis, mitral
incompetent
    i. aortic valve
    i. foramen ovale valve

incompetent *(continued)*
    i. mitral valve
    i. pulmonic valve
    i. tricuspid valve
incomplete
    i. abortion
    i. amnion
    i. amputation
    i. antibody
    i. compound fracture
    i. conjoined twins
    i. differentiation, cardiac valve
    i. dislocation
    i. dominance
    i. fracture
    i. hernia
    i. regeneration
    i. transposition
incontinence
    fecal i.
    urinary i.
incontinentia
    i. pigmenti
incoordination
increased
    i. appetite
    i. basal metabolism
    i. capillary fragility
    i. density
    i. flexion reflex
    i. flow
    i. libido
    i. metabolism
    i. potency
    i. pressure
    i. specific gravity
    i. stretch reflex
    i. turbidity
    i. viscosity
    i. volume

increment
incrementing
   i. response
incrustation
incubate
incubation
   i. period
incubator
incurable
incus
indanedione
independent
   i. assortment
   i. variable
index
   acidophilic i.
   Broders' i.
   i. case
   hematopneic i.
   hemolytic i.
   icteric i.
   Krebs' leukocyte i.
   maturation i.
   phagocytic i.
   pyknotic i.
   i. of refraction
   Reid's i.
   sedimentation i.
Index Medicus
Indian rat flea
indican
indicator
   i. organism
   i. tube
indices
indigenous
   i. bacterium
indigestion
indigo
indigoid dye
indirect
   i. addressing

indirect *(continued)*
   i. agglutination
   i. fluorescent antibody
   i. hemagglutination
   i. hernia
   i. transport
indium
indocyanine green
indole
indoleacetic acid
indoleaceturia
indoleaceturic acid
indolelactic acid
indoluria
indomethacin
indophenol
   i. dye
   i. test
indoprofen
indoxyl
   i. sulfate
indoxyluria
induced
   i. abortion
   i. allergic encephalomyelitis
   i. allergic neuritis
   i. aspermatogenesis
   i. glomerulonephritis
   i. thyroiditis
   i. uveitis
inducer
inducible
inductance
induction
inductor
induration
indusium griseum
INE — infantile necrotizing encephalomyelopathy
Inermicapsifer
   I. madagascariensis
inert

inertia
- colonic i.
- uterine i.

in extremis

inf — inferior
- infusion

infancy

infantile
- i. amaurotic familial idiocy
- i. hemangioma
- i. muscular atrophy
- i. paralysis
- i. progressive spinal muscular dystrophy
- i. respiratory distress syndrome
- i. spasm
- i. type coarctation
- i. uterus

infantilism

infarct
- acute i.
- anemic i.
- bland i.
- cerebral i.
- focal i.
- healed i.
- hemorrhagic i.
- microscopic i.
- old i.
- pale i.
- pulmonary i.
- recent i.
- red i.
- ruptured myocardial i.
- septic i.
- uric acid i.
- Zahn's i.

infarction
- atrial i.
- cerebral i.
- intestinal i.

infarction *(continued)*
- mesenteric i.
- myocardial i.
- pulmonary i.
- renal i.

infect

infection
- airborne i.
- colonization i.
- cryptogenic i.
- endogenous i.
- exogenous i.
- focal i.
- inapparent i.
- nosocomial i.
- pyogenic i.

infectious
- i. agent
- i. arteritis
- i. disease
- i. hepatitis
- i. mononucleosis
- i. parotitis
- i. wastes

infective

infectivity

inferior
- i. alveolar nerve
- i. aperture
- i. brachium
- i. cardiac branch
- i. cardiac nerve
- i. cerebellar peduncle
- i. cerebral vein
- i. cervical ganglion
- i. colliculus
- i. complete closed dislocation
- i. complete compound dislocation
- i. dislocation
- i. displacement

inferior *(continued)*
- i. division, oculomotor nerve
- i. epigastric artery
- i. esophageal sphincter
- i. frontal gyrus
- i. frontomarginal sulcus
- i. fronto-occipital fasciculus
- i. ganglion
- i. genicular artery
- i. gluteal nerve
- i. hemorrhoidal artery
- i. hemorrhoidal vein
- i. horn, lateral ventricle
- i. left pulmonary vein
- i. lingular bronchus
- i. longitudinal fasciculus
- i. medullary velum
- i. mesentery
- i. nasal turbinate
- i. nucleus, pulvinar
- i. oblique muscle
- i. occipital gyrus
- i. olivary nucleus
- i. pancreaticoduodenal artery
- i. parietal lobule
- i. peduncular interstitial nucleus
- i. petrosal sinus
- i. phrenic artery
- i. phrenic vein
- i. preoptic nucleus
- i. rectal artery
- i. rectal vein
- i. rectus muscle
- i. right pulmonary vein
- i. sagittal sinus
- i. segment
- i. striate vein
- i. temporal gyrus

inferior *(continued)*
- i. temporal sulcus
- i. thyroid artery
- i. vena cava

inferolateral
inferomedian
inferoposterior
inferosuperior
infertility
infestation
infiltrate
- acute inflammatory i.
- eosinophil leukocytic i.
- inflammatory i.
- leukocytic i.
- lymphocytic inflammatory i.
- monocytic inflammatory i.
- neutrophilic i.
- plasma cell i.
- polymorphonuclear leukocytic i.

infiltrating
- i. comedocarcinoma
- i. duct adenocarcinoma
- i. duct carcinoma
- i. lobular carcinoma

infiltration
- fatty i.
- glycogen i.
- lymphocytic i. of skin
- sanguineous i.
- tuberculous i.

infiltrative fasciitis
infinite
infinitesimal
infinity
infirm
infirmity
inflammable
inflammation
- active chronic i.

INFLAMMATION – INFLAMMATORY

inflammation *(continued)*
    acute i.
    acute and chronic i.
    blenorrhagic i.
    bullous i.
    bullous granulomatous i.
    calcified granulomatous i.
    caseating i.
    caseating granulomatous i.
    caseous i.
    catarrhal i.
    cavitating i.
    chronic i.
    circumscribed i.
    confluent i.
    cystic i.
    cystic granulomatous i.
    diffuse i.
    disseminated i.
    erosive i.
    exanthematous i.
    exudative i.
    exudative granulomatous i.
    fibrinoid necrotizing i.
    fibrinopurulent i.
    fibrinous i.
    fibrocaseous i.
    focal granulomatous i.
    follicular i.
    gangrenous i.
    gangrenous granulomatous i.
    gelatinous i.
    granulomatous i.
    gummatous i.
    hemorrhagic i.
    interstitial i.
    localized i.
    membranous i.
    miliary granulomatous i.
    multifocal i.
    necrotizing i.

inflammation *(continued)*
    necrotizing granulomatous i.
    non-necrotizing granulomatous i.
    obliterative i.
    organizing i.
    ossifying i.
    proliferative i.
    pseudomembranous i.
    purulent i.
    pustular i.
    recurrent i.
    serous i.
    subacute i.
    subsiding i.
    suppurative i.
    suppurative granulomatous i.
    transudative i.
    ulcerative i.
    uremic i.
    vesicular i.
    vesicular granulomatous i.
inflammatory
    i. adenocarcinoma
    i. bowel disease
    i. carcinoma
    i. cavity
    i. cyst
    i. exudate
    i. fistula
    i. infiltrate
    i. infiltrate, lymphocytic
    i. infiltrate, monocytic
    i. membrane
    i. necrosis
    i. perforation
    i, polyp
    i. pseudomembrane
    i. pseudotumor
    i. reaction

inflammatory *(continued)*
   i. rupture
   i. sinus
   i. sinus tract
   i. transudate
inflation
inflow tract
influenza
   i. virus, Types A, B, C
information
   i. retrieval
   i. theory
infra-axillary
infraclavicular
infracostal
infradian
   i. rhythm
infrahyoid
inframammary
infraorbital
infraorbitomeatal
   i. line
infrapatellar
infrared
   i. analyzer
   i. radiation
   i. spectroscopy
infrascapular
infraspinatus muscle
infraspinous
infratentorial
infratrochlear
infundibular
infundibulum (infundibula)
infusion
Infusoria
ingestion
ingrown
   i. hair
   i. toenail
inguinal
   i. artery

inguinal *(continued)*
   i. canal
   i. hernia
   i. ligament
   i. lymph node
   i. region
   i. ring
INH — isoniazid
      isonicotinic acid hydrazide
inhalation
   isoproterenol sulfate i.
   i. pneumonia
inherent
   i. filter
inheritance
   alternative i.
   amphigonous i.
   autosomal dominant i.
   autosomal recessive i.
   biparental i.
   codominant i.
   complemental i.
   cytoplasmic i.
   dominant i.
   extrachromosomal i.
   holandric i.
   hologynic i.
   homochronous i.
   intermediate i.
   maternal i.
   mendelian i.
   multifactorial i.
   polygenic i.
   quantitative i.
   quasicontinuous i.
   quasidominant i.
   recessive i.
   sex-linked i.
   supplemental i.
   unit i.
   X-linked dominant i.

inheritance *(continued)*
    X-linked recessive i.
inhibin
inhibit
inhibition
    allosteric i.
    competitive i.
    enzyme i.
inhibitor
    i. assay
    inter-alpha-trypsin i.
inhibitory postsynaptic potential
iniencephaly
inion
initialization
initiation
    i. condon
    i. factor
inj — inject
injection
injury
    birth i.
    blast i.
    cold i.
    compression i.
    crush i.
    decompression i.
    radiation i.
    torsion i.
innate
inner
    i. cerebellar funiculus
    i. mesothelial cell
    i. nuclear layer
    i. nuclear membrane alteration
    i. plexiform layer
innervation
    double i.
    reciprocal i.
innidiation
innominate
    i. artery
    i. bone
    i. lymph node
    i. vein
inochondritis
inoculate
inoculation
inoculum (inocula)
inorganic
    i. phosphate
    i. pyrophosphatase
    i. pyrophosphate
inosinase
inosine
    i. cyclohydrolase
    i. dehydrogenase
    i. diphosphate
    i. monophosphate
    i. phosphate
    i. phophorylase
    i. pyrophosphorylase
    i. triphosphate
inosinic acid
inositol
    i. dehydrogenase
    i. hexanitrate
    i. hexaphosphate
    i. niacinate
inotropic
input
    i. terminal
input/output
INPV — intermittent negative-pressure assisted ventilation
INS — idiopathic nephrotic syndrome
insect bite
insecticides
    organochlorine i.
    organophosphate i.

INSERTION – INTERCELLULAR 273

insertion
    parasol i.
    i. sequence
    velamentous i.
insertional
    i. activity
    i. translocation
in situ
insoluble
insomnia
insonation
inspiration
inspiratory
    i. reserve capacity
    i. reserve volume
inspissated
inspissation
instability
instillation
instrument
instrumentation
insufficiency
    aortic i.
    circulatory i.
    coronary i.
    mitral i.
    pulmonary i.
    renal i.
    respiratory i.
    tricuspid i.
    velopharyngeal i.
    venous i.
insufflation
    cranial i.
    endotracheal i.
    perirenal i.
    presacral i.
    retroperitoneal gas i.
insula (insulae)
insulator
insulin
insulinase
insulin-dependent diabetes mellitus
insulinoma
insulinopenic
insulitis
integral
    i. proteins
integrate
integrated circuit
integration
integrator
integument
in tela
intensification factor
intensifying screen
intensity
intensive care unit
intention
interaction
    drug i.
    i. of radiation with matter
inter-alpha-globulin
interatrial
    i. septal defect
    i. septum
interband
intercalary
    i. deletion
intercalate
intercalated
    i. disk
    i. duct
intercapillary
intercapital
intercarpal
intercellular
    i. bridge
    i. canaliculus
    i. cement
    i. desmosome
    i. junction
    i. zonula occludens

interchange
interchondral
interchromosomal
   i. aberration
intercoronary
   i. anastomosis
intercostal
intercostobrachial
   i. nerve
intercristal
   i. space
intercurrent
Interdepartmental Committee on Nutrition in National Defense
interdigital
   i. space
interelectrode
   i. distance
interface
   dineric i.
interfacial
   i. canal
interference
   constructive i.
   destructive i.
   i. filter
   i. pattern
interferon
interhemispheric
interkinesis
interleukin
interlobar
interlobular
   i. bile duct
   i. duct
   i. mammary connective tissue
intermaxillary
intermediary
   i. metabolism

intermediate
   i. coliform bacteria
   i.-density lipoprotein
   i. olfactory striae
intermedin
intermittent
   i. claudication
   i. positive pressure breathing
intermuscular
internal
   i. arcuate fibers
   i. auditory artery
   i. auditory canal
   i. auditory meatus
   i. auditory vein
   i. capsule
   i. carotid
   i. cerebral vein
   i. conversion
   i. ear
   i. endometriosis
   i. hemorrhoids
   i. hydrocephalus
   i. hypogastric artery
   i. iliac artery
   i. iliac vein
   i. inguinal ring
   i. jugular vein
   i. limiting membrane
   i. mammary artery
   i. mammary lymphatics
   i. mammillary nucleus
   i. medicine
   i. medullary lamina
   i. nasal branch, nasociliary nerve
   i. nose
   i. os
   i. pudendal artery
   i. pudendal vein

internal *(continued)*
   i. reduction
   i. rotation
   i. standard
   i. thoracic artery
   i. thoracic vein
   i. urethral orifice
International Academy of Pathology
International Association of Geographic Pathology
International Atomic Energy Agency
International Classification of Diseases
International Committee for Standardization in Hematology
International Council of Societies of Pathology
International Federation of Clinical Chemistry
International Federation of Gynecology and Obstetrics FIGO Classification of Staging
International Research Information Service
International Society for Clinical Laboratory Technology
International Society of Comparative Pathology
International Society of Hematology
International Society of Microbiologists
International Standards Organization
International System
International Union of Pure and Applied Chemistry

interneuron
   inhibitory i.
internodal
   i. tracts
internode
interoanterodorsal nucleus
interoanteromedial nucleus
interoanteroventral nucleus
interoceptor
interocular
   i. distance
interorbital
interosseous
interphalangeal
interphase
interpolation
interproximal
interpubic
interpupillary
   i. distance
   i. line
interrupted
   i. respiration
interscapular
intersexuality
interspinal
interspinalis muscle
interstice
interstitial
   i. cell
   i. cell–stimulating hormone
   i. cell tumor
   i. deletion
   i. emphysema
   i. fibrosis
   i. fluid
   i. growth
   i. inflammation
   i. nephritis
   i. nephropathy
   i. pneumonia

interstitial *(continued)*
   i. tissue
interstitium
intertransversalis muscle
intertrigo
intertubercular
interval
   i. estimate
   H-V i.
   i. scale
intervening
   i. sequence
interventional
   i. radiology
interventricular
   i. foramen
   i. septal defect
   i. septum
intervertebral
   i. disc
   i. fibrocartilage
intervillous
intestinal
   i. branch, vagus nerve
   i. flora
   i. flow disorder
   i. fluke
   i. juice
   i. lipodystrophy
   i. lumen
   i. lymphangiectasia
   i. metaplasia
   i. mucous membrane
   i. myiasis
   i. obstruction
   i. tract
   i. vein
   i. villi
   i. vomitus
intestine
   large i.
   small i.

intima
intimal
   i. cell
intolerance
   hereditary fructose i.
intoxication
   acid i.
   alkaline i.
   roentgen i.
   serum i.
   vitamin D i.
   water i.
intra-arterial
intra-articular
intrabiventral
   i. fissure
intrabronchial
intracanalicular
intracellular
   i. fluid
intrachange
intrachromosal
   i. aberration
intracranial
   i. arachnoid
   i. subdural space
intracristal
   i. space
intraculminate
   i. fissure
intracystic
   i. hyperplasia
   i. papilloma
intradermal
   i. nevus
   i. test
intraductal
   i. carcinoma
   i. hyperplasia
   i. papilloma
   i. papillomatosis
intradural

intraepidermal
    i. basal cell epithelioma, Borst-Jadassohn
    i. carcinoma
    i. nevus
intragastric
intrahepatic
    i. bile duct
intralaminar nucleus
intralimbic gyrus
intralobular
    i. bile ductule
    i. duct
    i. mammary connective tissue
intraluminal
intramembranous
intramuscular
intraocular
    i. pressure
intraoral
intraorbital
intraosseous
intraparietal
intrapartum
intraperitoneal
    i. gas
intrapleural
    i. pressure
intrapulmonary
intrapyramidal
    i. fissure
intraspinal
intrastitial
intrathenar
intratubal
intrauterine
    i. death
    i. device
intravasation
intravenous
intraventricular
    i. pressure
intrinsic
    i. factor
    i. laryngeal muscle
    i. lingual muscle
    i. pathway
    i. tongue muscle branch
introitus
intron
intubate
intubation
    endotracheal i.
    gastrointestinal i.
    rapid duodenal i.
intumescent
intumescentia
intussusception
inulase
inulin
    i. clearance
in utero
in vacuo
invagination
invalid
invasin
invasion
invasive
invasiveness
inverse-square law
inversion
    carbohydrate i.
    chromosomal i.
    i. of uterus
    visceral i.
invertase
inverted
    i. follicular keratosis
    i. keratosis
    i. repeat
invertin

invertose
in vitro
in vivo
involucrum
involuntary
involution
    menstrual i.
    postlactation i.
    senile i.
involutional
    i. melancholia
    i. psychosis
IO — internal os
    intestinal obstruction
    intraocular
I/O — input/output
Io — ionium
iocarmate meglumine
iocetamic acid
iodamide meglumine
Iodamoeba
    I. bütschlii
    I. williamsi
iodate
iodemia
iodic acid
iodide
    i. assays
iodimetry
iodinase
iodine
    butanol-extractable i.
    i. escape peak
    imidecyl i.
    i.-131-iodomethyl-19-
      norcholesterol
    protein-bound i.
    radioactive i.
    i. solution
    i. staining
    i.-131 therapy

iodine *(continued)*
    tincture of i.
    i.-131 uptake test
iodipamide
    i. meglumine
    i. sodium
iodized oil
iodoalphionic acid
iodobismuthate
iodochlorhydroxyquin
iodocholesterol
iododeoxyuridine
iodoform
iodohippurate sodium
iodophilia
iodophor
iodophthalein sodium
iodoplatinate
iodoprotein
iodopsin
iodopyracet
iodothyronine
iodotyrosine
IOFB — intraocular foreign
      body
ion
    i. counter
    dipolar i.
    i.-exchange chromatog-
      raphy
    i.-exchange resin
    gram i.
    hydrogen i.
    hydronium i.
    i. pair
ionic
    i. charge
    i. strength
ionization
    avalanche i.
    i. chamber

ionization *(continued)*
   i. constant
   i. interference
   specific i.
ionize
ionizing radiation
ionophore
iontophoresis
IOP — intraocular pressure
iopanoic acid
iophendylate
iophenoxic acid
iota
iothalamate
   i. meglumine
   i. sodium
iothiouracil
IP — incisoproximal
     incubation period
     inosine phosphorylase
     instantaneous pressure
     interphalangeal
     intraperitoneally
     isoelectric point
I-para — primipara
IPC — isopropyl chlorophenyl
IPD — inflammatory pelvic disease
ipecac
IPG — impedance plethysmography
IPH — idiopathic pulmonary hemosiderosis
IPL — intrapleural
ipodate
   i. calcium
   i. sodium
ipomea
IPP — intermittent positive pressure
IPPB — intermittent positive-pressure breathing
IPPO — intermittent positive-pressure inflation with oxygen
IPPR — intermittent positive-pressure respiration
IPPV — intermittent positive-pressure ventilation
iproniazid
ipronidazole
IPS — initial prognostic score
IPSID — immunoproliferative small intestinal disease
ipsilateral
IPSP — inhibitory postsynaptic potential
IPV — inactivated poliovaccine
IR — immunoreactive
    index of response
    infrared
    internal resistance
IR drop
Ir — immune response
    iridium
Ir genes
IRBBB — incomplete right bundle branch block
IRC — inspiratory reserve capacity
IRDS — idiopathic respiratory distress syndrome
    infant respiratory distress syndrome
IRG — immunoreactive glucagon
IRHCS — immunoradioassayable human chorionic somatomammotropin

IRhGH — immunoreactive human growth hormone
IRI — immunoreactive insulin
iridium
iridocapsulitis
iridocorneal angle
iridocyclitis
    heterochromic i.
iridokeratitis
IRIS — International Research Information Service
iris (irides)
    i. bombé
    Florentine i.
    tremulous i.
    umbrella i.
iritis
IRMA — immunoradiometric assay
iron
    i. ammonium citrate
    i. assays
    i.-binding capacity
    i. carbohydrate complex
    i. clearance
    i. deficiency anemia
    i. dextran
    ferric i.
    ferrous i.
    i. isotope
    i. lung
    i. oxide
    i.-positive pigment demonstration
    i. salt
    i. storage disease
    i.-sulfide protein
irovirus
irr — irradiation
irradiation
    i. change

irradiation *(continued)*
    i. damage
    interstitial i.
    ultraviolet blood i.
    whole-body i.
irregular pulse
irreversible
irreversibly sickled cell
irrigation
irritability
irritable bowel syndrome
IRS — infrared spectrophotometry
IRV — inspiratory reserve volume
IS — intercostal space
    interspace
isatin
ISC — irreversibly sickled cell
ischemia
    myocardial i.
    i. retinae
ischemic
    i. cardiomyopathy
    i. heart disease
    i. necrosis
ischial bursa
    i. b. gluteus maximus muscle
    i. b. obturator internus muscle
ischiocavernosus muscle
ischiopagus
ischium (ischia)
ISCLT — International Society for Clinical Laboratory Technology
ISCP — International Society of Comparative Pathology
ISD or ISDN — isosorbide dinitrate

ISF — interstitial fluid
ISG — immune serum globulin
Is genes
ISH — icteric serum hepatitis
International Society of Hematology
islet
   i. alpha cell
   i. beta cell
   i. delta cell
   i. hormones
   i's of Langerhans
   pancreatic i's
islet cell
   i. c. adenoma
   i. c. carcinoma
   i. c. hyperinsulinism
   i. c. hyperplasia
ISM — International Society of Microbiologists
ISO — International Standards Organization
iso — isoproterenol
isoagglutination
isoagglutinin
isoallele
isoallelism
isoalloxazine
isoamyl
   i. acetate
   i. nitrate
   i. salicylate
isoanaphylaxis
isoantibody
isoantigen
isobar
isobaric
isobestic point
isobornyl thiocyanoacetate
isobutyl alcohol
isobutyric acid
isocarboxazid

isochromatid break
isochromosome
isochronal
   i. rhythm
isochronous
isocitrate
   i. dehydrogenase
   i. lyase
isocitric
   i. acid
   i. dehydrogenase
isocyanate
isodesmosine
isodose
Isodrin
isoelectric
   i. focusing
   i. point
isoenzyme
   Regan i.
isoetharine
isoflupredone acetate
isoflurophate
isogamy
isogenic
   i. graft
isograft
isohemagglutination
isohemagglutinin
isohydric
   i. shift
isoimmune hemolytic anemia
isoimmunization
   Rh i. syndrome
isolate
isolated
   i. dextrocardia
   i. levocardia
   i. sinistrocardia
isolation
isoleucine
isoleucyl-RNA synthetase

isomaltase
isomer
isomerase
isomeric
    i. transition
isomerism
    chain i.
    dynamic i.
    functional group i.
    geometric i.
    nuclear i.
    optical i.
    position i.
    spatial i.
    stereochemical i.
    structural i.
isomerization
isometheptene hydrochloride
isometric
isomicrogamete
isomorphous
isomuscarine
isomylamine hydrochloride
isoniazid
    i. assays
    i. phenotype test
isonicotinic acid hydrazide
iso-osmotic
Isoparorchis
    I. hypselobagri
    I. trisimilitubis
isopathy
isopentenyl
    i. diphosphate
isopentenylpyrophosphate
    isomerase
isopleth
isoprene
isoprenoid
isopropamide iodide
isopropanol
    i. assays

isopropyl
    i. acetone
    i. alcohol
    i. benzene
    i. cresol
    i. meprobamate
    i. myristate
bis-(isopropylamido) fluorophosphate
isopropyl-*N*-(3-chlorophenyl) carbamate
isopropylmethylpyrimidyl diethyl thiophosphate
isopropyl-*N*-phenylcarbamate
isoproterenol
    i. hydrochloride
    i. sulfate
isopyknic
isopyknotic
isosexual
isosmotic
isosorbide
    i. dinitrate
Isospora
    I. belli
    I. hominis
isosporiasis
isothermal
isotone
isotonic sodium chloride
isotope
    i. dilution–mass spectrometry
    radioactive i.
    stable i.
isotropic
isovaleric acid
isovalericacidemia
isovaleryl CoA dehydrogenase
isovolume pressure flow curve
isoxsuprine hydrochloride
isozyme

ISP — interspace
Israels'
    I. familial jaundice
    I. shunt
IST — insulin sensitivity test
    insulin shock therapy
isthmus (isthmi)
    i. of aorta
    i. of fallopian tube
    i. of fauces
    i. of thyroid gland
    i. of uterus
ISW — interstitial water
IT — implantation test
    inhalation test
    inhalation therapy
    intradermal test
    intrathecal
    intratracheal
    intratracheal tube
    intratumoral
    isomeric transition
Itaqui virus
ITC — imidazolyl-thioguanine chemotherapy
itch
    grain i.
    swimmer's i.
    winter i.
itching
iter
    i. of Sylvius
iteration
iterative process
ITLC — instant thin-layer chromatography
ITP — idiopathic thrombocytopenic purpura
    inosine triphosphate
ITT — insulin tolerance test
IU — immunizing unit
    international unit

IU *(continued)*
    intrauterine
IUCD — intrauterine contraceptive device
IUD — intrauterine death
    intrauterine device
IUDR — iododeoxyuridine
IUFB — intrauterine foreign body
IUGR — intrauterine growth rate
IUM — intrauterine fetally malnourished
IUPAC — International Union of Pure and Applied Chemistry
^{131}I (radioactive iodine) uptake test
IUT — intrauterine transfusion
IV — interventricular
    intervertebral
    intravascular
    intravenous
    intraventricular
    invasive
IVAP — in vivo adhesive platelet
IVC — inferior vena cava
    intravenous cholangiogram
IVCC — intravascular consumption coagulopathy
IVCD — intraventricular conduction defect
IVCP — inferior vena cava pressure
IVCV — inferior venacavography
IVD — intervertebral disk
IVF — intravascular fluid
IVGTT — intravenous glucose tolerance test

IVH — intraventricular hemorrhage
IVM — intravascular mass
IVP — intravenous pyelogram
IVPF — isovolume pressure flow curve
IVS — interventricular septum
IVSD — interventricular septal defect
IVT — intravenous transfusion
IVTTT — intravenous tolbutamide tolerance test
IVU — intravenous urography
Ivy's method of bleeding time
IWL — insensible water loss
IWMI — inferior wall myocardial infarction
Ixodes
   I. bicornis
   I. cavipalpus
   I. frequens
   I. holocyclus
   I. pacificus
   I. persulcatus
   I. rasus
   I. ricinus
   I. scapularis
ixodiasis
ixodic

J

J — Joule's equivalent
jacksonian
   j. epilepsy
   j. march
   j. motor seizure
Jacobson's organ
Jadassohn's nevus
Jakob-Creutzfeldt
   disease
   pseudosclerosis
jalap
Janeway's lesion
janiceps
janus
Japanese B encephalitis virus
jar
   Coplin j.
Jarisch-Herxheimer reaction
jaundice
   congenital familial nonhemolytic j.
   familial nonhemolytic j.
   hemolytic j.
jaundice *(continued)*
   hepatocellular j.
   Israels' familial j.
   obstructive j.
JBE — Japanese B encephalitis
JCAH — Joint Commission on Accreditation of Hospitals
J chain
jej — jejunum
jejunal
   j. artery
   j. juice
   j. lumen
   j. mesentery
   j. mucous membrane
   j. submucosa
jejunitis
jejunoileitis
jejunostomy
jejunum
Jenner-Giemsa stain
Jensen's classification
jervine

jet lesion
JG — juxtaglomerular
JGC — juxtaglomerular cell
JGI — juxtaglomerular granulation index
JH virus
jigger
Job's syndrome
jock itch
Jod-Basedow phenomenon
Johne's bacillus
joint
    acromioclavicular j.
    ankle j.
    astragaloid j.
    j. body
    carpometacarpal j.
    cartilaginous j.
    cervical vertebral j.
    Charcot's j.
    costotransverse j.
    costovertebral j.
    elbow j.
    fibrous j.
    hip j.
    humeroradial j.
    humeroscapular j.
    intercarpal j.
    interchondral j.
    interphalangeal j.
    intervertebral j.
    knee j.
    lower extremity j.
    lumbar vertebral j.
    lumbosacral j.
    metacarpal j.
    metacarpophalangeal j.
    metatarsal j.
    metatarsophalangeal j.
    midcarpal j.
    midtarsal j.
    j. mouse

joint *(continued)*
    radiocarpal j.
    radioulnar j.
    sacrococcygeal j.
    sacroiliac j.
    shoulder j.
    sternoclavicular j.
    sternocostal j.
    synovial j.
    talocalcaneonavicular j.
    talocrural j.
    tarsal j.
    tarsometatarsal j.
    temporomandibular j.
    thoracic vertebral j.
    tibiofibular j.
    trunk j.
    upper extremity j.
    vertebral j.
    wrist j.
Joint Commission on Accreditation of Hospitals
Jolly's bodies
Jones-Cantarow test
Jones' method
Jones-Mote reaction
joule
Joule's law
JRA — juvenile rheumatoid arthritis
jt — joint
jugular
    j. ganglion
    j. glossopharyngeal nerve
    j. lymph node
    j. tenth cranial nerve
    j. vagus nerve
    j. vein
    j. venous pulse
juice
    cancer j.
    duodenal j.

286 JUICE – KARYOCYTE

juice *(continued)*
    gastric j.
    ileal j.
    intestinal j.
    jejunal j.
    pancreatic j.
junction
    gap j.
    tight j.
junctional
    j. automaticity
    j. complex
    j. escape
    j. nevus
    j. rhythm
    j. tachycardia
Junin virus
juvenile
    j. angiofibroma
    j. diabetes mellitus
    j. fibroadenoma

juvenile *(continued)*
    j. melanoma
    j. pernicious anemia
    j. pilocytic astrocytoma
    j. polyposis
    j. rheumatoid arthritis
    j. xanthogranuloma
    j. xanthoma
juxta-articular nodule
juxtaglomerular
    j. apparatus
    j. cell
    j. granules
juxtanuclear
juxtaposition
juxtapulmonary-capillary receptor
juxtarestiform body
JV – jugular vein
    jugular venous
JVP – jugular venous pulse

K

K – absolute zero
    electrostatic capacity
    kathode (obs. for cathode)
    Kell blood system
    kelvin
    potassium
k – constant
KA – kathode (cathode)
    ketoacidosis
    King-Armstrong (units)
kabure
Kahler's disease
Kahn test
kala-azar
kaliopenia
kalium
kallidin

kallikrein
kallikreinogen
Kallmann's syndrome
Kanagawa phenomenon
kanamycin
kaolin
Kaposi's
    sarcoma
    varicelliform eruption
kappa
    k. chain
    k. rhythm
Karathane
Karmen units
Kartagener's syndrome
karyochrome
karyocyte

karyogamy
karyogen
karyokinesis
karyoklasis
karyolysis
karyomere
karyon
karyophage
karyoplast
karyopyknosis
karyopyknotic index
karyoreticulum
karyorrhectic
karyorrhexis
karyotype
karyozoic
Kasabach-Merritt syndrome
kat — katal
katal
Katayama's test
katharometer
katolysis
katzenjammer
KAU — King-Armstrong units
Kauffman-White classification
Kawasaki disease
Kayser-Fleischer ring
KB — ketone bodies
kb — kilobase
kbp — kilobase pair
KBr — potassium bromide
KC — kathodal (cathodal) closing
kc — kilocycle
kcal — kilocalorie
KCC — kathodal(cathodal)-closing contraction
K cells
KCG — kinetocardiogram
KCl — potassium chloride
kcps — kilocycles per second

KCT — kathodal (cathodal)-closing tetanus
KD — kathodal (cathodal) duration
KDT — kathodal(cathodal)-duration tetanus
KE — kinetic energy
kedani mite
Kell
  antigens
  blood system
keloid
  Addison's k.
kelp
Kelthane
Kelvin
  temperature scale
  thermometer
kerasin
keratan sulfate
keratin
keratinization
  metaplastic k.
keratinize
keratinocyte
keratinous
keratitis
  acne rosacea k.
  k. bullosa
  k. disciformis
  herpetic k.
  interstitial k.
  mycotic k.
  parenchymatous k.
  reticular k.
  sclerosing k.
  serpiginous k.
  suppurative k.
  vascular k.
  vesicular k.
  zonular k.

keratoacanthoma
keratoconjunctivitis
    phlyctenular k.
keratoconus
keratocyte
keratoderma
    k. acquisitum
    k. blennorrhagicum
    k. climactericum
keratoglobus
keratohyalin
keratomalacia
keratopathy
    band k.
keratosis
    actinic k.
    arsenical k.
    follicularis k.
    inverted k.
    inverted follicular k.
    pilaris k.
    seborrheic k.
    senile k.
    solar k.
keratotic
    k. papilloma
    k. precipitates
kerion
    k. celsi
Kerckring's valves
kernicterus
Kernig's sign
kerosene, kerosine
ketal
ketamine hydrochloride
ketene
ketimine
3-ketoacid coenzyme A-transferase
ketoacidosis
ketoaciduria
    branched-chain k.
3-ketoacyl-coenzyme A thiolase
11-ketoandrosterone
ketoconazole
11-ketoetiocholanolone
ketogenesis
ketogenic
    k. steroid
ketogluconokinase
ketoglutarate
    k. dehydrogenase
ketoglutaric acid
ketohexokinase
ketohexose
ketone
    k. body
    dimethyl k.
ketonemia
ketonuria
ketopentose
ketoprofen
β-ketoreductase
ketose
ketosis
17-ketosteroid
Ketostix
ketotetrosealdolase
ketothiolase
ketotic
ketotransferase
ketotriose
kev — kilo electron volts
Key-Retzius lateral aperture
KFAB — kidney-fixing antibody
KFS — Klippel-Feil syndrome
kg — kilogram
kg-cal — kilogram-calorie
KGS — ketogenic steroid
khellin
kHz — kilohertz
KI — karyopyknotic index
KIA — Kliger iron agar

kidney
    abdominal k.
    Armanni-Ebstein k.
    arteriosclerotic k.
    artificial k.
    atrophic k.
    cicatricial k.
    cystic k.
    Goldblatt's k.
    mural k.
    supernumerary k.
    thoracic k.
Kienböck's disease
kieselguhr
kilobase
    k. pair
kilocalorie
kilocycle
kilo electron volt
kilogram
kilohertz
kilohm
kilojoule
kilometer
kilopascal
kilovolt
    k.-ampere
kilovoltage
kilowatt
    k.-hour
Kimmelstiel-Wilson
    lesion
    syndrome
Kimura's disease
kinase
kinesis
kinetic
kinetochore
kinetocyte
kinetoplasm
kinetoplast
kinetosome

King-Armstrong unit
kingdom
Kingella
    K. denitrificans
    K. kingae
kinin
kininase II
kininogen
kinking
kinocilium (kinocilia)
Kinyoun carbol fuchsin stain
Kirchoff's law
KIU — kallikrein-inhibiting unit
kj — kilojoule
Kjeldahl's method
Klebsiella
    K. friedländeri
    K. oxytoca
    K. ozaenae
    K. pneumoniae
    K. rhinoscleromatis
Klebsielleae
Klebs-Löffler bacillus
Kleine-Levin syndrome
Klein's bacillus
Klenow fragment
KLH — keyhole-limpet hemocyanin
Kliger iron agar
Klinefelter's syndrome
Klippel-Feil
    deformity
    syndrome
Klippel-Trenaunay syndrome
KM — kanamycin
km — kilometer
KMnO — potassium permanganate
KMV — killed measles virus vaccine
knee
    k. cap

knee *(continued)*
   k. jerk
   k. joint
   septic k.
knee joint
   lateral meniscus of k. j.
   ligament of k. j.
   medial meniscus of k. j.
knizocyte
Knott's technique
Kobelt's cyst
KOC — kathodal(cathodal)-opening contraction
Koch's
   bacillus
   postulates
Koch-Weeks
   bacillus
   hemophilus
Kogoj's abscess
KOH — potassium hydroxide
Köhler's disease
Kohn pores
Kohn's one-step staining technique
koilocytotic
   k. atypia
koilonychia
Kolmer's test
Koplik's spots
Korsakoff's psychosis
KP — keratitic precipitates
kPa — kilopascal
KPTT — kaolin partial thromboplastin time
Kr — krypton
Krabbe's
   disease
   leukodystrophy
kraurosis
   k. vulvae

Krause's end bulb
KRB — Krebs-Ringer bicarbonate buffer
Krebs'
   cycle
   leukocyte index
Krebs-Henseleit cycle
KRP — Kolmer's test with Reiter protein
   Krebs-Ringer phosphate
Krukenberg's tumor
krypton
KS — ketosteroid
   Klinefelter's syndrome
   Kveim-Siltzbach (test)
KSC. *See* KCC.
KST. *See* KCT.
KU — Karmen units
KUB — kidney, ureter and bladder
Kufs' disease
Kumba virus
Kunkel's test
Kupffer's
   cells
   cell sarcoma
kurtosis
kuru
Kussmaul respiration
KV — killed vaccine
kV — kilovolt
kVa — kilovolt-ampere
Kveim
   antigen
   test
kvp — kilovolt peak
KW — Keith-Wagener
kW — kilowatt
kwashiorkor
KWB — Keith, Wagener, Barker (classification)

kW-hr — kilowatt-hour
Kyasanur Forest
   K. F. disease
   K. F. disease virus
kyestein

kynurenine
   k. aminotransferase
   k. 3-hydroxylase
kyphoscoliosis
kyphosis

L

L — coefficient of induction
   left
   length
   lethal
   ligament
   liter
   lumbar
L. — *Lactobacillus*
LA — lactic acid
   latex agglutination
   left atrium
   leucine aminopeptidase
   linguoaxial
LAA — leukocyte ascorbic acid
lab — laboratory
Labbé's anastomosing vein
label
   radioactive l.
labia
labia majora
   anterior commissure of l.m.
   posterior commissure of l.m.
labile
   heat l.
   l. factor
labiomycosis
labium (labia)
labor
   abnormal l.
   postmature l.
   premature l.
laboratory

labyrinth
   acoustic l.
   cortical l.
   ethmoidal l.
   membranous l.
   olfactory l.
   perilymphatic l.
   statokinetic l.
   l. vestibule
lac (lacta)
   l. femininum
   l. sulfuris
   l. vaccinum
laceration
lacrimal
   l. apparatus
   l. artery
   l. caliculus
   l. canaliculus
   l. duct
   l. gland
   l. nerve
   l. papilla
   l. sac
   l. secretion
   l. suture
lacrimation
lactalbumin
lactamase
Lactarius
   L. torminosus
lactase

lactate
- l. dehydrogenase
- l. dehydrogenase isoenzyme
- ferrous l.
- l. oxidase
- l. racemase

lactating
- l. adenoma
- l. breast

lactation

lacteal

lactic
- l. acid
- l. acid bacteria
- l. acidosis
- l. dehydrogenase

lactiferous
- l. duct
- l. sinus

Lactobacillaceae

Lactobacilleae

Lactobacillus
- *L. acidophilus*
- *L. arabinosus*
- *L. bifidus*
- *L. brevis*
- *L. bulgaricus*
- *L. casei*
- *L. catenaforme*
- *L. cellobiosus*
- *L. fermentans*
- *L. fermenti*
- *L. jensenii*
- *L. leichmannii*
- *L. plantarum*

lactobacillus
- l. of Boas-Oppler

Lactobacteriaceae

lactoferrin

lactogen
- human placental l.

lactoglobulin
- immune l.

lactone

lactoperoxidase radioiodination

lactophenol

lactose

lactosidosis
- ceramide l.

lactosuria

lactosyl ceramide

lactotrope

lactoyl-glutathione lyase

lactulose

lacuna (lacunae, lacunas)
- absorption l.
- cartilage l.
- cerebral l.
- Howship's l.
- osseous l.
- parasinoidal l's
- trophoblastic l.

lacunar
- l. cell
- l. resorption

LAD — left anterior descending
left axis deviation

Ladendorff's test

LAE — left atrial enlargement

Laelaps

Laennec's cirrhosis

LAF — laminar air flow

Lafora's bodies

LAG — labiogingival
lymphangiogram

Lagochilascaris minor

LAH — lactalbumin hydrolysate
left atrial hypertrophy

LAI — labioincisal

LAIT — latex agglutination-inhibition test

Laki-Lorand factor
lambda
    l. chain
    l. wave
lambdoid suture
Lambert's law
lambliasis
lamella (lamellae)
lamellar necrosis
lamina (laminae)
    Bowman's l.
    l. choriocapillaris
    l. cribrosa, sclera
    dental l.
    Descemet's posterior l.
    l. dura
    l. propria
    l. suprachoroidea
    l. terminalis
    l. vasculosa
laminar
laminarinase
laminectomy
lamp
    hollow cathode l.
    mercury-vapor l.
    tungsten l.
    tungsten halogen l.
lanatoside C
Lancefield classification
lancet
Landouzy-Dejerine progressive muscular dystrophy
Landry's paralysis
Langerhans'
    cell
    granules
    islets
    layer
Lange's colloidal gold test
Langhans'
    giant cell

Langhans' *(continued)*
    layer
    type of giant cell reaction
Lansing virus
lanthanide
lanthanoid
lanthanum
LAO — left anterior oblique
LAP — left atrial pressure
           leucine aminopeptidase
           leukocyte alkaline phosphatase
           lyophilized anterior pituitary
laparotomy
lapinization
Laplace's law
large intestine
larva (larvae)
    fly l.
    lepidopterid l.
    l. migrans
laryngeal
    l. aperture
    l. branch
    l. cartilage
    l. cavity
    l. gland
    l. mucus
    l. muscle
    l. nerve
    l. nodule
    l. polyp
    l. prominence
laryngectomy
laryngismus
    l. stridulus
laryngitis
laryngotracheitis
laryngotracheobronchitis
larynx (larynges)
    fibroelastic membrane of l.

294 LARYNX (LARYNGES) – LATISSIMUS DORSI MUSCLE

larynx (larynges) *(continued)*
    ligament of l.
    lymphatics of l.
    mucous membrane of l.
    submucosa of l.
    ventricular fold of l.
LAS – linear alkylate sulfonate
LASER – light amplification by stimulated emission of radiation
laser
Lash's casein hydrolysate-serum medium
Lasiodiplodia theobromae
Lassa virus
lassitude
lat – lateral
latency
latent
    l. image
    l. porphyria
lateral
    l. aperture
    l. basal branch
    l. basal segment
    l. cerebral fissure
    l. circumflex femoral artery
    l. collateral ligament
    l. column
    l. corticospinal tract
    l. costal branches
    l. displacement
    l. femoral cutaneous nerve
    l. femoral cutaneous vein
    l. fornix
    l. funiculus
    l. geniculate body
    l. gray column
    l. horn
    l. lemniscus
    l. lemniscus nucleus

lateral *(continued)*
    l. ligament
    l. lobe, prostate
    l. mammillary nucleus
    l. margin
    l. medullary lamina
    l. meniscus
    l. nasal cartilage
    l. nucleus
    l. occipital gyrus
    l. occipital sulcus
    l. olfactory gyrus
    l. olfactory striae
    l. plantar artery
    l. proper fasciculus
    l. pterygoid nerve
    l. recess
    l. rectus muscle
    l. rectus nerve
    l. sacral artery
    l. sacral vein
    l. segment
    l. spinorubral tract
    l. spinothalamic tract
    l. striate perforating branches
    l. sural cutaneous nerve
    l. thoracic artery
    l. thoracic vein
    l. tuberal nucleus
    l. ventricle
    l. ventricular vein
    l. wall, hypopharynx
    l. wall, oropharynx
late replicating X chromosome
lateromedial
latex
    l. agglutination test
    l. fixation test
lathyrism
lathyrus protein
latissimus dorsi muscle

Latrodectus
   L. bishopi
   L. geometricus
   L. mactans
LATS — long-acting thyroid stimulator
laudanum
Laurell technique
Laurence-Moon-Biedl syndrome
lauric acid
lauryl
   l. isoquinolinium bromide
   l. thiocyanate
lavage
   bronchopulmonary l.
   gastric l.
   peritoneal l.
law
   Angström's l.
   Beer's l.
   Bell-Magendie l.
   Bouguer's l.
   Boyle's l.
   Charles' l.
   Coulomb's l.
   Courvoisier's l.
   Dalton's l.
   Einthoven's l.
   Faraday's l. of electrolysis
   Fick's l.
   Gay-Lussac's l.
   Graham's l.
   Hardy-Weinberg l.
   Henry's l.
   Hooke's l.
   Joule's l.
   Kirchoff's l.
   Lambert's l.
   Laplace's l.
   Mendel's l.
   Newton's l. of cooling

law *(continued)*
   Ohm's l.
   Planck's radiation l.
   Poiseuille's l.
   Raoult's l.
   Snell's l.
   Starling's l.
   Stefan-Boltzmann l.
   Stokes' l.
lawrencium
layer
   Langerhans' l.
   Langhans' l.
   nerve fiber l.
   Nitabuch's l.
   nuclear l.
   palisade l.
   plexiform l.
   subendocardial l.
   visceral l.
LBB — left bundle branch
LBBB — left bundle branch block
LBCD — left border of cardiac dullness
LBF — *Lactobacillus bulgaricus* factor
LBI — low serum-bound iron
LBM — lean body mass
LBNP — lower-body negative pressure
LBW — low birth weight
LBWI — low birth weight infant
LC — lethal concentration
       lipid cytosomes
LCA — left coronary artery
LCAT — lecithin-cholesterol acyltransferase
LCD — liquor carbonis detergens
LCFA — long-chain fatty acid
L chain

LCL — Levinthal-Coles-Lillie
      (bodies)
   lymphocytic leukemia
   lymphocytic lympho-
      sarcoma
LCM — left costal margin
   lymphatic choriomen-
      ingitis
   lymphocytic chorio-
      meningitis
LCM virus
LCT — long-chain triglyceride
LD — labyrinthine defect
   lactate dehydrogenase
   lactic dehydrogenase
   left deltoid
   legionnaires' disease
   lethal dose
   linguodistal
   living donor
   lymphocyte-defined
L-D — Leishman-Donovan
      (bodies)
LDA — left dorsoanterior
   linear displacement
      analysis
LDD — light-dark discrimina-
      tion
LDH — lactate dehydrogenase
LDL — low-density lipoprotein
LDLP — low-density lipopro-
      tein
L-dopa
LDP — left dorsoposterior
LDV — lactic dehydrogenase
      virus
LE — leukoerythrogenetic
   lupus erythematosus
lead
   l. acetate
   l. arsenate
   l. arsenite

lead *(continued)*
   l. chromate
   l. oxide
   l. tetraethyl
   l. tetramethyl
leakage
learning disorder
least
   l. significant bit
   l. significant digit
   l. squares regression
Leber's optic atrophy
LE cell
lecithin
   l.-cholesterol acyltransfer-
      ase
   l.-sphingomyelin ratio
lecithinase
lectin
lectotype
LED — lupus erythematosus
      disseminatus
leech
Lee-White clotting time method
left
   l. anterior oblique
   l. axis deviation
   l. bundle branch block
   l. posterior oblique
   l. ventricular ejection time
   l. ventricular hypertrophy
Legg-Calvé-Perthes disease
Legionella longbeacha
   L. pneumophila
legionellosis
legionnaires' disease
Leigh's disease
leiomyoblastoma
leiomyofibroma
leiomyoma
   vascular l.
leiomyosarcoma

Leishman-Donovan bodies
Leishmania
- *L. braziliensis*
- *L. caninum*
- *L. donovani*
- *L. infantum*
- *L. nilotica*
- *L. peruviana*
- *L. tropica*
- *L. tropica mexicana*

leishmaniasis
- l. americana
- cutaneous l.
- lupoid l.
- mucocutaneous l.
- naso-oral l.
- nasopharyngeal l.
- l. recidivans
- visceral l.

leishmanicidal
Leishman's stain
lemniscus (lemnisci)
- lateral l.
- medial l.
- optic l.
- spinal l.
- trigeminal l.

Lendrum's inclusion body stain
Lennert's lymphoma
lens
- capsule of l.
- cortex of l.
- crystalline l.
- l. plate
- suspensory ligament of l.
- l. vesicle

lenticular
- l. fasciculus
- l. nucleus
- l. opacities

lenticulostriate arteries

lentigo (lentigines)
- malignant l.

Lentivirinae
leonine facies
Leon virus
Lepidoptera
lepidopterid larva
Lepiota
- *L. morgani*

lepra
- l. cell
- l. manchada

leprechaun facies
lepromin
leprosy
- l. bacillus
- dimorphous l.
- lazarine l.
- lepromatous l.
- macular l.
- murine l.
- trophoneurotic l.
- tuberculoid l.

leptocyte
leptocytosis
leptokurtic
leptomeninges
leptomeningitis
Leptomitus
- *L. epidermidis*
- *L. urophilus*
- *L. vaginae*

leptomonad
Leptomonas
leptonema
Leptopsylla
- *L. segnis*

Leptosphaeria
- *L. senegalensis*

Leptospira
- *L. australis*

Leptospira (continued)
   L. autumnalis
   L. biflexa
   L. canicola
   L. grippotyphosa
   L. hebdomidis
   L. hyos
   L. icterohaemorrhagiae
   L. interrogans
   L. pomona
leptospirosis
   l. icterohemorrhagica
leptotene
Leptothrix
Leptotrichia
   L. buccalis
   L. placoides
Leptotrombidium
   L. akamushi
   L. deliense
Leptus
Leriche's syndrome
Lesch-Nyhan syndrome
lesion
   bird's nest l.
   central l.
   coin l.
   gross l.
   histologic l.
   impaction l.
   indiscriminate l.
   initial syphilitic l.
   irritative l.
   Janeway's l.
   jet l.
   Kimmelstiel-Wilson l.
   molecular l.
   onion scale l.
   organic l.
   peripheral l.
   precancerous l.
   primary l.

lesion *(continued)*
   ring-wall l.
   structural l.
   systemic l.
   trophic l.
   wire-loop l.
lesser
   l. alar cartilage
   l. curvature, stomach
   l. Galen's vein
   l. omentum
   l. peritoneal sac
   l. saphenous vein
   l. splanchnic nerve
   l. superficial petrosal nerve
LET — linear energy transfer
LE test
lethal
   l. equivalent
Lethane
lethargy
Letterer-Siwe disease
leucine
   l. aminopeptidase
   l. aminotransferase
leucofuchsin
leucovorin
   l. calcium
leucyl-RNA synthetase
leukapheresis
leukemia
   acute granulocytic l.
   acute lymphocytic l.
   acute megakaryoblastic l.
   acute monocytic l.
   acute myelogenous l.
   aleukemic granulocytic l.
   aleukemic lymphocytic l.
   aleukemic monocytic l.
   basophilic l.
   blast l.
   chronic granulocytic l.

leukemia *(continued)*
- chronic lymphocytic l.
- chronic monocytic l.
- chronic myelogenous l.
- compound l.
- eosinophilic l.
- granulocytic l.
- histiocytic l.
- lymphoblastic l.
- lymphocytic l.
- lymphosarcoma cell l.
- mast cell l.
- megakaryocytic l.
- monoblastic l.
- monocytic l.
- monomyelocytic l.
- myeloblastic l.
- myelocytic l.
- myelogenous l.
- myelomonocytic l.
- Naegeli type of monocytic l.
- plasmacytic l.
- promyelocytic l.
- Schilling-type monocytic l.
- stem cell l.
- subleukemic granulocytic l.
- subleukemic lymphocytic l.
- subleukemic monocytic l.
- thrombocytic l.

leukemic
- l. reticuloendotheliosis

leukemogenesis

leukemoid reaction

leukoagglutinins

leukocidin

leukocyte
- l. acid phosphatase stain
- l. alkaline phosphatase
- l. alloantibodies
- l. antigens
- basophilic l.

leukocyte *(continued)*
- l. differential count
- eosinophilic l.
- granular l.
- heterophilic l.
- mast l.
- neutrophilic l.
- polymorphonuclear l.
- transitional l.

leukocytic
- l. margination
- l. maturation
- l. nuclear hypersegmentation
- l. nuclear hyposegmentation

leukocytic infiltrate
- eosinophil l. i.
- polymorphonuclear l. i.

leukocytoblast

leukocytogenesis

leukocytosis
- basophilic l.
- eosinophilic l.
- neutrophilic l.

leukoderma

leukodystrophy
- Krabbe's l.
- metachromatic-type l.
- spongy degenerative-type l.
- sudanophilic l.

leukoencephalitis

leukoencephalopathy
- progressive multifocal l.

leukoerythroblastic
- l. anemia

leukoerythroblastosis

leukoerythrogenetic

leukogram

leukokeratosis

leukokinin

leukoma

leukonychia
leukoparakeratosis
leukopenia
    autoimmune l.
leukophoresis
leukoplakia
leukopoiesis
leukopoietin
leukorrhea
Leukosporidium
leukostasis
leukotaxis
leukotriene
Levaditi's method
levallorphan tartrate
levamphetamine
levan
levarterenol
    l. bitartrate
levator
    l. ani muscle
    l. glandulae thyroideae muscle
    l. muscle of scapula
    l. muscle of thyroid gland
    l. palpebrae branch, oculomotor nerve
    l. scapulae muscle
levatores costarum muscles
level
    barbiturate l.
    ethanol l.
    isoelectric l.
    lead l.
    salicylate l.
Levinson test
levoatrio-cardinal vein
levocardia
    isolated l.
levodopa
levonordefrin
levopropoxyphene
levorotatory
levorphanol
levothyroxine sodium
levulose
Lewis antibodies, Le^a, Le^b
lewisite
Lewy body
Lexosceles
    L. reclusus
Leydig cell hyperplasia
Leydig-Sertoli cell tumor
Leydig's interstitial cells
LF — laryngofissure
    limit flocculation
LFA — left femoral artery
    left frontoanterior
LFN — lactoferrin
LFP — left frontoposterior
LFT — latex flocculation test
    left frontotransverse
    liver function test
LG — left gluteal
    linguogingival
LGB — Landry-Guillain-Barré (syndrome)
LGN — lateral geniculate nucleus
LGV — lymphogranuloma venereum
LH — luteinizing hormone
LHL — left hepatic lobe
LHRF — luteinizing hormone–releasing factor
LI — linguoincisal
LIAFI — late infantile amaurotic familial idiocy
LIBC — latent iron-binding capacity
libido
Libman-Sacks endocarditis
LIC — limiting isorrheic concentration

lichen
- l. nitidus
- l. pilaris
- l. planopilaris
- l. planus
- l. planus, atrophic
- l. planus, bullous
- l. planus, hypertrophic
- l. sclerosus et atrophicus
- l. scrofulosorum
- l. simplex chronicus
- l. striatus

lichenase
lichenification
lichenoid
- l. dermatitis
- pigmented purpuric l. dermatitis

Lichtheimia corymbifera
lid
- granular l.
- l. lag

lidocaine
Lieberkühn's crypts
Liebermann-Burchardt reaction
LIF — left iliac fossa
lig — ligament
ligament
- acromioclavicular joint l.
- alar l.
- ankle joint l.
- annular l.
- arcuate l.
- arteriosum l.
- broad l.
- capsular l.
- carpometacarpal joint l.
- clitoral l.
- coccygeal l.
- conoid l.
- Cooper's suspensory l's
- coronary l.

ligament *(continued)*
- cruciate l.
- deltoid l.
- dentate l.
- denticulate l.
- diaphragmatic l.
- distal tibiofibular joint l.
- elbow joint l.
- epididymal l.
- falciform l.
- flaval l.
- gastrocolic l.
- gastrohepatic l.
- gastrophrenic l.
- gastrosplenic l.
- hepatoduodenal l.
- hepatorenal l.
- hip joint l.
- iliolumbar l.
- inguinal l.
- interphalangeal joint l.
- intraarticular l.
- ischiofemoral l.
- knee joint l.
- laryngeal l.
- lens l.
- liver l.
- lower extremity l.
- lumbosacral joint l.
- lung l.
- metacarpophalangeal joint l.
- metatarsophalangeal joint l.
- midcarpal joint l.
- midtarsal joint l.
- neck l.
- nuchal l.
- omental l.
- ossicular l.
- ovarian l.
- patellar l.
- pectinate l.

ligament *(continued)*
- l. of penis
- l. of perineum
- phrenicocolic l.
- proximal tibiofibular joint l.
- l. of pubic symphysis
- pulmonary l.
- radiocarpal joint l.
- round l.
- sacrococcygeal joint l.
- sacroiliac joint l.
- shoulder l.
- sternoclavicular joint l.
- superior radioulnar joint l.
- suspensory l.
- talocalcaneonavicular joint l.
- talocrural joint l.
- tarsometatarsal joint l.
- tracheal l.
- trapezoid l.
- triangular l.
- trunk l.
- umbilical l.
- upper extremity l.
- uterine l.
- uterosacral l.

ligamentum (ligamenta)
- l. arteriosum
- l. denticulatum
- l. flavum
- l. nuchae
- l. teres
- l. venosum

ligand
ligandin
ligase
ligate
ligation
ligature

light
- actinic l.
- l. chain
- coherent l.
- cold l.
- idioretinal l.
- infrared l.
- intrinsic l.
- l. microscope
- monochromatic l.
- polarized l.
- l. reflex
- refracted l.
- transmitted l.
- ultraviolet l.

lignoceric acid
ligroin
ligula
- l. intestinalis

Lillie's
- allochrome method
- hematoxylin

limb
- anacrotic l.
- l. bud
- catacrotic l.
- flail l.
- girdle-type progressive muscular dystrophy l.
- phantom l.
- thoracic l.

limbic system
limbus (limbi)
limen insulae
limit
- assimilation l.
- l. dextrinosis
- l. of flocculation
- quantum l.
- l. of resolution
- saturation l.

Limnatis
    L. granulosa
    L. mysomelas
    L. nilotica
limonene
Limulus
    L. polyphemus
lincomycin
lindane
Lindau–von Hippel disease
line
    absorption l.
    Beau's l's
    cervical l.
    l. filter
    l. focus
    Gennari's l.
    Hunter-Schreger l's
    M l.
    Reid's base l.
    l.-spread function
    Ullmann's l.
    Zahn's l's
linear
    l. accelerator
    l. attenuation coefficient
    l. energy transfer
    l. equation
    l. focus
    l. fracture
    l. regression
Lineweaver-Burke equation
lingual
    l. artery
    l. branch
    l. gyrus
    l. muscle
    l. nerve
    l. papillae
    l. thyroid
    l. tonsil

Linguatula
    L. serrata
linguatuliasis
linguatulid
lingula (lingulae)
lingular
    l. branch
    l. bronchus
linitis
    l. plastica
linkage
    chromosomal l.
    l. disequilibrium
linoleate
linoleic acid
linseed
Linstowiidae
liothyronine
liotrix
lip
    cleft l.
    rhombic l.
lipase
lipedema
lipemia
    alimentary l.
    l. retinalis
lipid
    aggregate alteration l., extracellular
    aggregate l., nuclear
    l. degeneration
    l. depletion
    l. disorder
    l. histiocytosis
    l. nephrosis
    l. peroxidation
    l. pneumonia
    l. storage disease
    l. transport
lipidase

lipidemia
lipidosis
    cerebroside l.
lipiduria
lipiodol
lipoamide dehydrogenase
lipoate acetyltransferase
lipoatrophy
lipoblastomatosis
lipochondrodystrophy
lipochrome pigmentation
lipocyte
lipodystrophy
    congenital l.
    inferior l.
    insulin l.
    intestinal l.
    progressive l.
lipofuscin
lipofuscinosis
lipogenesis
lipogranuloma
lipogranulomatosis
    Farber's l.
lipoic acid
lipoid
    l. degeneration
    l. dystrophy
    l. granuloma
    l. nephrosis
    l. pneumonia
    l. proteinosis
lipoidosis
lipolysis
lipoma
    fetal l.
    fetal fat cell l.
lipomatosis
lipomelanotic reticuloendo-
    thelial cell hyperplasia
liponisus. *See Lyponyssus.*

lipoprotein
    l. chylomicron
    l. lipase
lipoproteinemia
liposarcoma
liposome
lipotrophic
lipotropic
β-lipotropin
lipoxygenase
LIQ — lower inner quadrant
liquefaction
liquefactive
    l. degeneration
    l. necrosis
liquid
    l. chromatography
    l. crystal
    l. junction potential
    l. scintillation counter
LIS — lobular in situ
Lison-Dunn method
Lissauer's tract
lissencephaly
Listeria
    L. monocytogenes
listerosis
liter
lithic acid
lithium
    l. carbonate
    l. citrate
lithocholic acid
lithopedion
lithotomy
lithotroph
litmus
Little's disease
liver
    caudate lobe of l.
    l. cell adenoma

liver *(continued)*
    l. cell carcinoma
    central veins of l.
    l. fluke
    l. grooves
    left lobe of l.
    ligament of l.
    lymphatics of l.
    quadrate lobe of l.
    right lobe of l.
livor mortis
lixiviation
LJM — Löwenstein-Jensen medium
LK — left kidney
LL — left leg
    left lung
    lower lobe
    lysolecithin
LLF — Laki-Lorand factor
LLL — left lower lobe
LLM — localized leukocyte mobilization
LLQ — left lower quadrant
LM — light microscopy
    linguomesial
LMA — left mentoanterior
LMD, LMDX — low molecular weight dextran
LMP — left mentoposterior
LMT — left mentotransverse
LMW — low molecular weight
LMWD — low molecular weight dextran
LN — lipoid nephrosis
    lupus nephritis
    lymph node
LNPF — lymph node permeability factor
LO — linguo-occlusal
LOA — left occipitoanterior

Loa
    L. loa
lobar
    l. cerebral atrophy
    l. pneumonia
    l. pulmonary atrophy
lobe
    azygos l.
    cerebellar l.
    cruciate l.
    cuneiform l.
    digastric l.
    flocculonodular l.
    frontal l.
    hepatic l's
    occipital l.
    parietal l.
    Riedel's l.
    temporal l.
lobectomy
lobeline
Loboa loboi
lobomycosis
Lobo's disease
lobster claw deformity
lobular
    l. adenocarcinoma
    l. carcinoma
    l. carcinoma, infiltrating
    l. carcinoma in situ
    l. duct
    l. glomerulonephritis
    l. pneumonia
lobulation
    fetal l.
lobule
lobulus simplex
lobus (lobi)
localization
lochia
lockjaw

locomotor
   l. ataxia
locus coeruleus
Löffler's
   blood serum
   myocarditis
logarithm
   napierian l.
logarithmic
   l. curve
   l. phase
logit
lognormal distribution
loiasis
longissimus muscle
longitudinal
   l. caudate vein
   l. cerebral fissure
   l. duct of epoophoron
   l. fasciculi of pons
longus
   l. capitis muscle
   l. colli muscle
loop
   capillary l's
   Henle's l.
   ventricular l.
LOP – left occipitoposterior
lophotrichous
LOQ – lower outer quadrant
lorazepam
lordoscoliosis
lordosis
lordotic
LOT – left occipitotransverse
louping ill
louping ill virus
louse (lice)
   body l.
   l.-borne typhus
   chicken l.
   head l.

louse (lice) *(continued)*
   pubic l.
low density lipoprotein
Löwenstein-Jensen medium
lower
   l. extremity
   l. nephron nephrosis
   l. respiratory fluids
   l. respiratory spaces
   l. respiratory tract
   l. third of vagina
   l. trunk
   l. uterine segment
loxapine
   l. hydrochloride
   l. succinate
Loxosceles
   L. laeta
   L. reclusa
LP – latency period
   leukocyte-poor
   light perception
   linguopulpal
   lipoprotein
   low protein
   lumbar puncture
   lymphoid plasma
L/P – lactate-pyruvate ratio
LPA – left pulmonary artery
LPC – late positive component
LPE – lipoprotein electrophoresis
LPF – leukocytosis-promoting factor
   localized plaque formation
   low-power field
   lymphocytosis-promoting factor
LPH – lipotropin
LPL – lipoprotein lipase
lpm – liters per minute

LPO – left posterior oblique
LPS – lipopolysaccharide
LPV – left pulmonary veins
LR – laboratory references
  lactated Ringer's (solution)
  light reaction
L/R – left to right ratio
L & R – left and right
L → R – left to right
Lr – lawrencium
LRF – luteinizing hormone-releasing factor
LRH – luteinizing hormone-releasing hormone
LRQ – lower right quadrant
LRS – lactated Ringer's solution
LRT – lower respiratory tract
LS – lumbosacral
  lymphosarcoma
LSA – left sacroanterior
  lymphosarcoma
LSA/RCS – lymphosarcoma-reticulum cell sarcoma
LSB – left sternal border
LScA – left scapuloanterior
LScP – left scapuloposterior
LSCS – lower segment cesarean section
LSD – lysergic acid diethylamide
LSH – lymphocyte-stimulating hormone
LSM – late systolic murmur
LSP – left sacroposterior
L/S ratio – lecithin-sphingomyelin ratio
LST – left sacrotransverse
LSV – left subclavian vein
LT – levothyroxine
  lymphotoxin

LTB – laryngotracheobronchitis
LTH – lactogenic hormone
  luteotropic hormone
lt lat – left lateral
LTPP – lipothiamide pyrophosphate
LU – left upper
  lutetium
L & U – lower and upper
Lubarsch's crystals
lucanthone hydrochloride
Lucilia
lückenschädel
Ludwig's angina
lues
Lugol's solution
LUL – left upper lobe
lumbago
lumbar
  l. artery
  l. lymph node
  l. myotome
  l. nerve
  l. plexus
  l. spinal cord
  l. splanchnic nerve
  l. sympathetic nervous system
  l. vein
  l. vertebra
lumbosacral
  l. plexus
  l. spinal cord
lumbricales pedis muscles
lumbrical muscle
lumbricosis
lumbricus (lumbrici)
lumen (lumina)
  bronchial l.
  colonic l.
  duodenal l.

lumen (lumina) *(continued)*
   epididymal l.
   esophageal l.
   fallopian tube l.
   gastric l.
   ileal l.
   intestinal l.
   jejunal l.
   rectal l.
   seminal vesicle l.
   tracheal l.
   ureteral l.
   urethral l.
   vas deferens l.
luminescence
luminophore
luminous
   l. flux
   l. flux density
   l. intensity
lunate bone
lung
   bilobed right l.
   eosinophilic l.
   l. fluke
   hyperlucent l.
   rudimentary l.
   shock l.
Lunyo virus
lupinine
lupoid
   l. hepatitis
lupus
   hydralazine l.
   laryngeal l.
   l. nephritis
   l. pernio
   l. tumidus
   l. vulgaris
lupus erythematosus
   acute disseminated l. e.
   cell l. e.

lupus erythematosus *(continued)*
   chronic discoid l. e.
   disseminated l. e.
   systemic l. e.
LUQ — left upper quadrant
Luschka's
   crypts
   ducts
   foramen
luteal
   l. cyst
   l. phase
lutein
luteinization
luteinized follicular cyst
luteinizing hormone
Lutembacher's syndrome
luteoma
luteotropic
   l. hormone
luteotropin
lutetium
lututrin
luxation
Luys' nucleus
LV — left ventricle
   leukemia virus
   live virus
LVDP — left ventricular diastolic pressure
LVE — left ventricular enlargement
LVEDP — left ventricular end-diastolic pressure
LVEDV — left ventricular end-diastolic volume
LVET — left ventricular ejection time
LVF — left ventricular failure
   low-voltage fast
   low-voltage foci

LVH — large vessel hematocrit
    left ventricular hypertrophy
LVP — left ventricular pressure
    lysine vasopressin
LVS — left ventricular strain
LVSP — left ventricular systolic pressure
LVSV — left ventricular stroke volume
LVSW — left ventricular stroke work
LVW — left ventricular work
LVWI — left ventricular work index
LW — Lee-White (method)
LX — local irradiation
lyase
lycopene
lycopenemia
Lymnaea
lymph
    aplastic l.
    corpuscular l.
    euplastic l.
    glycerinated l.
    intercellular l.
    plastic l.
    vaccine l.
lymphadenitis
    dermatopathic l.
lymphadenopathy
    dermatopathic l.
lymphangiectasis
lymphangioendothelial sarcoma
lymphangioma
lymphangiosarcoma
lymphangitis
lymphatic
    l. cord
    l. duct
    l. follicle

lymphatic *(continued)*
    l. system
    l. trunks
    l. vessels
lymphedema — tardum
lymphmonocyte
lymph node
    Cloquet's l. n.
    Rosenmüller's l. n.
lymphoblast
lymphoblastic
    l. leukemia
    l. lymphosarcoma
lymphoblastoma
lymphoblastomid
lymphoblastosis
lymphocytapheresis
lymphocyte
    atypical l.
    circulating atypical l.
    Downey-type l.
    plasmacytoid l.
lymphocytic
    l. cells
    l. choriomeningitis
    l. choriomeningitis virus
    l. inflammatory infiltrate
    l. leukemia
    l. lymphoma
    l. lymphosarcoma
    l. thyroiditis
    l. tissue
lymphocytoblast
lymphocytolysis
lymphocytoma
lymphocytopenia
lymphocytopoiesis
lymphocytorrhexis
lymphocytosis
    neutrophilic l.
    l.-promoting factor
lymphocytotoxicity

lymphocytotoxin
lymphoepithelial
lymphoepithelioma
lymphogranuloma
   l. venereum
   l. venereum virus
lymphoid
   l. hyperplasia
   l. hypoplasia
   l. leukocyte
   l. polyp
   l. stem cell
lymphoid nodule
   appendiceal l. n.
   colonic solitary l. n.
   rectal solitary l. n.
   small intestine l. n.
lymphokine
lymphokinesis
lymphoma
   benign l.
   follicular l.
   giant follicle l.
   histiocytic l.
   Lennert's l.
   lymphocytic l.
   macrofollicular l.
   malignant l., lymphosarcoma type
   nodular l.
   stem cell l.
lymphomatoid
   l. granulomatosis
   l. papulosis
lymphomatous
lymphopathia venereum
lymphopenia
lymphoplasmapheresis
lymphoproliferative syndrome
lymphoreticular
lymphorrhea
lymphosarcoma
   cell leukemia l.
   lymphoblastic l.
   lymphocytic l.
   reticulum cell l.
lymphotoxin
lymphs — lymphocytes
Lyon hypothesis
lyophilization
lyophilize
Lyponyssus
lysate
lyse
lysemia
lysergic acid diethylamide
lysin
lysine
   l. dehydrogenase
   l. intolerance
   l. ketoglutarate reductase
   l. oxidoreductase
   l. oxoglutaryl reductase
   l. racemase
lysing
lysis
lysochrome
lysogeny
lysokinase
lysolecithin
   l. acylmutase
lysophosphatidate
lysophosphatidyl choline
lysophosphatidylethanolamine
lysophospholipase
lysosomal
   l. storage disease
lysosome
   l. alteration
   primary l.
   secondary l.
lysostaphin

MAC Mycobaterium avium complex

lysozyme
lysyl-RNA synthetase

lzm — lysozyme

M

M — macerate
  male
  maximal
  mega
  minim
  molar
  mucoid
  multipara
  murmur
  muscle
  myopia
  permanent molar
  strength of pole
  thousand (mil, milli)
M_1 — mitral first sound
M. — *Micrococcus*
  Microsporum
  Mycobacterium
  Mycoplasma
m — meter
μ — micron
  mu
MA — mandelic acid
  mean arterial (blood pressure)
  Miller-Abbott (tube)
Ma — masurium
ma — milliampere
MAA — macroaggregated albumin
MABP — mean arterial blood pressure
MAC — maximum allowable concentration
  minimum alveolar concentration

MacCallum's patch
Macchiavello's stain
MacConkey agar
macerated
  m. fetus
  m. stillbirth
maceration
Machado-Guerreiro test
Mache unit
machine
  m. language
Macracanthorhynchus
  M. hirudinaceus
macroaggregate
macroaleuriospore
macroamylase
macroamylasemia
Macrobdella
macroblast
macrocephaly
macroconidium (macroconidia)
macrocyte
macrocythemia
  hyperchromatic m.
macrocytic
  m. anemia
macrocytosis
macrodystrophia
macrofollicular
  m. adenoma
  m. lymphoma
macrogamete
macrogametocyte
macrogenitosomia
macroglia
macroglobulin

312 MACROGLOBULINEMIA – MAGNESIUM

macroglobulinemia
   Waldenström's m.
macroglossia
macrogyria
macrohomology
macrolide
macromastia
macromethod
   m. of Wintrobe
macromolecular
macromolecule
   m. aggregate alteration, extracellular
   crystalline m. alteration
   nuclear m's
Macromonas
   M. bipunctata
   M. mobilis
macromonocyte
macromyeloblast
macronormoblast
macronucleus
macrophage
   m. activation factor
   m. agglutination factor
   m. chemotactic factor
   m. migration inhibition factor
Macrophoma
macropolycyte
macroreticulocyte
macroscopic
macrosomia
Macrostoma mesnili
macrostomia
macrothrombocyte
macula (maculae)
   acoustic m.
   m. adherens
   maculae caeruleae
   m. cribrosa
   m. densa

macula (maculae) *(continued)*
   m. lutea
   m. occludens
   m. retinae
macular
   m. atrophy
macule
maculopapular
MAD – maximal acid output
Madura foot
Madurella
   M. grisea
   M. mycetomi
maduromycetoma
maduromycosis
maduromycotic mycetoma
maedivirus
MAF – macrophage activation factor
mafenide
Maffucci's syndrome
MAFH – macroaggregated ferrous hydroxide
magaldrate
Magendie's foramen
magenta
   acid m.
   basic m.
   m. O
   m. I, II, III
MAggF – macrophage agglutination factor
maggot
   Congo floor m.
magnesia
   m. alba
   m. calcinata
   m. carbonatada
   m. usta
magnesium
   m. ammonium phosphate
   m. carbonate

magnesium *(continued)*
- m. citrate
- m. hydrate
- m. hydroxide
- m. isotope
- m. oxide
- m. phosphate
- m. salt
- m. sulfate
- m. trisilicate

magnet

magnetic
- m. core memory
- m. field
- m. field strength
- m. flux
- m. induction
- m. moment
- m. susceptibility

magnetization

magneton
- Bohr m.

magnification

magnify

Majocchi's
- disease
- granuloma

major histocompatibility complex

malabsorption syndrome

malachite green

malacia

malacoplakia
- m. vesicae

maladie
- m. de Roger

maladjustment

malaise

malakoplakia

malaria
- algid m.
- bilious remittent m.

malaria *(continued)*
- bovine m.
- falciparum m.
- gastric m.
- hemolytic m.
- hemorrhagic m.
- ovale m.
- pernicious m.
- vivax m.

malariacidal

malarial
- m. pigment deposition

Malassezia
- *M. furfur*
- *M. macfadyani*
- *M. tropica*

malate
- decarboxylating m. dehydrogenase
- m. dehydrogenase
- m. oxidase

malathion

Malayan filariasis

male
- m. genital fluids
- m. genital spaces
- m. genitalia
- m. pseudohermaphroditism
- m. sex chromatin pattern
- m. urethra

maleic hydrazide

maleylacetoacetate isomerase

malformation
- Arnold-Chiari m.
- congenital m.
- Ebstein's m.

malfunction

Malherbe's calcifying epithelioma

malic
- m. acid
- m. enzyme

malignancy
malignant
   m. giant cell tumor of bone
   m. hypertension
   m. lymphocytoma
   m. lymphoma
   m. lymphoma, lymphosarcoma type
   m. melanoma
   m. meningioma
   m. neoplasm
   m. tumor
mallein
malleolar
   m. artery
   m. bursa
malleolus (malleoli)
Malleomyces
   M. mallei
   M. pseudomallei
   M. whitmori
malleomycosis
malleus
Mallophaga
Mallory's
   bodies
   collagen stain
Mallory-Weiss syndrome
Malmejde's test
malnutrition
malocclusion
malonate coenzyme A-transferase
malonic acid
malonyl-coenzyme A decarboxylase
malpighian follicle
malposition
malrotation
   intestinal m.
Malta fever
malt agar

maltase
maltose
   m. 4-glucosyltransferase
maltoside
maltosuria
MAM — methylazomethanol
M+Am — myopic astigmatism
mam — milliampere-minute
mamillary
   m. bodies
   m. peduncle
   m. peduncular nucleus
mammal
mammalgia
Mammalia
mammalian
mammary
   m. artery
   m. connective tissue
   m. duct
   m. duct ectasia
   m. dysplasia
   m. fluids
   m. gland lymphatics
   m. lobule
   m. lymphatics
   m. Paget's disease
mammography
mammotropic
mammotropin
Mandelin's reagent
mandible
mandibular
   m. arch
   m. cyst
   m. gingiva
   m. lymph node
   m. nerve
   m. torus
mandibulofacial dysostosis
maneuver
   Valsalva's m.

manganese
   m. ethylene bis-dithiocarbamate
   m. isotope
   m. salt
manganic
manganism
manganous
manifestation
mannans
mannitol
   m. dehydrogenase
   m. hexanitrate
   m.-1-phosphate dehydrogenase
mannoheptulose
mannoheptulosuria
mannokinase
mannose
mannosephosphate isomerase
alpha-mannosidase
mannosidosis (mannosidoses)
manometer
MANOVA — multivariate analysis of variance
Mansonella ozzardi
mansonelliasis
Mansonia
Mansonioides
mantle layer, embryonic
Mantoux
   conversion
   diameter
   skin test
manubrium (manubria)
MAO — maximal acid output
      monoamine oxidase
MAOI — monoamine oxidase inhibitor
MAP — mean aortic pressure
      mean arterial pressure

MAP *(continued)*
      megaloblastic anemia of pregnancy
      methylacetoxyprogesterone
      methylaminopurine
      muscle-action potential
MAPF — microatomized protein food
maple
   m. bark strippers' disease
   m. syrup urine disease
Maragiliano body
marantic
   m. atrophy
   m. endocarditis
   m. thrombus
marasmus
marble bone disease
Marburg
   agent
   virus disease
march
Marchiafava-Bignami disease
Marchiafava-Micheli syndrome
marcy agent
Marfan's syndrome
margin
marginal
   m. gyrus
   m. insertion of umbilical cord
   m. layer, embryonic
   m. sulcus
   m. venous sinus
margination
   leukocytic m.
Marie's disease
Marie-Strumpell disease
marihuana
Marituba virus

marker
  m. chromosome
  genetic m.
Marochetti's blisters
Maroteaux-Lamy syndrome
Marquis reagent
marrow
  basophilic m.
  bone m.
  eosinophilic m.
  erythrocytic m.
  leukocytic m.
  lymphocytic m.
  monocytic m.
  neutrophilic m.
  m. platelets
  reticulocytic m.
marsupial
marsupialization
Martin-Lester agar
mas — milliampere-second
masculinization
  ovarian m.
masculinovoblastoma
MASER — microwave amplification by stimulated emission of radiation
  molecular application by stimulated emission of radiation
mask
  Venturi m.
mass
  m. action law
  m. attenuation coefficient
  m. concentration
  m. fragmentography
  m. number
  m. reflex
  m. spectrograph
  m. spectrometer
  m. spectrometry

mass *(continued)*
  m. storage
massage
  cardiac m.
  m. effect
massa intermedia
masseter
  m. fascia
  m. muscle
masseteric
massive
  m. embolus
Masson
  stain
  trichrome method
mastadenovirus
mastalgia
mast cell
  m. c. hyperplasia
  m. c. leukemia
  m. c. sarcoma
  m. c. tumor
mastectomy
Master two-step test
mastication
Mastigophora
mastigophorous
mastigote
mastitis
  chronic cystic m.
  fibrocystic m.
  plasma cell m.
mastocytoma
mastocytosis
mastodynia
mastography
mastoid
  m. antrum
  m. cells
mastoiditis
mastopathy
  fibrocystic m.

Masugi-type nephrotoxic serum nephritis
mathematical logic
matrilineal
matrix alteration
  bone m. a.
  cartilage m. a.
  extracellular m. a.
  fibrocartilage m. a.
matt
maturation alteration
  hematopoietic m. a.
  leukocytic m. a.
maturation arrest, hematopoietic
mature
  m. abnormal chorion
  m. abnormal chorionic villi
  m. abnormal placenta
  m. ovarian follicle
maturity
Maurer's dots
max. — maximum
maxilla (maxillae)
maxillary
  m. antrum
  m. artery
  m. gingiva
  m. nerve
  m. process
  m. sinus
maximal
  m. acid output
  m. breathing capacity
  m. expiratory flow rate
  m. expiratory flow volume
  m. midexpiratory flow rate
  m. voluntary ventilation
maximum (maxima)
maxwell
Mayaro virus
Mayer's
  acid alum hematoxylin stain
  hematoxylin
May-Grünwald-Giemsa stain
May-Hegglin anomaly
mazoplasia
Mazzotti test
MB — mesiobuccal
  methylene blue
  microbiological assay
Mb — myoglobin
m.b. — mix well
MBA — methylbovine albumin
M band
MBAS — methylene blue active substance
MBC — maximal breathing capacity
  minimal bactericidal concentration
MBD — methylene blue dye
  minimal brain damage
  minimal brain dysfunction
  Morquio-Brailsford disease
MBF — myocardial blood flow
MBK — methyl butyl ketone
MBL — minimal bactericidal level
MBO — mesiobucco-occlusal
MBP — antigen prepared from *Brucella melitensis*, *B. bovis* and *B. suis*
  mean blood pressure
  mesiobuccopulpal
MBSA — methylated bovine serum albumin
MC — mast cell
  maximum concentration

MC *(continued)*
    metacarpal
    mineralocorticoid
    myocarditis
    mytomycin-C
Mc — megacurie
    megacycle
mC — millicoulomb
mc, mCi or MCU — millicurie
MCA — methylcholanthrene
    middle cerebral artery
    multichannel analyzer
McArdle-Schmid-Pearson disease
McArdle's syndrome
MCB — membranous cytoplasmic body
MCBR — minimum concentration of bilirubin
MCC — mean corpuscular hemoglobin concentration
    minimum complete-killing concentration
McCallum's plaque
MC concentration
MCD — mean cell diameter
    mean of consecutive differences
    mean corpuscular diameter
    medullary cystic disease
MCF — macrophage chemotactic factor
MCFA — medium-chain fatty acid
mcg or μg — microgram
MCH — mean corpuscular hemoglobin
mch — millicurie-hour
MCHC — mean corpuscular hemoglobin concentration
MCHg — mean corpuscular hemoglobin
MCI — mean cardiac index
mCi — millicurie
MCL — midclavicular line
    midcostal line
McLeod phenotype
McMaster technique
M colony
M component
MCP — metacarpophalangeal
    mitotic-control protein
mc p s — megacycles per second
MCR — metabolic clearance rate
MCT — mean cell threshold
    mean circulation time
    mean corpuscular thickness
    medium-chain triglyceride
MCTD — mixed connective tissue disease
MCV — mean corpuscular volume
MD — malic dehydrogenase
    Mantoux diameter
    Marek's disease
    movement disorder
    muscular dystrophy
    myocardial damage
    myocardial disease
Md — mendelevium
MDA — mentodextra anterior
    methylenedioxyamphetamine
    motor discriminative acuity

MDC — minimum detectable concentration
MDF — mean dominant frequency
myocardial depressant factor
MDH — malic dehydrogenase
MDHV — Marek's herpesvirus disease
MDP — mentodextra posterior
MDT — median detection threshold
mentodextra transversa
MDTR — mean diameter-thickness ratio
MDUO — myocardial disease of unknown origin
ME — mercaptoethanol
M/E — myeloid-erythroid ratio
Me — methyl
MEA — mercaptoethylamine
multiple endocrine adenomatosis

mean
    arithmetical m.
    m. arterial pressure
    m. cell diameter
    m. cell threshold
    m. of consecutive differences
    m. corpuscular diameter
    m. corpuscular hemoglobin
    m. corpuscular hemoglobin concentration
    m. corpuscular volume
    m. deviation
    m. effective life
    geometric m.
    m. square deviation
    m. time between failures
    trimmed m.
    windsorized m.

measles
    German m. virus
    virus m.
measure
meatus (meattus, meatuses)
    external auditory m.
    internal acoustic m.
    nasal m.
    urethral m.
    urinary m.
mebutamate
mecamylamine
mechanical
    m. ileus
    m. ventilation
mechanism
    countercurrent m.
    Frank-Starling m.
    oculogyric m.
    somatic m.
    splanchnic m.
mechlorethamine
mecillinam
Mecistocirrhus
Meckel's
    cartilage
    diverticulum
meclizine hydrochloride
meconium
    m. extravasation
    m. ileus
    m. peritonitis
    m. retention
MED — minimal erythema dose
med — median
medial
    m. cystic necrosis
    m. degeneration
    m. fasciculus
    m. lemniscus
    Mönckeberg's m. calcification

medial *(continued)*
- m. necrosis of aorta
- m. nucleus

median
- m. aperture
- m. cubital vein
- m. eminence
- m. forebrain
- m. lobe branch
- m. nerve

mediastinal
- m. artery
- m. emphysema
- m. lymph node
- m. pleura
- m. shift
- m. vein

mediastinitis
mediastinopericarditis
mediastinoscopy
mediastinum (mediastina)
Medical Internal Radiation Dose
medina infection
mediolateral
medionecrosis
- m. aortae idiopathica cystica
- cystic m.

Mediterranean
- anemia
- fever

medium (media)
- Apathy's gum syrup m.
- Balamuth's culture m.
- Boeck-Drbohlav-Locke egg serum m.
- clearing m.
- contrast m.
- culture m.
- differential m.
- dispersive m.

medium (media) *(continued)*
- Farrant's m.
- glycerol gelatin m.
- Lash's casein hydrolysate-serum m.
- Löwenstein-Jensen m.
- Novy, MacNeal and Nicolle's m.
- nutrient m.
- oxidation-fermentation m.
- PVA-lacto-phenol m.
- radiopaque m.
- Rees's culture m.
- refracting m.
- separating m.
- thioglycollate m.
- Tobie, von Brand and Mehlman's diphasic m.
- transport m.
- Weinman's m.

medium-chain triglycerides
medroxyprogesterone
medulla (medullae)
- adrenal m.
- kidney m.
- ovary m.
- renal m.
- spinal m.
- suprarenal m.
- thymic m.

medulla oblongata
- arcuate nucleus of m. o.
- dorsal lateral sulcus of m. o.
- dorsal median sulcus of m. o.
- dorsal spinocerebellar tract of m. o.
- dorsal spinothalamic tract of m. o.
- external arcuate fibers of m. o.

medulla oblongata *(continued)*
   fasciculus cuneatus of m. o.
   fasciculus gracilis of m. o.
   internal arcuate fibers of m. o.
   lateral nucleus of m. o.
   medial lemniscus of m. o.
   medial longitudinal fasciculus of m. o.
   raphe of m. o.
   reticular formation of m. o.
   tectospinal tract of m. o.
   ventral lateral sulcus of m. o.
   ventral median fissure of m. o.
   ventral spinocerebellar tract of m. o.
   ventral spinothalamic tract of m. o.
medullary
   m. adenocarcinoma
   m. carcinoma
   m. cystic disease
   m. fibrosarcoma
   m. histiocytic reticulosis
   m. lamina
   m. necrosis
   m. reticulosis
medulloblast
medulloblastoma
medulloepithelioma
MEF – maximal expiratory flow
MEFR – maximal expiratory flow rate
MEFV – maximal expiratory flow volume
MEG – megakaryocytes
megacolon
   aganglionic m.
   chronic idiopathic m.

megacolon *(continued)*
   toxic m.
megacycle
megaelectron volt
megaesophagus
megahertz
megakaryoblast
megakaryocyte
megakaryocytic
   m. aplasia
   m. cells
   m. hyperplasia
   m. hypoplasia
   m. leukemia
   m. myelosis
megakaryocytopoiesis
   extramedullary m.
megakaryocytosis
megalencephaly
megaloblast
megaloblastic
   m. anemia
   m. erythropoiesis
megaloblastoid
megaloblastosis
megalocyte
megaloureter
Megaselia
Megasphaera
megathrombocyte
megavolt
megestrol acetate
meglumine
   m. diatrizoate
   m. iodipramide
megohm
meibomian
   m. cyst
   m. gland
Meigs' syndrome
Meinicke turbidity reaction
meiocyte

meiosis
meiotic
Meissner's
   corpuscle
   nerve plexus
MEK — methyl ethyl ketone
melancholia
   involutional m.
melanin
   m. pigmentation
melanoameloblastoma
melanoblast
melanocarcinoma
melanocyte
   m.-inhibiting hormone
   m.-stimulating hormone
melanocytic
   m. nevus
melanoderma
melanogen
melanoglossia
Melanoides
Melanolestes
   M. picipes
melanoma
   acral lentiginous m.
   amelanotic m.
   desmoplastic m.
   epithelioid cell m.
   juvenile m.
   lentigo maligna m.
   malignant m.
   nodular m.
   spindle cell m.
melanophage
melanophore
melanoplakia
melanosarcoma
melanosis
   m. coli
   Riehl's m.
   vagabond's m.

melanosome
melanotic
   m. freckle of Hutchinson
   m. progonoma
melanuria
melarsonyl potassium
melarsoprol
melasma
melatonin
melena
melioidosis
melitose
melituria
   glycosuric m.
   m. inosita
   nondiabetic glycosuric m.
Melkersson's syndrome
Meloidae
Meloidogyne
   M. javanica
melon seed body
melorheostosis
melphalan
MEM — minimum essential medium
membrane
   acute inflammatory m.
   acute pyogenic m.
   Bowman's m.
   Bruch's basal m.
   cloacal m.
   Descemet's m.
   diphtheritic m.
   exocelomic m.
   fetal m's
   hyaline m.
   inflammatory m.
   mucous m.
   placental m.
   pupillary m.
   pyogenic m.
   Reissner's m.

membrane *(continued)*
    Shrapnell's m.
    spiral m.
    synovial m.
    tectorial m.
    tympanic m.
membranelle
membranoproliferative glomerulonephritis
membranous
    m. acute inflammation
    m. ampulla
    m. glomerulonephritis
    m. labyrinth
    m. nephropathy
MEN — multiple endocrine neoplasia
menadiol sodium diphosphate
menadione reductase
menaquinone
menarche
mendelevium
mendelian
Mendel's law
Menetrier's disease
Mengo virus
Meniere's disease
meningeal
    m. artery
    m. sarcoma
    m. sarcomatosis
    m. spaces
meninges
meningioma
    angiomatous m.
    fibroblastic m.
    malignant m.
    meningothelial m.
    psammomatous m.
meningiomatosis
    diffuse m.
meningismus

meningitis (meningitides)
    amebic m.
    aseptic m.
    bacterial m.
    cryptococcal m.
    meningococcal m.
    mycotic m.
    pyogenic m.
    syphilitic m.
    torular m.
    tuberculous m.
    viral m.
meningocele
meningocerebritis
meningococcal
meningococcemia
meningoccin
meningococcus (meningococci)
meningocyte
meningoencephalitis
meningoencephalocele
meningoencephalomyelitis
meningoencephalopathy
    carcinomatous m.
meningomyelitis
meningomyelocele
meningomyeloradiculitis
meningothelial meningioma
meniscocyte
meniscus (menisci)
Menkes' syndrome
menometrorrhagia
menopausal
    m. endometrium
    m. gonadotropin
    m. syndrome
menopause
menorrhagia
menostasis
menses
menstrual
    m. cycle

menstrual *(continued)*
   m. disorder
   m. endometrium
   m. fluid
   m. involution
menstruation
   vicarious m.
mental
   m. deficiency
   m. disturbance
   m. retardation
mentalis muscle
menthol
Menzies' method
mep — meperidine
meparfynol
mepazine acetate
mepenzolate
meperidine
mephenesin
mephenoxalone
mephentermine
mephenytoin
mephobarbital
mepivacaine hydrochloride
MEPP — miniature end-plate potential
meprobamate
meprylcaine hydrochloride
mEq or meq — milliequivalent
MER — mean ejection rate
        methanol-extruded residue
MER-29 — triparanol
meralluride
merbromin
mercaptan
mercaptoacetic acid
mercaptoethanol
mercaptoethylamine
mercaptoethylguanidine
mercaptomerin sodium
mercaptopurine
3-mercaptopyruvate sulfurtransferase
mercocresols
mercumatilin
mercuriacetate
mercurialism
mercuric
   m. acetate
   m. chloride
   m. cyanoguanidine
   m. dicyanodiamine
   m. iodide
   m. oxide
   m. phosphate
   m. salt
mercurichloride, hydroxyphenyl
mercurous chloride
mercury
   ammoniated m.
   m. bichloride
   m. chloride
   m. isotope
   m. oxycyanide
   m. phosphate
merethoxylline procaine
Merkel's
   cell
   corpuscle
   tactile disc
mermithid
Mermithidae
Mermithoidea
merocrine
Merodicein
merogony
   diploid m.
   parthenogenetic m.
meromelia
meromyarial
merozoite

merozygote
mersalyl
Merulius
   M. lacrimans
Merzbacher-Pelizaeus disease
mesangial
   m. proliferative glomerulopathy
mesangium
   extraglomerular m.
   glomerular m.
mesaxon
mescaline
mesencephalic
mesencephalitis
mesencephalon
mesenchymal
   m. tumor
   m. villous core
mesenchyme
mesenchymoma
mesenteric
   m. artery
   m. cyst
   m. hyperplasia
   m. lymph node
   m. plexus
   m. thrombosis
   m. vein
mesentery
   dorsal m.
   ileal m.
   jejunal m.
   sigmoid colon m.
   small intestinal m.
mesiodistal
mesion
mesoappendix
mesobacterium
mesoblast
mesoblastic nephroma
mesocardia

Mesocestoides
   M. variabilis
Mesocestoididae
mesocolon
   sigmoid m.
   transverse m.
mesoderm
mesodermal
mesogastric
mesogastrium
Mesogastropoda
mesometanephric
mesometrium
meson
mesonephric
   m. adenocarcinoma
   m. cyst
   m. rest
mesonephroma
mesonephros (mesonephroi)
mesophile
mesoridazine besylate
mesosalpinx
mesosome
mesotendineum
mesothelial
   m. cell
   m. cyst
   m. sarcoma
mesothelioma
   fibrous m.
mesothelium
   pericardial m.
   peritoneal m.
   pleural m.
mesovarium
messenger RNA
Met or M — methionine
metabiosis
metabolic
   m. acidosis
   m. alkalosis

metabolic *(continued)*
   m. insufficiency
metabolism
   aerobic m.
   anaerobic m.
   basal m.
   inborn errors of m.
   intermediary m.
metabolite
metabutethamine
metabutoxycaine
metacarpal
metacarpophalangeal
metacarpus (metacarpi)
metacentric
metacercaria (metacercariae)
metachromasia
metachromatic leukodystrophy
metachronous
metacresylacetate
metagenesis
metagglutinin
metaglobulin
metagonimiasis
Metagonimus
   M. ovatus
   M. yokogawai
metaldehyde
metalloenzyme
metalloflavoprotein
metalloprotein
metamorphosis
   fatty m.
metamyelocyte
   basophilic m.
   eosinophilic m.
   neutrophilic m.
metanephrine
metanephros (metanephroi)
metaphase
metaphosphoric acid
metaphysis

metaplasia
   agnogenic myeloid m.
   apocrine m.
   cartilaginous m.
   chondroid m.
   decidual m.
   endothelial m.
   epidermoid m.
   glandular m.
   Hürthle cell m.
   intestinal m.
   myeloid m.
   osseous m.
   squamous m.
metaplastic keratinization
metaraminol
metarubricyte
metastasis
metastasize
metastatic
   m. calcification
   m. carcinoma
   m. neoplasm
   m. tumor
Metastrongylus
   M. elongatus
metatarsal
metatarsalgia
metatarsophalangeal
metatarsus
metazoa (metazoon)
metazoan
   m. parasite
metencephalon
meteorism
meter
meter-kilogram-second system
methacholine
methacycline
methadone hydrochloride
methallenestril
methamphetamine

methandrostenolone
methane
Methanobacterium
Methanococcus
methanol
methantheline
methapyrilene
methaqualone
metharbital
methazolamide
MetHb — methemoglobin
methdilazine
    m. hydrochloride
methemalbumin
methemalbuminemia
methemalbuminuria
metheme
methemoglobin
methemoglobinemia
    hereditary enzymatic-type m.
methemoglobinuria
methenamine
    m. hippurate
    m. mandelate
    m. silver
methenyltetrahydrofolate cyclohydrolase
methicillin
methimazole
methine dye
methiodal sodium
methionine
    m. adenosyltransferase
    m. malabsorption syndrome
    m. synthase
methionyl-RNA synthetase
methisazone
methitural
methixene hydrochloride
methocarbamol
methocycline
method
    Ashby's differential agglutination m.
    Ayoub-Shklar m.
    Baker's Sudan black m.
    Barrnett-Seligman dihydroxydinaphthyl disulfide m.
    Barrnett-Seligman indoxyl esterase m.
    Barroso-Moguel and Costero silver m.
    Baumgartner m.
    Beaver direct smear m.
    Bengston's m.
    Bennett's sulfhydryl m.
    Bennhold's Congo red m.
    Bensley's aniline–acid fuchsin methyl green m.
    benzo sky blue m.
    Berg's chelate removal m.
    Bielschowsky's m.
    Bodian's m.
    Borchgrevink m.
    Brecher-Cronkite m.
    Cajal's gold-sublimate m.
    Cajal's uranium silver m.
    Caldwell-Moloy m.
    Camp-Gianturco m.
    cellophane tape m.
    Chang's aniline-acid fuchsin m.
    Chiffelle and Putt m.
    chloranilate m.
    chrome alum-hematoxylin-phloxine m.
    chromolytic (dyed-starch) m.
    Ciaccio's m.
    clean-catch collection m.
    cobaltinitrite m.

method *(continued)*
    Colcher-Sussman m.
    constitutive heterochromatin m.
    Cope m. of bronchography
    Craigie's tube m.
    Credé's m.
    Crippa's lead tetraacetate m.
    cysteic acid m.
    Dale-Laidlaw's clotting time m.
    Dane's m.
    De Galantha's m. for urates
    diazo staining m.
    Dieterle's m.
    Duke's m. of bleeding time
    Fite's m.
    Fontana-Masson staining m.
    Foot's reticulin m.
    formaldehyde-induced fluorescence m.
    formalin-ether sedimentation m.
    freeze-cleave m.
    freeze-etch m.
    freeze-fracture-etch m.
    frozen section m.
    glass-bead retention m.
    Gomori's m. for chromaffin
    Granger m.
    Grimelius argyrophil m.
    Grocott-Gomori methenamine-silver m.
    Hall's m.
    Highman's m. for amyloid
    Holmes' m.
    Holzer's m.
    Ivy's m. of bleeding time
    Jones' m.

method *(continued)*
    Kjeldahl's m.
    Lee-White clotting time m.
    Levaditi's m.
    Lillie's allochrome m.
    Lison-Dunn m.
    Masson trichrome m.
    Menzies' m.
    Monte Carlo m.
    Movat's pentachrome m.
    Penfield's m.
    Pfeiffer-Comberg m.
    Pizzolato's peroxide-silver m.
    plasma-thrombin clot m.
    Puchtler's alkaline Congo red m.
    Puchtler's Sirius red m.
    PVA fixative m.
    Reese-Ecker m.
    Salzman m.
    Schales and Schales m. for chloride
    Stovall-Black m.
    Sweet m.
    Thoms m.
    von Kossa's m.
methodology
methohexital
methotrexate
methotrimeprazine
methoxamine
methoxsalen
methoxyamphetamine
methoxychlor
methoxyethyl mercuriacetate
methoxyflurane
methoxyphenamine
methoxypromazine
methscopolamine
methsuximide

methyclothiazide
methyl
  m. acetate
  m. alcohol
  m. bromide
  m. butyl ketone
  m. chloride
  m. chloroform
  m. chlorophenoxyacetic acid
  m. cyclohexane
  m. demeton
  m. ethyl ketone
  m. formate
  m. *p*-hydroxybenzoate
  m. hydroxybutyric acid
  m. iodide
  m. isobutyl ketone
  m. mercuric cyanoguanidine
  m. mercuric dicyanodiamine
  m. mercury
  m. methacrylate
  m. parathion
  m. phenol
  m. phenylethylhydantoin
  m. polysiloxane
  m. salicylate
N-methyl-aminoacid oxidase
methylaminoheptane
p-methylaminophenol hydrochloride
p-methylaminophenol sulfate
methylaspartate mutase
methylated naphthalene
methylation
methylbenzethonium
methylcellulose
methylcholanthrene
methylcrotonoyl-coenzyme A carboxylase
methyldopa
methylene
  m. blue
  m. chloride
methylenedioxyamphetamine
methylergonovine
methylformamide
methylglutaconyl–coenzyme A hydratase
1-methyl-histidine
3-methyl-histidine
methylmalonic acid
methylmalonyl-CoA decarboxylase
methylmalonyl-CoA mutase
methylmercaptan
methylmercury
α-methylmetatyrosine
methylmorphine
methylnicotinamide
α-methylnorepinephrine
methylparaben
methylparafynol
methylphenidate
methylprednisolone
methylrosaniline
methyltestosterone
methylthiouracil
methyltransferase
methyprylon
methysergide
metocurine iodide
Metopirone test
metoprolol tartrate
metoxenous
metoxeny
metraterm
metritis
metrizamide
metrizoate
metrocele
metromalacia

metronidazole
metrorrhagia
Mets — metastases
metyrapone
MeV — megaelectron volt
mev — million electron volts
mevaldate reductase
mevalonate kinase
Meyenburg's complex
Meynet's nodes
MF — medium frequency
    mycosis fungoides
    myelin figures
mF — millifarad
mf — microfilaria
μf or μfd — microfarad
MFB — metallic foreign body
MFP — monofluorophosphate
MFR — mucus flow rate
MG — menopausal gonadotropin
    mesiogingival
    methyl glucoside
    Michaelis-Gutmann (bodies)
    muscle group
    myasthenia gravis
Mg — magnesium
mg — milligram
mg% — milligrams per 100 milliliters; milligrams per deciliter
Mg agglutinin
MGGH — methylglyoxal guanylhydrazone
MGH or mgh — milligram-hour
mgm — milligram
MGN — membranous glomerulonephritis
MGP — marginal granulocyte pool
MGR — modified gain ratio
mgtis — meningitis
MH — mammotropic hormone
mH — millihenry
MHA — methemalbumin
    microangiopathic hemolytic anemia
    mixed hemadsorption
MHA-TP — micro-hemagglutination–*Treponema pallidum*
MHb — methemoglobin
MHC — major histocompatibility complex
MHD — mean hemolytic dose
    minimum hemolytic dose
mHg — millimeters of mercury
MHN — massive hepatic necrosis
MHP — 1-mercuri-2-hydroxypropane
MHPG — methoxyhydroxyphenylglycol
MHR — maximal heart rate
MHz — megahertz
MI — mercaptoimidazole
    mitral incompetence
    mitral insufficiency
    myocardial infarction
Mibelli's porokeratosis
MIC — minimal isorrheic concentration
    minimum inhibitory concentration
micelle
Michaelis-Gutmann bodies
Michaelis-Menten equation
miconazole
microabscess
    Munro m.
    Pautrier m.

microaerophile
microaerophilic
   m. streptococcus
microaleuriospore
microampere
microaneurysm
microangiopathic
   m. hemolytic anemia
microangiopathy
   diabetic m.
   thrombotic m.
Microbacterium
microbar
microbe
microbial
microbioassay
microbiol. — microbiological
microbiologic
microbiology
microbiotic
microbody
microbroth
microburet
microcephaly
microchemistry
microchromosome
microcirculation
Micrococcaceae
Micrococcus
   M. flavus
   M. intracellularis
   M. pyogenes var. *aureus*
   M. tetragenus
microcolony
microconidium (microconidia)
microcoulomb
microcrystalline
microcurie
microcyte
microcythemia
microcytic
   m. anemia

microcytic *(continued)*
   m. hypochromic anemia
microcytosis
microdensitometer
microdiffusion analysis
microdrepanocytic
microelectrophoresis
microfibril
microfiche
microfilament
microfilaremia
Microfilaria
   M. bancrofti
   M. streptocerca
microfilariasis
microflora
microfollicular
   m. adenoma
microgamete
microgametocyte
microglia
microgliocyte
microglioma
microglobulin
microglossia
micrognathia
microgram
micrograph
microgyria
micro-hemagglutination–
   Treponema pallidum
microhematocrit
microhistology
microhomology
microinfarct
microinvasive carcinoma
microliter
microlithiasis
micromelia
micrometer
micromethod
micrometry

micromole
Micromonospora
   M. faeni
Micromonosporaceae
micron (microns, micra). Abbreviated μ.
microne
micronucleus (micronuclei)
microorganism
microphage
microphthalmia
micropolygyria
Micropolyspora
   M. faeni
micropredation
microprobe
   laser m.
microprotein
microscope
   binocular m.
   color-contrast m.
   comparison m.
   compound m.
   darkfield m.
   darkground m.
   electron m.
   fluorescent m.
   infrared m.
   integrating m.
   interference m.
   laser m.
   light m.
   Nomarski m.
   operating m.
   Oto-Microscope
   phase-contrast m.
   polarizing m.
   reflecting m.
   simple m.
   slit-lamp m.
   stereoscopic m.
   trinocular m.

microscope *(continued)*
   ultraviolet m.
   x-ray m.
microscopic
   m. infarct
microscopy
   electron m.
microsecond
microsomal
   m. antibodies
   m. enzyme system
   m. thyroid antibody
microsome
microsphere
microspherocyte
microspherocytosis
microspore
Microsporon
microsporosis
Microsporum
   M. audouini
   M. canis
   M. felineum
   M. ferrugineum
   M. fulvum
   M. furfur
   M. gypseum
   M. lanosum
   M. nanum
microstomia
microtome
microtubule
microunit
microvillus (microvilli)
microvolt
microwatt
microwave
MID — maximum inhibiting dilution
      mesioincisodistal
      minimum infective dose
midbody

midbrain
midcarpal
midcolic lymph node
Middlebrook-Dubos hemagglutination test
Middlebrook's
    agar
    broth
midge
midline
    m. lethal granuloma
    m. nucleus
midlobular region
midpalmar space
midsagittal plane
midsternal line
midtarsal
midzonal
    m. necrosis
Miescheria
MIF — macrophage-inhibiting factor
        melanocyte-stimulating hormone–inhibiting factor
        migration inhibition factor
        mixed immunofluorescence
MIFR — maximal inspiratory flow rate
migraine
migrating thrombophlebitis
migration
    m. inhibition factor
Mikulicz's disease
miliaria
    m. profunda
    m. rubra
miliary
    m. aneurysm

miliary *(continued)*
    m. granulomatous inflammation
    m. tuberculosis
milieu
milium (milia)
    colloid m.
    m. cyst
milk
    m. alkali syndrome
    biundulant m. fever
    m. spot
Milkman's syndrome
Miller-Abbott tube
milliammeter
milliamperage
milliampere
    m.-second
millicoulomb
millicurie
milliequivalent
millifarad
milligram
millihenry
millilambert
milliliter
millimeter
    m. of mercury
millimole
milliosmole
millirad
millirem
milliroentgen
millisecond
milliunit
millivolt
milliwatt
Millon's reagent
Milroy's disease
Mima
    M. polymorpha

Mimeae
min. — minute(s)
Minamata disease
mineral
    m. foreign body
    m. oil foreign body
mineralization
mineralocorticoid
minicell
minify
minimal bactericidal concentration
minimum inhibitory concentration
minocycline
minor
    m. calyx
    m. histocompatibility complex
    m. inferior aperture
    m. pelvis
    m. salivary gland
    m. sublingual duct
    m. superior aperture
    m. vestibular gland
minoxidil
minuthesis
miosis
MIP — maximum inspiratory pressure
miracidium (miracidia)
MIRD — Medical Internal Radiation Dose
miscarriage
miscibility
miscible
MIT — monoiodotyrosine
mite
    parasitoid m.
    red m.
    trombiculid m.
mithramycin

mitochondrial
    m. cristae alteration
    m. matrix alteration
    m. membrane alteration
    m. myopathy
mitochondrion (mitochondria)
mitogen
mitogillin
mitokinetic
mitomalcin
mitomycin
mitoplasm
mitosis (mitoses)
mitotane
mitotic
    m. arrest
mitral
    m. orifice
    m. regurgitation
    m. ring
    m. stenosis
    m. valve calcification
    m. valve prolapse
mittelschmerz
Mittendorf's dots
mixed
    m. connective tissue disease
    m. lymphocyte reaction
    m. tumor
mixoploid
mixoploidy
mixotrophic
Miyagawanella
    M. illinii
    M. louisianae
    M. lymphogranulomatosis
    M. ornithosis
    M. pneumoniae
    M. psittaci
MK — monkey kidney
MKS — meter-kilogram-second
MKV — killed-measles vaccine

ML — mesiolingual
M:L — monocyte-lymphocyte ratio
mL — millilambert
ml — milliliter
μl — microliter
MLA — mentolaeva anterior
mesiolabial
monocytic leukemia, acute
MLAI — mesiolabioincisal
MLAP — mean left atrial pressure
MLC — minimum lethal concentration
mixed leukocyte culture
mixed lymphocyte culture
multilamellar cytosome
myelomonocytic leukemia, chronic
MLD — metachromatic leukodystrophy
minimum lethal dose
MLI — mesiolinguoincisal
M line
MLO — mesiolinguo-occlusal
MLP — left mentoposterior (*mento-laeva posterior*)
mesiolinguopulpal
MLR — mixed lymphocyte reaction
MLS — myelomonocytic leukemia, subacute
MLT — left mentotransverse (*mento-laeva transversa*)
MLV — Moloney's leukemogenic virus
mouse leukemia virus

MM — malignant melanoma
Marshall-Marchetti
medial malleolus
mucous membrane
multiple myeloma
muscularis mucosa
myeloid metaplasia
mM — millimolar
millimole
mm — millimeter
mμ — millimicron
$\mu\mu$ — micromicron
MMA — methylmalonic acid
MMC — minimal medullary concentration
mμc — millimicrocurie (nanocurie)
$\mu\mu$c — micromicrocurie (picocurie)
MMD — minimal morbidostatic dose
MMEF — maximal midexpiratory flow
MMEFR — maximal midexpiratory flow rate
MMF — maximal midexpiratory flow
MMFR — maximal midexpiratory flow rate
maximal midflow rate
mμg — millimicrogram (nanogram)
μmg — micromilligram
$\mu\mu$g — micromicrogram (picogram)
mmHg — millimeter(s) of mercury
mM/L or mM/l — millimols per liter
MMM — myeloid metaplasia with myelofibrosis

MMM *(continued)*
    myelosclerosis with myeloid metaplasia
μmm — micromillimeter
M-mode echo
mmol — millimole
mmpp — millimeters partial pressure
MMPR — methylmercaptopurine riboside
MMR — mass miniature radiography
    myocardial metabolic rate
MMTV — mouse mammary tumor virus
MM virus
MN — multinodular
    myoneural
Mn — manganese
mN — millinormal
MNCV — motor nerve conduction velocity
mnemonic
    m. code
MNU — methylnitrosourea
MO — mesio-occlusal
    no evidence of distant metastases
Mo — molybdenum
mo — month(s)
Moberg's arthrodesis
mobile
    m. cecum
    m. genes
mobilization
    m. test
mobilometer
Möbius' disease
MOD — mesio-occlusodistal
modality
mode
    B-m.

moderator band
modiolus
modular
modulation
    antigenic m.
    m. transfer function
module
moiety
molal
molality
molar
    deciduous m.
    mandibular m.
    maxillary m.
molarity
mold
mole
    Breus m.
    hydatid m.
    hydatidiform m.
    invasive m.
molecular
    m. biology
    m. exclusion chromatography
    m. layer
    m. mass
    m. sieve
    m. sieve chromatography
    m. weight
molecule
molindone hydrochloride
Mollicutes
Moll's gland
molluscum (mollusca)
    m. contagiosum
    m. contagiosum virus
    m. sebaceum virus
mollusk
Moloney's
    leukemogenic virus
    sarcoma virus
mol wt — molecular weight

molybdenum
   m. isotope
molybdic
MOMA — methoxyhydroxymandelic acid
monad
Monadina
monamide
monaminergic
monarthritis
Monas
monaster
Mönckeberg's
   arteriosclerosis
   medial calcification
Mondor's disease
Monge's disease
mongolian
   m. idiot
   m. spot
mongolism
mongoloid
monilethrix
Monilia
   M. sitophila
monilial
moniliasis
moniliform
Moniliformis
   M. moniliformis
moniliid
monitor
monkey B virus
monoamine oxidase
monoaminodicarboxylic acid
monoaminomonocarboxylic acid
monobasic acid
monobenzone
monoblast
monoblastic leukemia

monobutyl
   m. biphenyl sodium monosulfonate
   m. phenyl phenol sodium monosulfonate
monocentric
monocephalus
   m. tetrapus dibrachius
   m. tripus dibrachius
monochromatism
monochromator
monoclonal
   m. antibodies
   m. band
   m. gammopathy
   m. immunoglobulin
monocyte
monocytic
   m. cells
   m. inflammatory infiltrate
   m. leukemia
   m. tissue
monocytopenia
monocytopoiesis
monocytosis
5-monodeiodinase
monofluoroacetate salt
monoglyceride
monohistiocytic
monohydric
monoiodothyronine
3-monoiodo-L-tyrosine
monolayer
monomer
monomeric
monomethyl-*p*-aminophenol sulfate
monomorphic
monomyelocytic leukemia
monomyositis
Mononchus

mononeuritis
   m. multiplex
mononeuropathy
mononuclear
   m.-phagocyte system
mononucleate
mononucleosis
   infectious m.
mononucleotide
monooxygenase
monophosphate
monophosphoglyceromutase
monoplegia
monopolar
monoptychial
Monos — monocytes
monosaccharide
monosodium glutamate
monosome
monosomic
monosomy G, X
Monosporium
   M. apiospermum
Monospot test
monostotic fibrous dysplasia
Monotospora
monotreme
Monotricha
monotrichous
monovalent
monozygotic
Monro's
   abscesses
   foramen
mons (montes)
   m. pubis
   m. ureteris
   m. veneris
monster
   anencephalic m.
Monte Carlo method
Montevideo unit

MOPP — nitrogen mustard, Oncovin, prednisone, procarbazine
MOPV — monovalent oral poliovirus vaccine
Morax-Axenfeld
   bacillus
   diplococcus
   hemophilus
Moraxella
   M. kingae
   M. lacunata
   M. liquefaciens
   M. lwoffi
   M. nonliquefaciens
   M. osloensis
   M. phenylpyruvica
   M. urethralis
morbidity
morbillivirus
mordant
Morgagni's
   crypt
   cyst
   hernia
   hydatid
   nodules
   syndrome
Morganella
   M. morganii
Morgan's bacillus
morococcus
morphea
morphine
morphodifferentiation
morphogenesis
morpholine
morphologic
morphology
morphometry
Morquio-Brailsford disease
Morquio's disease

mortality
Mortierella
Morton's
    disease
    neuralgia
    toe
morula
mOs — milliosmolal
mosaicism
Mosenthal's test
mOsm — milliosmol, milliosmole
most significant bit
most significant digit
motile
motilin
motility
    gastrointestinal m.
motoneuron
motor
    m. aphasia
    m. cortex
    m. end plate
    m. hyperactivity
    m. neuron
    m. nucleus, trigeminal nerve
    m. root
Mott cell
mottled
Motulsky dye reduction test
mouse
    m. mammary tumor virus
    m. unit
mouth
    tapir m.
    trench m.
Movat's pentachrome method
movements
    athetoid m.
MP — mean pressure
    melting point
    menstrual period

MP *(continued)*
    mercaptopurine
    mesiopulpal
    metacarpophalangeal
    monophosphate
    mucopolysaccharide
    multiparous
MPA — main pulmonary artery
    medroxyprogesterone acetate
    methylprednisolone acetate
MPAP — mean pulmonary arterial pressure
MPC — marine protein concentrate
    maximum permissible concentration
    meperidine, promethazine, chlorpromazine
    minimum mycoplasmacidal concentration
MPD — maximal permissible dose
MPEH — methylphenylethylhydantoin
MPGN — membranoproliferative glomerulonephritis
M phase
MPJ — metacarpophalangeal joint
MPL — mesiopulpolingual
MPLA — mesiopulpolabial
MPO — myeloperoxidase
MPP — mercaptopyrazidopyrimidine
M protein
MPS — mononuclear-phagocyte system
    mucopolysaccharide
MR — metabolic rate

MR *(continued)*
    methyl red
    mitral reflux
    mitral regurgitation
    mortality rate
    mortality ratio
    muscle relaxant
mR — milliroentgen
mrad — millirad
MRAP — mean right atrial pressure
mrem — millirem
MRF — melanocyte-stimulating hormone releasing factor
    mesencephalic reticular formation
    mitral regurgitant flow
mRNA — messenger RNA
MRVP — mean right ventricular pressure
MS — mass spectrometry
    mitral stenosis
    morphine sulfate
    mucosubstance
    multiple sclerosis
    musculoskeletal
MSA — multiplication-stimulating activity
MSB — most significant bit
MSD — most significant digit
msec — millisecond
MSER — mean systolic ejection rate
MSG — monosodium glutamate
MSH — melanocyte-stimulating hormone
    melanophore-stimulating hormone
MSK — medullary sponge kidney
MSL — midsternal line
MSLA — mouse-specific lymphocyte antigen
MSU — monosodium urate
MSUD — maple syrup urine disease
MSV — Moloney's sarcoma virus
    murine sarcoma virus
MT — malignant teratoma
    membrana tympani
    metatarsal
    methyltyrosine
MTBF — mean time between failures
MTF — maximum terminal flow
    modulation transfer function
MTHF — methyltetrahydrofolic acid
MTI — malignant teratoma intermediate
MTP — metatarsophalangeal
MTR — Meinicke turbidity reaction
MTT — malignant trophoblastic teratoma
    monotetrazolium
MTU — methylthiouracil
MTV — mammary tumor virus
MTX — methotrexate
MU — Mache unit
    Montevideo unit
mU — milliunit
mu — micron
    mouse unit
MUC — maximum urinary concentration
mucase
mucicarmine stain

mucin
    m. clot test
mucinosis
mucinous
    m. adenocarcinoma
    m. atrophy
    m. carcinoma
    m. cyst
    m. cystadenocarcinoma
    m. cystadenoma
    m. degeneration
mucocele
mucocutaneous
mucoenteritis
mucoepidermoid
    m. carcinoma
    m. tumor
mucoid
mucolipidosis (mucolipidoses)
mucopeptide
mucopolysaccharidase
mucopolysaccharide
mucopolysaccharidosis (mucopolysaccharidoses)
mucoprotein
mucopurulent exudate
Mucor
    M. corymbifer
    M. mucedo
    M. pusillus
    M. racemosus
    M. ramosus
    M. rhizopodiformis
Mucoraceae
mucormycosis
mucosa
    buccal m.
    gallbladder m.
    gastric m.
    gastrointestinal m.
    seminal vesicle m.
    vas deferens m.

mucosal neuroma syndrome
mucous
    m. cast
    m. colitis
    m. connective tissue
    m. cyst
    m. gland
    m. membrane
    m. membrane gland
    m. neck cell
    m. plug
mucoviscidosis
mucus
    accessory sinus m.
    bronchial m.
    cervical m.
    colonic m.
    endocervical m.
    epiglottic m.
    esophageal m.
    m. extravasation
    laryngeal m.
    lower respiratory tract m.
    nasal m.
    nasopharyngeal m.
    pharyngeal m.
    rectal m.
    m. retention
    tracheal m.
    upper respiratory tract m.
Mueller-Hinton
    agar
    broth
Mueller's
    arteries
muliebria
Müller duct
müllerian
    m. duct
    m. rest
    m. tumor
multicellular

Multiceps
   M. glomeratus
   M. multiceps
   M. serialis
multichannel analyzer
multifactorial
multifocal
   m. fibrosis
   m. inflammation
   m. progressive leukoencephalopathy
multiform
multigravida
multilamellar
multilobar
multilobate placenta
multilobular
multilocular
   m. cyst
multinodular
multip — pregnant woman who has borne two or more children
multipara
multiplane tomographic scanner
multiple
   m. adenomatous polyps
   m. endocrine neoplasia
   m. fractures
   m. hemorrhagic sarcoma
   m. meningiomas
   m. myeloma
   m. neurofibromatosis
   m. polyposis
   m. sclerosis
   m. spike complex
   m. spike foci
multiplex
multipolar
multitrichous
multivalent
multivesicular
multiwire proportional chamber
mummification
mumps
   m. antibody titer
   iodine m.
   meningoencephalitis m.
   metastatic m.
   m. virus
Münchausen's syndrome
Munro microabscess
mural
   m. thrombosis
muralium
muramic acid
muramidase
muriatic acid
murine
   m. typhus
murmur
   aortic m.
   apical m.
   Austin Flint m.
   basal m.
   cardiac m.
   cardiovascular m.
   continuous m.
   diastolic m.
   ejection m.
   holosystolic m.
   regurgitant m.
   systolic m.
   venous m.
   ventricular filling m.
   vesicular m.
Murphy-Pattee test
Murray Valley encephalitis virus
Musca
   M. domestica
   M. volitans

muscarine
  m. receptor
muscle
  cardiac m.
  constrictor m.
  extrafusal fiber of m.
  m. fiber
  intermediate fiber of striated m.
  intrafusal fiber of m.
  m. palsy
  skeletal m.
  smooth m.
  m. spindle
muscular
  m. fibrillation
  m. rigidity
muscular atrophy
  Charcot-Marie-Tooth m. a.
  hypertrophic polyneuritic-type m. a.
  infantile m. a.
  peroneal m. a.
  progressive m. a.
muscular dystrophy
  distal-type m. d.
  Duchenne-type m. d.
  facioscapulohumeral-type m. d.
  Landouzy-Dejerine progressive m. d.
  limb girdle–type m. d.
  ophthalmoplegic-type m. d.
muscularis
  tunica m.
musculoaponeurotic fibromatosis
musculocutaneous
musculophrenic
musculoskeletal
musculotendinous
mushroom poisoning
mustard
  m. gas
  nitrogen m.
  uracil m.
mutagen
  chromosomal m.
mutagenesis
mutagenic
mutant
mutarotation
mutase
mutation
  auxotrophic m.
  clear plaque m.
  cold-sensitive m.
  conditional lethal m.
  constitutive m.
  deletion m.
  feedback inhibition m.
  forward m.
  frameshift m.
  host-range m.
  insertion m.
  lethal m.
  missense m.
  nonsense m.
  ochre m.
  phage-resistant m.
  pleiotropic m.
  rapid-lysis m.
  reverse m.
  somatic m.
  spontaneous m.
  subvital m.
  suppressor m.
  temperature-sensitive m.
  transition m.
  transversion m.
  ultraviolet light–induced m.
mutism
  akinetic m.
muton

mutualism
MUU – mouse uterine units
MV – megavolt
   minute volume
   mitral valve
   mixed venous
mv – millivolt
MVM – microvillose membrane
MVP – mitral valve prolapse
MVR – massive vitreous retraction
MVV – maximal voluntary ventilation
MW – molecular weight
mW – milliwatt
mw – microwave
M wave
Mx – maxwell
My – myopia
my – mayer (unit of heat capacity)
myalgia
myasthenia gravis
myatrophy
Mycelia
   M. sterilia
mycelium (mycelia)
mycetismus
   m. cerebris
   m. choleriformis
   m. gastrointestinalis
   m. nervosus
   m. sanguinarius
mycetoma
mycetosis
mycoagglutinin
mycobacteria
   anonymous m.
   atypical m.
   Group I–IV m.
   nonphotochromogenic m.
   photochromogenic m.

mycobacteria *(continued)*
   scotochromogenic m.
Mycobacteriaceae
mycobacteriosus
Mycobacterium
   M. abscessus
   M. aquae
   M. avium-intracellulare
   M. balnei
   M. berolinenis
   M. borstelense
   M. bovis
   M. butyricum
   M. chelonei
   M. flavescens
   M. fortuitum
   M. gastri
   M. gordonae
   M. habana
   M. haemophilum
   M. intracellularis
   M. johnei
   M. kansasii
   M. leprae
   M. leprae murium
   M. luciflavum
   M. malmoense
   M. marinum
   M. microti
   M. nonchromogenicum
   M. paratuberculosis
   M. peregrinum
   M. phlei
   M. scrofulaceum
   M. simiae
   M. smegmatis
   M. szulgai
   M. terrea-nonchromogenicum-triviale
   M. triviale
   M. tuberculosis
   M. tuberculosis var. *avium*

Mycobacterium (continued)
    M. tuberculosis var. *bovis*
    M. tuberculosis var. *hominis*
    M. tuberculosis var. *muris*
    M. ulcerans
    M. xenopi
mycobacterium (mycobacteria)
    Battey-type m.
mycobactin
Mycocandida
Mycococcus
Mycoderma
    M. aceti
    M. dermatitidis
    M. immite
mycolic acids
mycology
mycomyringitis
Myconostoc
    M. gregarium
Mycoplana
    M. bullata
    M. dimorpha
Mycoplasma
    M. buccale
    M. faucium
    M. fermentans
    M. hominis
    M. orale
    M. pharyngis
    M. pneumoniae
    M. salivarium
mycoplasma
    T-strain m.
Mycoplasmataceae
Mycoplasmatales
mycoside
mycosis
    m. fungoides
mycotic
    m. aneurysm

mycotic *(continued)*
    m. keratitis
mycotoxicosis
mydriasis
myelapoplexy
myelencephalon
myelin
    m. degeneration
    m. sheath
myelinated
myelinolysis
    central pontine m.
myelitis
    transverse m.
myeloblast
myeloblastic leukemia
myelocele
myeloclast
myelocystocele
myelocystomeningocele
myelocyte
    basophilic m.
    eosinophilic m.
    neutrophilic m.
myelocytic leukemia
myeloencephalitis
myelofibrosis
myelogenous
    m. leukemia
myelography
    gas m.
    opaque m.
    radionuclide m.
myeloid
    m. hyperplasia
    m. metaplasia
    m. metaplasia, agnogenic
myelolipoma
myeloma
    plasma cell m.
    plasmacytic m.
myelomalacia

myelomatosis
myelomeningitis
myelomeningocele
myelomonocytic
    m. leukemia
myelopathy
    transverse m.
myeloperoxidase
myelophthisic
myelophthisis
myelopoiesis
    extramedullary m.
myelopoietic
myeloproliferative
myeloradiculitis
myelorrhagia
myelosarcoma
myeloschisis
myelosclerosis
myelosis
    aleukemic m.
    erythremic m.
    megakaryocytic m.
    nonleukemic m.
myelosyringosis
myenteric
    m. plexus
myenteron
MyG — myasthenia gravis
myiasis
Mylar capacitor
mylohyoid muscle
Mylone
myoblastoma
    granular cell m.
myocardial
    m. infarct
    m. infarction
    m. ischemia
myocarditis
    Fiedler's m.
    Löffler's m.

myocarditis *(continued)*
    rheumatic m.
myocardium
myocele
myoclonic
    m. epilepsy
myoclonus
myocyte
    Anichkov's (Anitschkow's) m.
myocytolysis
myoepithelial
myoepithelioma
myoepithelium
myofibril
myofibroblast
myofibroma
myofibrosis
myofibrositis
myofilament
myoglobin
myoglobinemia
myoglobinuria
    acute paroxysmal m.
myoglobinuric
    m. nephrosis
myo-inositol oxygenase
myokinase
myokymia
myolipoma
myolysis
myoma (myomas, myomata)
myomalacia
myometritis
myometrium
myonecrosis
myoneme
myoneural
myopathy
    alcoholic m.
    congenital m.
    corticosteroid m.

myopathy *(continued)*
   endocrine m.
   nemaline m.
myopericarditis
myophosphorylase
myopia
myorrhexis
myosarcoma
myoseism
myosin
myosis
   endolymphatic stromal m.
myositis
   clostridial m.
   m. ossificans
   m. ossificans progressiva
   ossifying interstitial m.
myotome
   caudal m.
   cervical m.
   lumbar m.
   occipital m.
   sacral m.
   thoracic m.
myotonia
   m. acquisita
   m. atrophica
   m. congenita
   m. dystrophica
   m. neonatorum
myotonic
   m. dystrophy
myotubular
Myriapoda
myringitis
   bullous m.
myringomycosis
myristic acid
myrmecia
myrosulfatase

Myrtophyllum
   M. hepatis
myxadenitis
myxedema
   m. coma
   pituitary m.
   pretibial m.
myxochondroma
myxofibroma
myxofibrosarcoma
myxoid
   m. cyst
   m. degeneration
   m. fibroma
myxolipoma
myxoliposarcoma
myxoma (myxomas, myxomata)
   atrial m.
   cardiac m.
   cystic m.
   endochondromatous m.
   erectile m.
   infectious m.
   lipomatous m.
   odontogenic m.
   vascular m.
myxomatosis
   cardiac valve m.
myxomatous
   m. degeneration
myxopapillary
   m. ependymoma
myxopod
myxosarcoma
Myxosporidia
myxovirus
Myzomyia
Myzorhynchus
MZ — monozygotic

N

N — newton
   nitrogen
   normal
   unit of neutron dosage
N. — *Neisseria*
   Nocardia
n — index of refraction
   neutron
   normal
NA — neutralizing antibody
   Nomina Anatomica
   noradrenalin
   numerical aperture
Na — sodium
NAA — neutron activation analysis
NAACLS — National Accrediting Agency for Clinical Laboratory Sciences
nabam
nabothian
   n. cyst
   n. gland
NaBr — sodium bromide
NAC-EDTA — *N*-acetyl-L-cysteine ethylenediaminetetraacetic acid
NaCl — sodium chloride
NaClO — sodium hypochlorite
NaClO$_3$ — sodium chlorate
Na$_2$CO$_3$ — sodium carbonate
Na$_2$C$_2$O$_4$ — sodium oxalate
NAD — nicotinamide-adenine dinucleotide
   normal axis deviation
NADH — nicotinamide-adenine dinucleotide (reduced form)
NADH methemoglobin reductase
nadolol
NADP — nicotinamide adenine dinucleotide phosphate
NADPH — nicotinamide adenine dinucleotide phosphate (reduced form)
Naegeli type of monocytic leukemia
Naegleria
naepaine
nafcillin
Naffziger's syndrome
nafoxidine hydrochloride
Nagler's reaction
NaI — sodium iodide
nail-patella syndrome
nalbuphine hydrochloride
nalidixic acid
nalorphine
   n. hydrochloride
naloxone hydrochloride
NANA — *N*-acetylneuraminic acid
nandrolone
nanism
Nannizzia
   N. cajetani
   N. grubia
   N. gypsea
   N. incurvata
   N. obtusa
nanocurie
nanofarad
nanogram

nanoliter
nanometer
nanomole
nanosecond
NAPA — *N*-acetyl-*p*-aminophenol
naphazoline hydrochloride
naphtha
naphthalene
naphthol
N-1-naphthyl phthalmic acid
N-1-naphthyl sodium salt
1(1-naphthyl)-2-thiourea
Napier formol-gel test
napierian logarithm
naproxen
narceine
narcolepsy
narcosis
    carbon dioxide n.
    nitrogen n.
narcotic
nares
NAS — National Academy of Sciences
nasal
    n. glioma
    n. lymphoepithelioma
    n. plasmacytoma
    n. polyp
    n. turbinate
nascent
nasion
nasociliary nerve
nasolabial fold
nasolacrimal
nasopalatine
nasopharyngeal
    n. cavity
    n. gland
    n. mucus
    n. pituitary gland

nasopharyngeal *(continued)*
    n. submucosa
nasopharyngitis
nasopharyngography
nasopharynx
nasosinusitis
nasotracheal
National Academy of Sciences
National Accrediting Agency for Clinical Laboratory Sciences
National Association of Medical Examiners
National Cancer Institute
National Certification Agency for Medical Laboratory Personnel
National Council of Health Laboratory Services
National Formulary
National Institutes of Health
National Registry in Clinical Chemistry
National Registry of Microbiologists
National Society for Histotechnology
natremia
natrium
natriuresis
nausea
navicular
    n. cells
NB — newborn
    nitrous oxide–barbiturate
Nb — niobium
NBS — normal blood serum
NBT — nitroblue tetrazolium
NBTE — nonbacterial thrombotic endocarditis
NBW — normal birth weight

nc — nanocurie
NCA — neurocirculatory asthenia
NCAMLP — National Certification Agency for Medical Laboratory Personnel
NCHLS — National Council of Health Laboratory Services
NCI — National Cancer Institute
nCi — nanocurie
NCV — nerve conduction velocity
ND — neonatal death
Newcastle disease
Nd — neodymium
n_D — refractive index
NDA — no data available
no demonstrable antibodies
NDGA — nordihydroguaiaretic acid
NDI — nephrogenic diabetes insipidus
NDMA — nitrosodimethylaniline
NDP — net dietary protein
NDV — Newcastle disease virus
NE — nerve ending
neurologic examination
nonelastic
norepinephrine
Ne — neon
nearsightedness
nebulizer
Necator
N. americanus
necatoriasis
neck
bull n.
wry n.
Necrobacterium necrophorum

necrobiosis
n. lipoidica diabeticorum
necrophagocytosis
necrophilic
necropsy
necrosis
acute inflammatory n.
aseptic n.
avascular n.
caseous n.
central n.
centrilobular n.
coagulative n.
cortical n.
cystic medial n.
cytodegenerative n.
cytotoxic n.
diffuse n.
fat n.
fibrinoid n.
focal n.
gangrenous n.
hyaline n.
inflammatory n.
ischemic n.
lamellar n.
liquefactive n.
massive hepatic n.
medial n.
medullary n.
midzonal n.
papillary n.
peripheral n.
periportal n.
postpartum pituitary n.
radiation n.
radium n.
renal medullary n.
renal papillary n.
sclerosing hyaline n.
septic n.
tumor n.

NECROSIS – NEOPLASTIC 351

necrosis *(continued)*
    zonal n.
necrotic
necrotizing
    n. angiitis
    n. arteriolitis
    n. bronchopneumonia
    n. glomerulonephritis
    n. inflammation
    n. lobar pneumonia
    n. pancreatitis
    n. papillitis
    n. vasculitis
NED – no evidence of disease
needle
    aneurysm n.
    aspirating n.
    n. aspiration cytology
    n. biopsy
    hypodermic n.
    ligature n.
    Menghini n.
    spinal n.
NEFA – nonesterified fatty acid
neg. – negative
negative
    n. interference
    n. pressure
    n. pressure lavage
negatron
    n. beta decay
Negri bodies
Neisseria
    N. catarrhalis
    N. caviae
    N. flava
    N. flavescens
    N. gonorrhoeae
    N. intracellularis
    N. lactamicus

Neisseria (continued)
    N. meningitidis
    N. mucosa
    N. ovis
    N. perflava
    N. pharyngis
    N. sicca
    N. subflava
Neisseriaceae
Neisser
    diplococcus of N.
Neivamyia
Nelson's syndrome
NEM – *N*-ethylmaleimide
nema
nemathelminth
Nemathelminthes
nematocide
Nematoda
nematode
nematodiasis
Nematomorpha
nematosis
neocerebellum
neocinchophen
neocyte
neocytosis
neodymium
neogenesis
neomycin
neon
neonatal
neonate
neoplasia
neoplasm
    adrenal n.
    benign n.
    epithelial n.
    malignant n.
    metastatic n.
neoplastic

neostigmine
   n. bromide
   n. methylsulfate
Neotestudina
Neotran
neotype
nephelometric
   n. immunoassays
   n. inhibition assay
nephelometry
nephrectomy
nephritides
nephritis
   bacterial n.
   interstitial n.
   lupus n.
   Masugi-type nephrotoxic serum n.
   transfusion n.
   tubular n.
nephroblastoma
nephrocalcinosis
nephrogenic
nephrogenous
nephrolithiasis
nephrology
nephroma
   embryonal n.
   mesoblastic n.
nephron
nephronophthisis
nephropathy
   acute uric acid n.
   analgesic n.
   Balkan n.
   diabetic n.
   gouty n.
   hemoglobinuric n.
   IgA n.
   membranous n.
   myoglobinuric n.
   sickle cell n.

nephropathy *(continued)*
   tubulointerstitial n.
nephroptosis
nephropyelitis
nephrorrhagia
nephrosclerosis
   arteriolar n.
   hyaline n.
   hyperplastic n.
   intercapillary n.
   malignant n.
   senile n.
nephrosis (nephroses)
   amyloid n.
   bile n.
   cholemic n.
   hemoglobinuric n.
   hypokalemic n.
   lipid n.
   lipoid n.
   lower nephron n.
   myoglobinuric n.
   osmotic n.
   toxic n.
   tubular n.
   vacuolar n.
nephrostomy
nephrotic syndrome
nephrotomography
nephrotoxic serum nephritis, Masugi type
nephrotoxin
nephrotuberculosis
nephrourography
neptunium
Nernst equation
nerve
   n. block
   n. cord
   n. fiber
   Hering's n.
   Wrisberg's n.

nervonic acid
nervous system
    aminergic n. s.
    autonomic n. s.
    central n. s.
    parasympathetic n. s.
    peptidergic n. s.
    peripheral n. s.
    sympathetic n. s.
nervus (nervi)
nesidioblast
nesidioblastoma
nesidioblastosis
nesslerization
Nessler reaction
nest
    Brunn's epithelial n's
net
    achromatic n.
    chromidial n.
    n. protein ratio
    n. protein utilization
network
    Chiari's n.
neural
    n. cell
    n. crest
    n. tube
neuralgia
    cardiac n.
    cervicobrachial n.
    cervico-occipital n.
    cranial n.
    geniculate n.
    glossopharyngeal n.
    idiopathic n.
    intercostal n.
    mammary n.
    mandibular joint n.
    migrainous n.
    Morton's n.
    nasociliary n.

neuralgia *(continued)*
    peripheral n.
    postherpetic n.
    sphenopalatine n.
    stump n.
    supraorbital n.
    trifacial n.
    trigeminal n.
    vidian n.
    visceral n.
neuralgic
    n. amyotrophy
neuraminic acid
neuraminidase
neurapraxia
neurasthenia
neurectoderm
neurilemma
neurilemmitis
neurilemoma
    ameloblastic n.
    malignant n.
neurilemosarcoma
neurinoma
neuritic atrophy
neuritis
neuroarthropathy
neuroastrocytoma
neuroblast
neuroblastic
neuroblastoma
    olfactory n.
neurochoroiditis
neurocirculatory asthenia
neurocutaneous
neurocytoma
neurodermatitis
neuroencephalomyelopathy
neuroendocrine
neuroendocrinology
neuroepithelial
neuroepithelioma

neuroepithelium
neurofibril
neurofibroma
   plexiform n.
neurofibromatosis
neurofibrosarcoma
neurofilament
neurogenic
   n. bladder
   n. sarcoma
neuroglia
neurohypophysis
neuroleptanalgesia
neuroleptanesthesia
neuroleptic
neurologic
neurology
neuroma
   acoustic n.
   amputation n.
   mucosal n.
   plexiform n.
   traumatic n.
neuromalacia
neuromere
neuromodulator
neuromuscular
neuromyelitis
   n. optica
neuromyositis
neuromyotonia
neuron
   afferent n.
   central n.
   efferent n.
   Golgi's n.
   intercalary n.
   motor n.
   multiform n.
   multipolar n.
   polymorphic n.
   postganglionic n.

neuron *(continued)*
   preganglionic n.
   pyramidal n.
   sensory n.
   unipolar n.
neuronal
neuronevus
neuronophagia
neuroparalysis
neuropathic
neuropathology
neuropathy
   amblyopia n.
   amyloid n.
   diabetic n.
   entrapment n.
   hereditary sensory radicular n.
   hypertrophic interstitial n.
   peripheral n.
   retrobulbar n.
   vincristine n.
neuropeptide
neurophysin
neurophysiology
neuropil
neuroretinitis
neuroretinopathy
neurosarcoma
neurosclerosis
neurosecretion
neurosis
   anxiety n.
   compensation n.
   obsessive-compulsive n.
   phobic n.
neuroskeletal
Neurospora
   N. sitophila
neurosyphilis
neurotensin
neurotoxin

neurotransducer
neurotransmitter
neurotrophic
neurotubule
neurovascular
neutral
neutralism
neutralizing
    n. antibody
neutrino
neutron
    n. activation analysis
    epithermal n.
    intermediate n.
    thermal n.
neutropenia
neutrophil
    band n.
    filamented n.
    giant n.
    juvenile n.
    mature n.
    polymorphonuclear n.
    rod n.
    segmented n.
    stab n.
neutrophilia
neutrophilic
    n. hyperplasia
    n. infiltrate
    n. leukemia
    n. leukocytosis
    n. metamyelocytes
    n. myelocytes
    n. promyelocytes
nevocarcinoma
nevoxanthoendothelioma
nevus (nevi)
    araneus n.
    bathing trunk n.
    blue n.
    cellular blue n.

nevus (nevi) *(continued)*
    compound n.
    dermal n.
    dermal-epidermal n.
    epithelioid cell n.
    n. flammeus
    giant blue n.
    intradermal n.
    intraepidermal n.
    Jadassohn's n.
    junctional n.
    lymphatic n.
    melanocytic n.
    nevocytic n.
    pigmented n.
    sebaceous n.
    spider n.
    spindle cell n.
    Spitz n.
    spongy n.
    n. unius lateris
    vascular n.
newborn
    n. hemolytic disease
    n. hemorrhagic disease
    icterus gravis of n.
    n. respiratory syndrome
Newcastle disease
    N. d. virus
Newcastle-Manchester bacillus
newton
Newton's law of cooling
New World hookworm
nexus (nexus, nexuses)
Nezelof's syndrome
NF — National Formulary
nF — nanofarad
NFTD — normal full-term delivery
NG — nasogastric
ng — nanogram
NGF — nerve growth factor

NGU — nongonococcal urethritis
NHA — nonspecific hepatocellular abnormality
NHC — nonhistone chromosomal (protein)
NHS — normal horse serum
normal human serum
Ni — nickel
NIA — nephelometric inhibition assay
niacin
niacinamide
nialamide
niche
nickel
    n. carbonyl
Nickerson-Kveim test reaction
Nicollella
Nicol prism
nicotinamide
    n.-adenine dinucleotide
    n. methyltransferase
    n. mononucleotide adenylyltransferase
    n. mononucleotide pyrophosphorylase
    n. phosphoribosyltransferase
nicotinate
    n. 6-hydroxylase
    n. phosphoribosyltransferase
nicotine
nicotinic
    n. acid
    n. receptor
NIDDM — noninsulin-dependent diabetes mellitus
Niemann-Pick
    disease

Niemann-Pick *(continued)*
    type of histiocyte
nifuroxime
Nigrospora
NIH — National Institutes of Health
nikethamide
Nikolsky's sign
Nile blue sulfate
Ninhydrin
    N.-Schiff reaction
ninth cranial nerve
niobium
niridazole
Nissl
    bodies
    substance alteration
Nitabuch's layer
nitrate
    n. ester reductase
    n. reduction test
nitric
    n. acid
    n. oxide
nitrile
nitrite
nitroaniline
Nitrobacter
Nitrobacteraceae
nitrobenzene
nitroblue tetrazolium test
nitrochlorobenzene
Nitrocystis
nitro dye
nitroethane
nitrofurans
nitrofurantoin
nitrofurazone
nitrofurfuryl methylether
nitrogen
    amide n.
    n. dioxide

nitrogen *(continued)*
   n. fixation
   n. isotope
   n. mustard
   n. narcosis
   n. pentoxide
   n. phosphorus
   n. pressure
   n. tetroxide
   n. trioxide
   urea n.
nitroglycerin
nitromersol
nitromethane
nitrophenol
4-nitrophenylphosphate
nitropropane
nitroprusside
nitrosamine
nitroso dye
nitrosyl chloride
nitrous
   n. acid
   n. oxide
NIXIE tube
NKH — nonketotic hyperosmotic
Nl — normal
nl — nanoliter
NLA — neuroleptanalgesia
NLP — no light perception
NLT — normal lymphocyte transfer test
NM — neuromuscular
   not measurable
   nuclear medicine
nm — nanometer
NMA — neurogenic muscular atrophy
NMP — normal menstrual period

N:N — (indicates presence of) the azo group
NND — neonatal death
   New and Nonofficial Drugs
NNN — Novy, MacNeal and Nicolle's (medium)
NO — nitric oxide
N_2O — dinitrogen monoxide (nitrous oxide)
No — nobelium
nobelium
Nocardia
   N. asteroides
   N. brasiliensis
   N. caviae
   N. madurae
   N. minutissima
   N. pelletieri
   N. tenuis
Nocardiaceae
nocardiosis
Nocard's bacillus
nociceptive
nociceptor
nocturia
nocturnal
   n. dyspnea
   n. hemoglobinuria
nodal
node
   Aschoff-Tawara n.
   atrioventricular n.
   Bouchard's n's
   Delphian n.
   Dürck's n's
   Haygarth's n's
   Heberden's n.
   Hensen's n.
   Meynet's n's
   Osler's n's

node *(continued)*
  Ranvier's n's
  SA n.
  singer's n.
  sinoatrial n.
  Virchow's n.
nodose ganglion
nodular
  n. adrenal cortex
  n. calcific aortic stenosis
  n. calcific stenosis
  n. colloid goiter
  n. embryo
  n. fibrosis
  n. glomerulosclerosis
  n. goiter
  n. hidradenoma
  n. hyperplastic goiter
  n. lymphoma
  n. nonsuppurative panniculitis
  n. vasculitis
nodule
  Aschoff's n.
  Dalen-Fuchs n's
  fibrocalcific n.
  fibrosiderotic n.
  fibrous n.
  Gamna-Gandy n's
  juxta-articular n.
  laryngeal n.
  Morgagni's n's
  rheumatic n.
  rheumatoid n.
  Schmorl's n.
  subcutaneous n.
  thyroid n.
nodulus
Noguchia
  N. granulosus
noma
Nomarski microscope

nomenclature
  binomial n.
Nomina Anatomica
nominal
  n. variable
  n. wavelength
nomogram
  Radford n.
  Siggaard-Andersen alignment n.
nomograph
nonchromaffin paraganglioma
noncommunicating hydrocephalus
noncoronary cusp
nondisjunction
nonelectrolyte
nongonococcal urethritis
noninsulin-dependent diabetes mellitus
non-ionizing radiation
non-myelinated
nonnucleated
nonparametric
nonpathogenic
nonpituitary
nonprotein nitrogen
nonsecretor
nonsecretory
nonseptate
nonsuppressible insulin-like activity
nontropical sprue
nonunion
  n. fracture
nonviable
Noonan's syndrome
noradrenalin
noradrenergic
norbormide
norbornane
norcodeine

nordefrin hydrochloride
norepinephrine
norethandrolone
norethindrone
norethynodrel
normal
    n. distribution
    n. flora
    n. probability
    n. sinus rhythm
    n. values
normetanephrine
normoblast
    acidophilic n.
    basophilic n.
    intermediate n.
    orthochromatic n.
    orthochromatophilic n.
    polychromatophilic n.
normoblastic
normoblastosis
normocalcemia
normochromic
normocrinic
normocyte
normocytic
normocytosis
normoglycemia
normokalemia
normo-orthocytosis
normorphine
normothermia
normovolemia
nornicotine
norpropoxyphene
Norrie's disease
North American blastomycosis
nortriptyline
Norum's disease
Norwalk
    agent
    virus

NOS — not otherwise specified
noscapine
nosocomial
nosology
nosomycosis
Nosopsyllus
    N. fasciatus
notencephalocele
notencephalus
notochord
Notoedres
novobiocin
Novy, MacNeal and Nicolle's medium
noxious
NP — nasopharyngeal
    nasopharynx
    neuropathology
    neuropsychiatric
    nitrogen-phosphorus
    normal plasma
    nucleoplasmic index
    nucleoprotein
Np — neptunium
NPB — nodal premature beat
NPC — near point of convergence
NPD — Niemann-Pick disease
NP detector
NPDL — nodular, poorly differentiated lymphocytes
NPH — neutral protamine Hagedorn (insulin)
NPN — nonprotein nitrogen
4-NPP — 4-nitrophenylphosphate
NPR — net protein ratio
NPT — neoprecipitin test
NPU — net protein utilization
NR — nonreactive
    no radiation

NR *(continued)*
   no response
   normal
   not recorded
   not resolved
NRBC — nucleated red blood cell
NRC — National Research Council
   normal retinal correspondence
   Nuclear Regulatory Commission
NRCC — National Registry in Clinical Chemistry
NRD — nonrenal death
NREM — nonrapid eye movement
NREM sleep
NRM — National Registry of Microbiologists
NRS — normal rabbit serum
   normal reference serum
NS — nephrotic syndrome
   nervous system
   neurologic survey
   nonspecific
   nonsymptomatic
   normal saline
   not significant
   not sufficient
N/S — normal saline
ns, nsec — nanosecond
NSA — no serious abnormality
   no significant abnormality
NSC — no significant change
NSD — nominal single dose
   normal spontaneous delivery
   no significant defect
   no significant deviation

NSD *(continued)*
   no significant difference
   no significant disease
NSH — National Society for Histotechnology
NSILA — nonsuppressible insulin-like activity
NSM — neurosecretory material
NSND — nonsymptomatic, nondisabling
NSQ — not sufficient quantity
NSR — normal sinus rhythm
NSS — normal saline solution
   not statistically significant
NSU — nonspecific urethritis
NT — nasotracheal
   neutralization test
   neutralizing
   nontypable
NTAB — nephrotoxic antibody
Ntaya virus
NTG — nontoxic goiter
NTN — nephrotoxic nephritis
NTP — normal temperature and pressure
nuchal
   n. fascia
   n. hemangioma
   n. region
   n. rigidity
Nuck's canal
nuclear
   n. aggregate
   n. alteration
   n. crystalline aggregate
   n. cytoplasmic ratio alteration
   n. enlargement
   n. inclusion body
   n. lipid aggregate

nuclear *(continued)*
    n. macromolecules
    n. magnetic resonance
    n. magnetic resonance spectrometer
    n. magneton
    n. membrane alteration
    n. ploidy
    n. pore alteration
    n. reactor
    n. sap alteration
    n. shape alteration
    n. size alteration
    n. transplantation
    n. vacuolization
Nuclear Regulatory Commission
nuclease
nucleated
nucleic acid
nucleography
nucleohistone
nucleoid
nucleolar
    n. alteration
    n. satellite
nucleolinus (nucleolini)
nucleolonema
nucleolus (nucleoli)
nucleon
nucleophagocytosis
nucleophile
nucleoplasmic
nucleoprotein
nucleosidase
nucleoside
    n. diphosphatase
    n. phosphorylase
    n. triphosphate
nucleosidediphosphate kinase
nucleosidemonophosphate kinase
nucleosome
nucleotidase
    3-n.
    5-n.
nucleotide
    n. cyclase
    n. pyrophosphatase
nucleotidyl transferase
nucleus (nuclei)
    accessory n.
    n. ambiguus
    n. amygdalae
    Balbiani's n.
    caudate n.
    Clarke's n.
    cuneate n.
    Darkshevich's n.
    Deiters' n.
    dentate n.
    diploid n.
    Edinger-Westphal n.
    n. gracilis
    hypothalamic n.
    n. of Luys
    motor n.
    olivary n.
    pontine n.
    n. pulposus
    Roller's n.
    sensory n.
    n. thoracicus
    vesicular n.
    vestibular n.
nuclide
NUG — necrotizing ulcerative gingivitis
nullipara
number
    Avogadro's n.
    CT n.
    Reynold's n.
numbness

NUMERICAL APERTURE – OBLITERATIVE

numerical aperture
nummular
nutrient
nutrition
nutritional
nux vomica
NV – negative variation
NVD – Newcastle virus disease

nyad
nyctalopia
Nygmia
nylidrin hydrochloride
Nyssorhynchus
nystagmus
nystatin

O

O – oxygen
    respirations (anesthesia chart)
    suture size (zero)
O – nonmotile organism
OA – occipital artery
    osteoarthritis
    oxalic acid
OAAD – ovarian ascorbic acid depletion
OAD – obstructive airway disease
OAF – osteoclast-activating factor
O agglutination
O agglutinin
O antigen
O antistreptolysin
OAP – osteoarthropathy
oasthouse urine disease
oat cell
    o. c. carcinoma
OAV – oculoauriculovertebral dysplasia
O & B – opium and belladonna
Obermayer's test
Obermeier's spirillum
Obermüller's test
obesity

object
    o. code
objective
    achromatic o.
    aplanatic o.
    apochromatic o.
    flat-field o.
    fluorite o.
    immersion o.
    semiapochromatic o.
obl – oblique
obligate
    o. anaerobe
oblique
    o. fracture
    o. inferior branch, oculomotor nerve
    o. interlobar fissure
obliquus
    o. capitis muscle
    o. externus abdominis muscle
    o. internus abdominis muscle
obliteration
    fibrous o.
obliterative
    o. endocarditis
    o. inflammation

obliterative *(continued)*
    o. pleuritis
OBS — organic brain syndrome
obsession
obsessive-compulsive
    o.-c. neurosis
    o.-c. personality
    o.-c. psychoneurosis
obstetrical
obstipation
obstruction
    ball-valve o.
    complete o.
    intestinal o.
    mesenteric vascular o.
    partial o.
    urinary o.
obstructive
    o. cirrhosis
    o. diverticulitis
    o. emphysema
    o. hyperbilirubinuria
    o. jaundice
    o. pulmonitis
obturator
    o. artery
    o. internus muscle
    o. lymph node
    o. muscle
    o. nerve
    o. vein
OC — occlusocervical
    oral contraceptive
O_2cap — oxygen capacity
occipital
    o. artery
    o. bone
    o. gyrus
    o. horn
    o. lobe
    o. lymph node
    o. myotome

occipital *(continued)*
    o. nerve
    o. pole
    o. region
    o. sinus
    o. sulcus
    o. vein
occipitalization
occipitofrontal projection
occipitotemporal gyrus
occiput
occlusal
occlusion
    thrombotic o.
occult
occupational
    o. lung disease
OCG — oral cholecystogram
ochratoxin
Ochromyia
    O. anthropophaga
ochronosis
O colony
OCR — optical character recognition
OCT — ornithine carbamoyltransferase
    oxytocin challenge test
octachlorocyclohexenone
octamethyl pyrophosphoramide
octane
octanoic acid
Octomitus
    O. hominis
Octomyces
    O. etiennei
octopamine
N-octylbicycloheptene dicarboximide
octyl cresol
N-octyl isosafrole sulfoxide

ocular
- o. muscle
- o. muscle palsy

oculocardiac reflex
oculocerebrorenal syndrome
oculomotor
- o. nerve
- o. nucleus

oculomycosis
OD — optical density
    outside diameter
ODA — occipitodextra anterior
ODD — oculodentodigital dysplasia
Oddi's sphincter
ODM — ophthalmodynamometry
odontoameloblastoma
odontoblast
odontogenic
- o. cyst
- o. fibroma
- o. fibrosarcoma
- o. myxoma
- o. tumor

odontology
odontoma
- ameloblastic o.
- complex o.
- compound o.
- fibroameloblastic o.

ODP — occipitodextra posterior
ODT — occipitodextra transversa
odynophagia
OER — oxygen enhancement ratio
Oesophagostomum
- *O. apiostomum*
- *O. bifurcum*
- *O. stephanostomum*

Oestridae
Oestrus
- *O. hominis*
- *O. ovis*

OF — Ovenstone factor
OFC — occipitofrontal circumference
OFD — oral-facial-digital
OGTT — oral glucose tolerance test
Oguchi's disease
OH — hydroxyl group
Ohara's disease
17-OHCS — 17-hydroxycorticosteroid
ohm
ohmmeter
Ohm's law
OHP — oxygen under high pressure
17-OHP — 17-hydroxyprogesterone
Oidiomycetes
oidiomycosis
OIF — oil immersion field
OIH — orthoiodohippurate
oil immersion lens
oil-water ratio
ointment
- Credé's o.

Okazaki's segments
OKN — optokinetic nystagmus
OLA — occipitolaeva anterior
Old World hookworm
oleaginous
oleandomycin
oleandrin
oleate
olecranarthropathy
olecranon
olefin
oleic acid
- o. a. uptake test

oleoresin
    aspidium o.
    capsicum o.
oleovitamin A and D
olfactory
    o. bulb
    o. gland
    o. gyrus
    o. mucosa
    o. nerve
    o. neuroblastoma
    o. sensory epithelium
    o. striae
    o. sulcus
    o. system
    o. tract
    o. trigone
OLH — ovine lactogenic hormone
oligemia
oligocythemia
oligodactyly
oligodendroblastoma
oligodendrocyte
oligodendroglia
oligodendroglioma
    Grade I
    Grades II–IV
oligodynamic
oligo-1,6-glucosidase
oligohydramnios
oligomeganephronia
oligomenorrhea
oligomer
oligopeptide
oligophrenia
    phenylpyruvic o.
oligosaccharide
oligospermatism
oligospermia
oligotrophic
oliguria

oliva
    o. cerebellaris
olivary nucleus
olive
    cerebellar o.
    inferior o.
    spurge o.
    superior o.
olivocerebellar
    o. atrophy
    o. fibers
olivopontocerebellar atrophy
Ollier's disease
olophonia
OLP — occipitolaeva posterior
ol res — oleoresin
OM — otitis media
omagra
OMD — ocular muscle dystrophy
omental
omentum
    gastrocolic o.
    gastrohepatic o.
    gastrosplenic o.
    pancreaticosplenic o.
    splenogastric o.
OMI — old myocardial infarction
omitis
omohyoid muscle
OMPA — octamethylpyrophosphoramide
    otitis media, purulent, acute
Omphalalotus olearius
omphalelcosis
omphalitis
omphalocele
omphalomesenteric
    o. artery
    o. duct

omphalomesenteric *(continued)*
    o. vein
    o. vessels
Omsk hemorrhagic fever
Omsk hemorrhagic fever virus
onanism
Onchocerca
    O. caecutiens
    O. cervicalis
    O. lienalis
    O. volvulus
onchocerciasis
oncocyte
oncocytic adenoma
oncocytoma
oncofetal antigen
oncogene
oncogenesis
oncogenic
oncology
oncolysis
oncolytic
Oncomelania
oncornavirus
oncosphere
oncotic
Oncovirinae
Onthophagus
ontogeny
onychatrophia
onycholysis
onychomycosis
onychorrhexis
O'nyong-nyong fever
O'nyong-nyong fever virus
oocyst
oocyte
oogenesis
oogonium
oolemma
oophorectomy
oophoritis

Oospora
ootid
OP — opening pressure
       osmotic pressure
O & P — ova and parasites
opacities
    lenticular o.
opalgia
opaque
opening snap
open spina bifida
operand
operculum
operon
    arabinose o.
    lactose o.
    transfer o.
OPG — ocular plethysmography
        oxypolygelatin
ophiasis
ophidism
ophthalmia
    gonococcal o.
    gonorrheal o.
    o. neonatorum
    sympathetic o.
ophthalmic
    o. artery
    o. nerve
    o. vein
ophthalmitis
    sympathetic o.
ophthalmodynamometry
ophthalmology
ophthalmomycosis
ophthalmopathy
    infiltrative o.
ophthalmoplegia
ophthalmoplegic-type progressive muscular dystrophy
ophthalmoscopy
ophthalmosteresis

ophthalmotrope
opiate
opioid
opisthorchiasis
Opisthorchioidea
Opisthorchis
    O. felineus
    O. noverca
    O. viverrini
opisthorchosis
opisthotonos
opium
OPK — optokinetic
Oppenheim's disease
opponens
    o. digiti minimi muscle
    o. pollicis muscle
opportunist
opportunistic infection
opsin
opsoclonus
opsonin
opsonization
optic
    o. chiasm
    o. cup
    o. disc, disk
    o. nerve
    o. radiation
    o. recess
    o. stalk
    o. tract
    o. vesicle
optical
    o. character reader
    o. character recognition
    o. density
    o. isomer
    o. path
    o. rotary dispersion
    o. rotation
    o. scanner

optics
    fiber o. (fiberoptics)
    geometric o.
    physical o.
optimizing compiler
Optochin susceptibility test
OPV — oral poliovaccine
        oral poliovirus vaccine
ora (orae)
    o. serrata
oral
    o. cavity
    o. gland
    o. mucous membrane
    o. pharynx
    o. vestibule
orange
    acridine o.
    A. o.
    ethyl o.
    methyl o.
    victoria o.
orbicularis
    o. oculi muscle
    o. oris muscle
orbiculus (orbiculi)
orbit
orbital
    o. gyrus
    o. pneumotomography
    o. sulcus
orbitography
orbitomeatal
orbitoparietal
orbivirus
orcein
orchiectomy
orchioblastoma
orchiocele
orchitis
    autoimmune o.
    granulomatous o.

orcinol
ORD — optical rotary dispersion
ordinate
orexigenic
orf
    o. virus
organ
    Chievitz's o.
    Corti's o.
    Golgi's o.
    Jacobson's o.
    o. percussion
    spiral o.
    vestibulocochlear o's
    vomeronasal o.
    Zuckerkandl's o's
organelle
organic
    o. acid
    o. brain syndrome
    o. phosphate
organism
    Arizona o.
    Rickett's o.
    Vincent's o.
organization
organized
    o. hematoma
    o. pneumonia
    o. thrombus
organogenesis
organometallic compound
organon
organophosphate
organothiophosphate
organotroph
organotropism
organum vasculosum of the lamina terminalis
Oriboca virus

oriental
    o. body fluke
    o. lung fluke
    o. sore
orifice
origanum oil
Ormond's disease
ornithine
    o. aminotransferase
    o. carbamoyltransferase
    o. decarboxylase
    o.-ketoacid aminotransferase
    o. oxo-acid aminotransferase
    o. transcarbamylase
ornithinemia
Ornithodoros
    O. coriaceus
Ornithonyssus
ornithosis
    o. virus
orofaciodigital syndrome
orogenital syndrome
oropharyngeal
    o. isthmus
    o. membrane
oropharynx
Oropouche virus
orosomucoid
orotate phosphoribosyltransferase
orotic acid
oroticaciduria
orotidine-phosphate decarboxylase
orotidine-5'-phosphate pyrophosphorylase
orotidylate decarboxylase
Oroya fever
orphenadrine

Ortalidae
orthochlorobenzene
orthochromatic
   o. normoblast
orthodiagraphy
orthodromic conduction
orthoiodohippurate
orthomyxovirus
orthophosphoric
   o. acid
   o. ester monohydrolase
orthopnea
Orthopodomyia
orthopoxvirus
Orthoptera
orthoroentgenography
Orthorrhapha
orthostatic
   o. albuminuria
   o. hypertension
   o. hypotension
orthotopic
orthovoltage
Os — osmium
os (ossa)
   o. acromiale
   o. basilare
   o. calcis
   o. capitatum
   o. carpale
   o. coccygis
   o. coxae
   o. cuboideum
   o. cuneiforme
   o. ethmoidale
   o. frontale
   o. hamatum
   o. ilium
   o. interparietale
   o. lacrimale
   o. lunatum
   o. nasale

os (ossa) *(continued)*
   o. naviculare
   o. occipitale
   o. pubis
   o. sacrum
   o. unguis
   o. zygomaticum
oscillator
oscillopsia
oscilloscope
Osgood-Schlatter disease
Osler's
   disease
   erythema
   nodes
Osler-Vaquez disease
Osler-Weber-Rendu disease
OSM — oxygen saturation meter
Osm — osmole
osmic acid
osmicate
osmiophilic
osmium
   o. tetroxide
osmolality
osmolar
osmolarity
osmole
osmolute
osmometry
osmosis
osmotic
   o. coefficient
   o. fragility
   o. hemolysis
   o. nephrosis
   o. pressure
   o. shock
ossa
   o. carpi
   o. cranii

ossa *(continued)*
- o. digitorum
- o. faciei
- o. membri
- o. metacarpalia
- o. metatarsalia
- o. sesamoidea
- o. suprasternalia
- o. tarsi

osseous
- o. labyrinth
- o. metaplasia

ossicle
- auditory o.

ossicular
- o. ligament
- o. muscle

ossification

ossifying
- o. fibroma
- o. inflammation
- o. interstitial myositis

ostealgia

osteitis
- o. condensans
- o. deformans
- o. fibrosa cystica
- o. fibrosa disseminata
- sclerosing o.

osteoarthritis

osteoarthropathy
- hypertrophic o.
- hypertrophic pulmonary o.

osteoblast

osteoblastoma

osteocartilaginous exostosis

osteochondral

osteochondritis dissecans

osteochondrodystrophy

osteochondroma

osteochondrosarcoma

osteochondrosis

osteoclast
- o.-activating factor

osteoclastic resorption

osteoclastoma

osteocyte

osteodystrophy

osteofibroma

osteogenesis imperfecta

osteogenic sarcoma

osteoid

osteolysis

osteoma
- fibrous o.
- giant osteoid o.
- osteoid o.
- parosteal o.

osteomalacia

osteomere

osteomyelitis
- Garré's sclerosing o.
- pyogenic o.
- tuberculous o.

osteomyelodysplasia

osteomyelosclerosis

osteon

osteonecrosis

osteopathia

osteopathy
- alimentary o.
- disseminated condensing o.
- myelogenic o.

osteopenia

osteoperiostitis

osteopetrosis

osteophyte

osteopoikilosis

osteoporosis
- o. circumscripta

osteopsathyrosis

osteosarcoma
- parosteal o.

osteosclerosis

Ostertag
    streptococcus of O.
Ostertagia
ostium (ostia)
    o. primum
    o. secundum
    o. uteri
Ostwald viscosimeter
OT — occlusion time
        old tuberculin
        orotracheal
otalgia
OTC — ornithine transcarbamylase
        over-the-counter
        oxytetracycline
OTD — organ tolerance dose
otic
    o. ganglion
    o. vesicle
otitis
    o. desquamativa
    o. diphtheritica
    o. externa
    o. labyrinthica
    o. mastoidea
    o. media
    mucosis o., mucosus o.
    o. mycotica
    o. sclerotica
otoconia
otodynia
otolaryngology
otolith
Oto-Microscope
Otomyces
    O. hageni
    O. purpureus
otomycosis
    o. aspergillina
otorhinolaryngology
otorrhagia
otorrhea
otosclerosis
ototoxic
OTR — Ovarian Tumor Registry
ouabain
Ouchterlony immunodiffusion
Oudin immunodiffusion
OURQ — outer upper right quadrant
outer nuclear membrane alteration
ova
ovalbumin
ovalocyte
ovalocytosis
ovarialgia
ovarian
    o. artery
    o. cycle
    o. cyst
    o. follicle
    o. ligament
    o. masculinization
    o. tumor
    o. vein
ovaritis
ovary (ovaries)
oviduct
OVLT — organum vasculosum of the lamina terminalis
ovotestis
Ovotran
ovotransferrin
ovulation
ovulatory
ovum (ova)
    blighted o.
    pathologic o.
O/W — oil in water
        oil-water ratio

ox — oxymel
oxacillin sodium
oxalacetate transacetase
oxalate
    o. coenzyme A–transferase
oxalic acid
oxalism
oxaloacetate
    o. decarboxylase
oxaloacetic acid
oxalosis
oxalosuccinate
oxaluria
oxanamide
oxazepam
oxazine dye
oxazolidinedione compounds
oxethazaine
oxidant
oxidase
oxidation
    o.-fermentation test
    o.-reducing potential
oxidative
    o. phosphorylation
    o. phosphorylation inhibitors
    o. phosphorylation uncouplers
oxide
oxidize
oxidizing
    o. agent
    o. gas
oxidoreductase
oximinotransferase
3-oxo-adipate coenzyme A–transferase
3-oxobutyric acid
oxogluconate dehydrogenase
oxoglutarate dehydrogenase
oxoglutaric acid
oxohydroxybutyrate aldolase
oxoisovalerate dehydrogenase
oxolinic acid
oxonium ion
oxophenarsine hydrochloride
oxoprolinase
oxoproline
    o. reductase
oxoprolinuria
oxtriphylline
oxybiotin
oxycephaly
oxycodone hydrochloride
oxycyanide
oxygen
    o. affinity
    o. analyzer
    o.-hemoglobin dissociation curve
    o. poisoning
    o. pressure
    o. toxicity
    o. uptake
oxygenase
oxygenation
oxygenator
oxyhemoglobin
oxyhemogram
oxyhemograph
oxymel
oxymetholone
oxymorphone
oxyntic
oxyphenbutazone
oxyphencyclimine hydrochloride
oxyphenonium bromide
oxyphil
    o. adenoma
    o. cell
oxyphilic
oxyprocaine

oxypurinol
oxyquinoline
oxysteroid
oxytalan fiber
oxytalanolysis
oxytetracycline
oxytocin
   o. challenge
   o. hormone
   o. secretion
oxytropism
Oxyurata
oxyuriasis
Oxyuridae
Oxyuris
   O. incognita
   O. vermicularis
oz — ounce
ozena
ozolinone
ozone
ozonide
ozonophore

P

P — partial pressure
   pharmacopeia
   phosphorus
   plasma
   position
   postpartum
   premolar
   presbyopia
   pressure
   primipara
   probability
   protein
   pulse
   pupil
P. — *Pasteurella*
   Plasmodium
   Proteus
P_1 — parental generation
P_2 — pulmonic second sound
^{32}P — radioactive phosphorus
p- — para-
PA — paralysis agitans
   pathology
   pernicious anemia
   phakic-aphakic
   posteroanterior

PA *(continued)*
   pregnancy-associated
   primary amenorrhea
   primary anemia
   pulmonary artery
   pulpoaxial
Pa pascal
   protactinium
PAB or PABA — para-aminobenzoic acid
PAC — premature auricular contraction
pacchionian granulation
pacemaker
   wandering p.
pachyacria
pachycephaly
pachyderma
   p. laryngis
   p. oris
pachydermoperiostosis
pachygyria
pachymeningitis
   chronic adhesive p.
   fibrous hypertrophic p.
pachynema

pachyonychia
   p. congenita
pachytene
pacing
   cardiac p.
pacinian corpuscle
pack
packed
   p. cell volume
   p. red blood cells
Paecilomyces
paecilomycosis
PAF — platelet-activating factor
   pulmonary arteriovenous fistula
PAFIB — paroxysmal atrial fibrillation
Paget's disease
PAGMK — primary African green monkey kidney
PAH — para-aminohippuric acid
   polycyclic aromatic hydrocarbon
   pulmonary artery hypertension
PAHA — para-aminohippuric acid
pain
   fulgurant p's
   heterotopic p.
   homotopic p.
   ideogenous p.
   lancinating p.
   phantom limb p.
   referred p.
   terebrating p.
P-A interval
pairing
   base p.
   somatic p.

PAL — posterior axillary line
Palaemonetes
palatal
palate
   cleft p.
   gothic p.
   premaxillary p.
   soft p.
palatine
   p. arch
   p. bone
   p. gland
   p. mucous membrane
   p. muscle
   p. process
   p. tonsil
palatitis
palatognathous
palatography
pale infarct
paleocerebellum
palindromia
palladium
   p. chloride
pallium
pallor
palmar
   p. aponeurosis
   p. artery
   p. fibromatosis
   p. metacarpal artery
   p. skin
   p. vein
palmaris
   p. brevis muscle
   p. longus muscle
palmitate
palmitic acid
palmitin
palmitoleate
palmitoleic acid

handwritten note: p-ANCA per Dr. Settle (Hep) also c-ANCA

palmitone
palmitoyl–coenzyme A hydrolase
palpebra (palpebrae)
palpebral
    p. artery
    p. conjunctiva
palpitation
palsy
    Bell's p.
    bulbar p.
    cerebral p.
    Erb's p.
    facial p.
    ocular muscle p.
    progressive bulbar p.
    pseudobulbar p.
Paludina
paludism
PAM – crystalline penicillin G in 2 per cent aluminum monostearate
    phenylalanine mustard
    pralidoxime
    pulmonary alveolar macrophage(s)
    pulmonary alveolar microlithiasis
    pyridine aldoxime methiodide
pampiniform plexus
PAN – periodic alternating nystagmus
    peroxyacetyl nitrate
panacinar emphysema
panagglutination
Pancoast's tumor
pancreas (pancreata)
    aberrant p.
    accessory p.
    annular p.

pancreas *(continued)*
    Baggenstoss change in p.
    dorsal p.
    ventral p.
pancreatic
    p. acinus
    p. cholera
    p. duct
    p. fluid
    p. interstitial tissue
    p. islet cell antibody test
    p. islets
    p. islet stain
    p. lipase
    p. polypeptide
    p. tumor
pancreaticoduodenal
    p. artery
    p. vein
pancreatin
pancreatitis
    calcifying p.
    hemorrhagic p.
    necrotizing p.
    relapsing p.
pancreatography
pancreatolithiasis
pancreatopeptidase E
pancreatosplenic lymph node
pancrelipase
pancreozymin
pancuronium bromide
pancytopenia
    autoimmune p.
pandemic
Pándy's test
panencephalitis
    subacute sclerosing p.
Paneth's cells
panhematopoietic
panhemocytophthisis

panhypopituitarism
  postpuberal p.
  prepuberal p.
panmyelosis
panniculitis
  mesenteric p.
  metastatic p.
  nodular nonsuppurative p.
  relapsing febrile nodular p.
panniculus
  p. adiposus
  p. carnosus
pannus
panography
panophthalmitis
PANS — puromycin aminonucleoside
Panstrongylus
pantetheine
  p. kinase
pantetheinephosphate adenylyltransferase
pantomography
pantothenic acid
pantothenoylcysteine decarboxylase
PAO — peak acid output
PAOD — peripheral arterial occlusive disease
       peripheral arteriosclerotic occlusive disease
PAP — Papanicolaou (smear, stain, test)
    peroxidase-antiperoxidase
    positive airway pressure
    primary atypical pneumonia
    prostatic acid phosphatase

PAP *(continued)*
    pulmonary alveolar proteinosis
    pulmonary artery pressure
Papanicolaou's
  smear
  stain
  test
papaverine
  p. hydrochloride
papilla (papillae)
papillary
  p. adenocarcinoma
  p. adenoma
  p. adenomatous polyp
  p. carcinoma
  p. cystadenocarcinoma
  p. cystadenoma
  p. cystadenoma lymphomatosum
  p. duct
  p. ependymoma
  p. hidradenoma
  p. hyperplasia
  p. layer
  p. muscle
  p. necrosis
  p. serous cystadenocarcinoma
  p. serous cystadenoma
  p. syringadenoma
  p. transitional cell carcinoma
papillate
papilledema
papillitis
  anal p.
  chronic lingual p.
  necrotizing p.
  optic p.

papilloma
 basal cell p.
 choroid plexus p.
 fibroepithelial p.
 hyperkeratotic p.
 intracystic p.
 intraductal p.
 keratotic p.
 Shope p.
 squamous cell p.
 squamous p.
 transitional cell p.
 verrucous p.
 villous p.
papillomatosis
 intraductal p.
papillomatous
papillomavirus
Papoviridae
papovavirus
PAPP — para-aminopropiophenone
pappataci
 p. fever
 p. fever virus
Pappenheimer body
Pappenheim's stain
PAPS — phosphoadenosine diphosphosulfate
 phosphoadenosine phosphosulfate
 phosphoadenosylphosphosulfate
papule
 prurigo p.
papulonecrotic tuberculid
PAPVC — partial anomalous pulmonary venous connection
PAR — pulmonary arteriolar resistance
para-aminohippuric acid

para-aminosalicylic acid
para-aortic body
parabiosis
parabiotic
parabola
paracasein
paracentesis
paracentral
 p. lobule
 p. nucleus
 p. sulcus
parachlorophenol
Parachordodes
parachromatopsia
paracoagulation
Paracoccidioides
 P. brasiliensis
paracoccidioidomycosis
Paracolobactrum
 P. aerogenoides
 P. arizonae
 P. coliforme
 P. intermedium
paracolon bacilli
paracrine
paradichlorobenzene
paradidymis
paradoxical
 p. embolus
 p. infarct
parafascicular nucleus
Par. aff. — part affected
paraffin
paraffinoma
paraflocculus
parafollicular
paraformaldehyde
Parafossarulus
paraganglioma
 chromaffin p.
 nonchromaffin p.
paraganglion (paraganglia)

paragonimiasis
Paragonimus
   P. africanus
   P. caliensis
   P. heterotremus
   P. kellicotti
   P. mexicanus
   P. westermani
Paragordius
   P. cintus
   P. tricuspidatus
   P. varius
paragranuloma
   Hodgkin's p.
parahemophilia
parahormone
parainfluenza antibody test
parainfluenza virus, Types 1–4
parakeratosis
   p. scutularis
paralbuminemia
paraldehyde
parallax
paralysis
   p. agitans
   ascending p.
   bulbar p.
   familial periodic p.
   immunologic p.
   ischemic p.
   Landry's p.
   tick p.
   Volkmann's p.
   Werdnig-Hoffmann p.
paralytic
paramagnetic
paramammillary gray matter
Paramecium
   P. coli
paramecium (paramecia)
paramedian lobule

paramesonephric
   p. duct
   p. rest
parameter
paramethadione
paramethasone
parametrial lymph node
parametritis
parametrium
Paramphistomatidae
paramyloid
paramyotonia
   p. congenita
paramyxovirus
paranasal sinus
paraneoplastic syndrome
paraneuron
para-nitrophenylic acid
para-nitrosulfathiazole
paranoia
paranoid
   p. personality
   p. reaction
   p. schizophrenia
paraortic lymph node
paraoxon
paraparesis
parapepsin
paraphenylenediamine
paraphimosis
paraphyseal cyst
paraplegia
Paraponera
parapraxia
paraprotein
paraproteinemia
parapsoriasis
   p. en plaque
   p. lichenoides et varioliformis acuta
paraquat

pararosaniline
Parasaccharomyces
   P. ashfordi
parasellar
parasite
   ectozoic p.
   entozoic p.
   extracellular p.
   facultative p.
   intermittent p.
   intracellular p.
   malarial p.
   metazoan p.
   obligate p.
   protozoan p.
   spurious p.
parasitemia
parasitic
   p. ectopic pregnancy
   p. embolus
   p. fetus
   p. twin
parasiticide
parasitism
parasitoid
Parasitoidea
parasitology
parasomnia
paraspadias
parasternal lymph node
parasympathetic
   p. fiber
   p. nervous system
parasympatholytic
parasympathomimetic
parataenial nucleus
paraterminal body
parathion
parathormone
parathyrin
parathyroid
   p. chief cell

parathyroid *(continued)*
   p. extract
   p. gland
   p. hormone
   p. oxyphil cell
   p. transitional cell
   p. wasserhelle cell
parathyroidin
paratuberculous pneumonia
paratyphi S.C.
paratyphoid
   p. A and B.
   p. fever
   p. immunization
paraurethral
   p. duct
   p. gland
paraventricular nucleus
paravirus
parenchyma
parenchymal
parenchymatous
paresis
paresthesia
pargyline
parietal
   p. artery
   p. cell
   p. gyrus
   p. lobe
   p. lobule
   p. pericardium
   p. peritoneum
parietoacanthal projection
parietomastoid suture
parietooccipital
   p. artery
   p. fissure
   p. sulcus
parietoorbital projection
parietotemporal projection
Parinaud's syndrome

Paris
- P. classification
- P. green

parity

parkinsonism

Parkinson's
- disease
- facies

Park's aneurysm

parolfactory area

paromomycin
- p. sulfate

paronychia
- herpetic p.

paroophoron

parosmia

parosteal
- p. osteoma
- p. osteosarcoma

parotid
- p. duct
- p. fascia
- p. gland
- p. lymph node
- p. papilla

parotiditis

parotitis
- infectious p.

parovarian

paroxysmal
- p. auricular tachycardia
- p. cold hemoglobinuria
- p. dyspnea
- p. myoglobinuria
- p. nocturnal dyspnea
- p. nocturnal hemoglobinuria
- p. ventricular tachycardia

parrot fever

Parrot's disease

Parry's disease

pars (partes)
- p. distalis
- p. flaccida
- p. intermedia
- p. nervosa
- p. tuberalis

parthenogenesis

partial thromboplastin time test

particle
- alpha p's
- beta p's
- Dane's p.
- radioactive p's

particulate
- p. crystalline material
- settled p's
- suspended p's

partition
- p. coefficient
- oropharyngeal p.

parturition

Parvobacteriaceae

Parvoviridae

parvovirus

Paryphostomum
- *P. sufrartyfex*

PAS — para-aminosalicylic acid
periodic acid–Schiff (method, stain, technique, test)
pulmonary artery stenosis

PASA — para-aminosalicylic acid

PAS-C — para-aminosalicylic acid crystallized with ascorbic acid

pascal

PASM — periodic acid–silver methenamine

Passavant's bar
passive
    p. agglutination
    p.-aggressive personality
    p. anaphylaxis
    p. Arthus reaction
    p. congestion
    p. cutaneous anaphylaxis
    p. hemagglutination
    p. immunity
    p. transport
Passovoy factor
Past. — *Pasteurella*
Pasteurella
    P. haemolytica
    P. multocida
    P. pestis
    P. pneumotropica
    P. pseudotuberculosis
    P. septica
    P. tularensis
    P. ureae
pasteurellosis
pasteurization
Pasteur effect
PAT — paroxysmal atrial tachycardia
Patau's syndrome
patch
    gray p.
    herald p.
    MacCallum's p.
    mucous p.
    Peyer's p's
    salmon p.
    p. test
    white p.
Patein's albumin
patella
patent
    p. ductus arteriosus

patent *(continued)*
    p. foramen ovale
    p. urachus
Paterson-Kelly syndrome
path — pathology
pathogen
pathogenesis
pathognomonic
pathologic
    p. fracture
    p. ovum
pathology
    anatomic p.
    cellular p.
    clinical p.
    comparative p.
    dental p.
    experimental p.
    functional p.
    general p.
    humoral p.
    internal p.
    oral p.
    solidistic p.
    special p.
    speech p.
    surgical p.
pathophysiologic
pathophysiology
pathway
    alternative p.
    biosynthetic p.
    Embden-Meyerhof p.
    Entner-Doudoroff p.
    final common p.
    internuncial p.
    metabolic p.
    pentose phosphate p.
    reentrant p.
patient
Paul-Bunnell-Barrett test

KEY TO ENZYMES (CIRCLED NUMBERS)

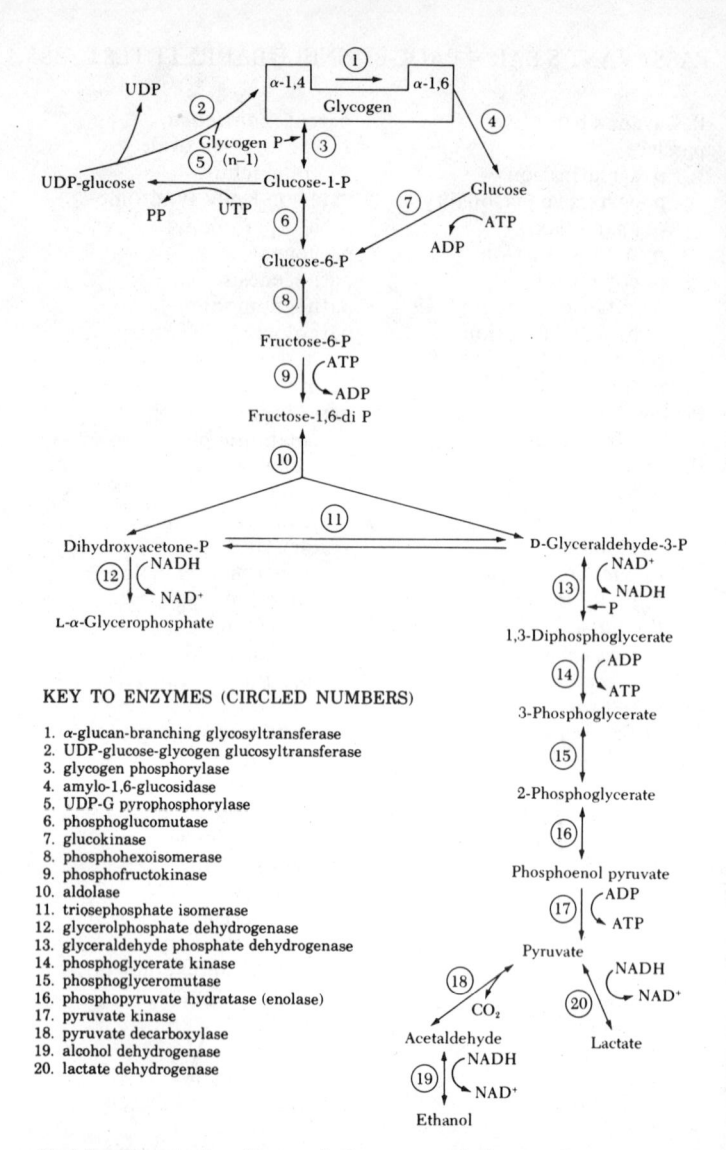

1. α-glucan-branching glycosyltransferase
2. UDP-glucose-glycogen glucosyltransferase
3. glycogen phosphorylase
4. amylo-1,6-glucosidase
5. UDP-G pyrophosphorylase
6. phosphoglucomutase
7. glucokinase
8. phosphohexoisomerase
9. phosphofructokinase
10. aldolase
11. triosephosphate isomerase
12. glycerolphosphate dehydrogenase
13. glyceraldehyde phosphate dehydrogenase
14. phosphoglycerate kinase
15. phosphoglyceromutase
16. phosphopyruvate hydratase (enolase)
17. pyruvate kinase
18. pyruvate decarboxylase
19. alcohol dehydrogenase
20. lactate dehydrogenase

Embden-Meyerhof pathway of glucose metabolism. (After Mazur and Harrow.) (From Dorland's Illustrated Medical Dictionary. 26th ed. Philadelphia, W. B. Saunders Company, 1981.)

Paul-Bunnell test
paurometabolous
Pautrier microabscess
Pavlov's pouch
PB — phenobarbital
phonetically balanced
protein binding
Pb — lead (plumbum)
PBA — pulpobuccoaxial
PBC — primary biliary cirrhosis
PBF — pulmonary blood flow
PBG — porphobilinogen
PBI — protein-bound iodine
P blood group
PBN — paralytic brachial neuritis
PBO — penicillin in beeswax
placebo
PBS — phosphate-buffered saline
PBT_4 — protein-bound thyroxine
PBV — predicted blood volume
pulmonary blood volume
PBZ — pyribenzamine
PC — pentose cycle
phosphate cycle
phosphatidylcholine
phosphocreatine
platelet concentrate
platelet count
portacaval
printed circuit
pubococcygeus
pulmonic closure
pc — picocurie
PCA — passive cutaneous anaphylaxis
PCB — paracervical block
polychlorinated biphenyl

PcB — near point of convergence
PCc — periscopic concave
PCD — phosphate-citrate-dextrose
polycystic disease
posterior corneal deposits
PCF — posterior cranial fossa
PCG — phonocardiogram
PCH — paroxysmal cold hemoglobinuria
pCi — picocurie
PCM — protein-calorie malnutrition
PCN — penicillin
PCO_2 or pCO_2 — carbon dioxide pressure
PCP — parachlorophenate
pentachlorophenol
phencyclidine
PCPA — parachlorophenylalanine
PCS — portacaval shunt
pcs — preconscious
PCT — plasmacrit
porphyria cutanea tarda
portacaval transposition
prothrombin consumption time
PCV — packed cell volume
polycythemia vera
PCV-M — myeloid metaplasia with polycythemia vera
PCx — periscopic convex
PD — papilla diameter
Parkinson's disease
patent ductus
phosphate dehydrogenase
plasma defect
prism diopter

PD *(continued)*
   pulmonary disease
   pulpodistal
   pupillary distance
Pd — palladium
PDA — patent ductus arteriosus
PDAB — para-dimethylamino-benzaldehyde
PDD — pyridoxine-deficient diet
PDH — phosphate dehydrogenase
pdl — pudendal
PDLL — poorly differentiated lymphocytic lymphoma
PDP — piperidino-pyrimidine
PE — pharyngoesophageal
   phenylephrine
   phosphatidylethanolamine
   photographic effect
   pleural effusion
   polyethylene
   pulmonary edema
   pulmonary embolism
peak
   p. acid output
   p. amplitude
   p. area
   p. broadening
   p. expiratory flow rate
   p. height
   p. kilovoltage
pearl
   epithelial p's
PEBG — phenethylbiguanide
peccary
pectenosis
pectin
pectinate
   p. body

pectinate *(continued)*
   p. ligament
pectinesterase
pectineus muscle
Pectinibranchiata
Pectobacterium
   P. carotovorum
pectoral
   p. fascia
   p. lymph node
   p. muscle
pectus
   p. carinatum
   p. excavatum
   p. gallinatum
   p. recurvatum
pederin
pediatrics
pedicle
Pediculoides
   P. ventricosus
pediculosis
Pediculus
   P. humanus capitis
   P. humanus corporis
   P. inguinalis
   P. pubis
pedigree chart
pedogenesis
pedophilia
peduncle
   cerebellar p.
   cerebral p.
   p. of flocculus
   inferior p.
   mammillary p.
pedunculated
PEEP — positive end-expiratory pressure
PEF — peak expiratory flow
PEFR — peak expiratory flow rate

PEG — pneumoencephalography
polyethylene glycol
PEI — phosphate excretion index
physical efficiency index
pelargonic acid
Pel-Ebstein fever
Pelecypoda
Pelger-Huët nuclear anomaly
peliosis
   p. hepatis
Pelizaeus-Merzbacher disease
pellagra
Pellegrini's disease
pelletierine
pellicle
pelvic
   p. bones
   p. endometriosis
   p. fascia
   p. kidney
   p. lymph node
   p. organs
   p. peritoneal cavity
   p. peritoneum
   p. plexus
pelvicephalography
pelvicephalometry
pelvimetry
pelvioradiography
pelviradiography
pelvis (pelves)
   p. major
   p. minor
   renal p.
Pemberton's sign
pemphigoid
   bullous p.
pemphigus
   benign mucous membrane p.

pemphigus *(continued)*
   p. erythematosus
   familial benign p.
   p. foliaceus
   p. neonatorum
   p. vegetans
   p. vulgaris
pen — penicillin
Pendred's syndrome
penetrance
penetrating
   p. ulcer
   p. wound
penetrometer
Penfield's method
penicillamine
penicillin
penicillinase
penicillinosis
Penicillium
   P. barbae
   P. bouffardi
   P. minimum
   P. montoyai
   P. notatum
   P. patulum
   P. spinulosum
penicillus (penicilli)
penile
   p. artery
   p. fascia
   p. vein
penis
   corpus cavernosum of p.
   glans of p.
   ligament of p.
   radix p.
   raphe p.
pent — pentothal
pentachloroethane
pentachloronitrobenzene
pentachlorophenol

pentaene
pentaerythritol tetranitrate
pentagastrin
pentamer
pentamidine
pentane
pentasodium tripolyphosphate
Pentastoma
   P. constrictum
   P. denticulatum
   P. taenioides
pentastomiasis
Pentatrichomonas
   P. ardin delteili
pentatrichomoniasis
pentavalent
pentazocine
   p. hydrochloride
   p. lactate
pentene
penthienate bromide
pentobarbital
pentolinium tartrate
pentolysis
pentosan
pentosazon
pentose
   p. phosphate pathway
pentosealdolase
pentoside
pentosuria
pentosyltransferase
pentylenetetrazol
PEO — progressive external ophthalmoplegia
PEP — phosphoenolpyruvate pre-ejection period
PEPP — positive expiratory pressure plateau
pepsin
pepsinogen

peptic
   p. esophagitis
   p. ulcer
peptidase
   leucine amino p.
peptide
   p. hormone
   p. hydrolase
   p. peptidohydrolase
   p. synthetase
peptidergic
   p. nervous system
peptidoglycan
Peptococcaceae
Peptococcus
   P. anaerobius
   P. asaccharolyticus
   P. constellatus
   P. magnus
   P. prevotii
peptone
Peptostreptococcus
   P. anaerobius
   P. intermedius
   P. lanceolatus
   P. micros
   P. productus
PER — protein efficiency ratio
peracetic acid
peracid
perbromate
percentile
perception
perchlorate
   p. discharge test
perchloric acid
perchlormethane
perchloroethane
perchloroethylene
percolation
percussion wave

percutaneous
perforated
    p. diverticulitis
    p. gastric ulcer
    p. ulcer
perforating
    p. fibers of Sharpey
    p. wound
perforation
    inflammatory p.
performic acid
    p. a.–Schiff reaction
perfuse
perfusion
perianal
periaortic
periapical
    p. abscess
    p. granuloma
periappendiceal
periappendicitis
periarteritis
    p. gummosa
    p. nodosa
    syphilitic p.
pericanalicular
    p. fibroadenoma
pericardial
    p. artery
    p. cavity
    p. fluid
    p. friction rub
    p. mesothelium
    p. sac
    p. tamponade
    p. vein
pericardiocentesis
pericardiophrenic
pericarditis
    adherent p.
    adhesive p.
    bacterial p.

pericarditis *(continued)*
    carcinomatous p.
    constrictive p.
    fibrinous p.
    fungal p.
    hemorrhagic p.
    idiopathic p.
    mediastinal p.
    obliterative p.
    purulent p.
    rheumatic p.
    serofibrinous p.
    suppurative p.
    tuberculous p.
    uremic p.
    viral p.
pericardium
    fibrous p.
    parietal p.
    serofibrinous effusion p.
    serous p.
    visceral p.
pericholangitis
perichondrium
pericolic
pericyte
    Rouget's p.
    p. of Zimmermann
periductal mastitis
periesophageal
perifornical nucleus
perihepatic
perihepatitis
perikaryon
perilymph
perilymphatic
perimetrium
perimysium (perimysia)
perinatal
perineal
    p. artery
    p. nerve

perinephric
    p. abscess
perinephritis
perineum
perineural
    p. fibroblastoma
perineurium
perineuronal satellite cell
perinuclear
    p. cisterna
periodate
periodic
    p. disease
    p. paralysis, familial
periodicity
periodontal
    p. cyst
    p. tissues
periodontitis
periodontium
periodontology
perionychium
perioophoritis
periorbital
periosteal
    p. fibroma
    p. fibrosarcoma
    p. sarcoma
periosteitis
    p. fibrosa
periosteum
    alveolar p.
periostitis
periostosis
peripancreatic
peripeduncular nucleus
peripheral
    p. circulatory failure
    p. edema
    p. lobule
    p. motor structure
    p. necrosis

peripheral *(continued)*
    p. nerve
    p. nervous system
    p. neuropathy
    p. odontogenic fibroma
    p. perfusion scan
    p. resistance unit
    p. sensory structure
    p. vascular disease
periplasmic
periplast
periportal
    p. bile ductule
    p. cardiomyopathy
    p. necrosis
periprostatic
perirectal
perirenal
perisplenic
perisplenitis
    hyaline p.
peristalsis
    reverse p.
    ureteral p.
peristaltic
peritendineum
perithecium
perithelioma
peritoneal
    p. cavity
    p. fluid
    p. hemodialysis
    p. lavage
    p. mesothelium
    p. sac
peritoneography
    positive contrast p.
peritoneopathy
peritoneoscopy
peritoneum
peritonitis
    acute diffuse p.

peritonitis *(continued)*
    fibrinous p.
    gonogoccal p.
    localized p.
    meconium p.
    septic p.
peritonsillar
    p. abscess
    p. tissue
peritracheal
peritrichous
periureteral
periurethral
perivasculitis
periventricular
    p. arcuate nucleus
    p. gray matter
perivesical
perlèche
Perls' reaction
permanent
permanganate
permeability
permeable
permease
permutation
pernicious
    p. anemia
    p. malaria
pernio (perniones)
peroneal
    p. artery
    p. longus plantaris muscle tendon
    p. muscle
    p. muscular atrophy
    p. nerve
    p. vein
peroxidase
    p.-antiperoxidase
peroxide
    hydrogen p.

peroxisome
peroxyacetic acid
peroxyacetyl nitrate
peroxyacylnitrate
perpad — perineal pad
perpendicular fasciculus
perphenazine
perseveration
personality
    compulsive p.
    cyclothymic p.
    hypomanic p.
    inadequate p.
    obsessive-compulsive p.
    paranoid p.
    passive-aggressive p.
    phobic p.
    psychopathic p.
    schizoid p.
perspiration
PERT — program evaluation and review technique
pertechnetate
Perthane
pertussis
perversion
pes (pedes)
    p. cavus
    p. valgus
pesticide
PET — positron-emission tomography
    pre-eclamptic toxemia
petechia (petechiae)
petechial
    p. hemorrhage
petit mal epilepsy
PETN — pentaerythritol tetranitrate
petrichloral
Petri dish

petriellidiosis
Petriellidium
  P. boydii
Petri's test
petrolatum
  hydrophilic p.
petroleum
  p. ether
  p. jelly
petrosal sinus
petrositis
petrosooccipital synchondrosis
petrous ganglion
PETT — positron emission transverse tomography
Peutz-Jeghers syndrome
Peyer's patches
peyote
Peyronie's disease
PF — peritoneal fluid
  platelet factor
pF — picofarad
PFAS — performic acid–Schiff reaction
PFC — plaque-forming cell
Pfeiffer-Comberg method
Pfeiffer's
  bacillus
  disease
  phenomenon
PFIB — perfluoroisobutylene
PFK — phosphofructokinase
PFO — patent foramen ovale
PFP — platelet-free plasma
PFR — peak flow rate
PFT — posterior fossa tumor
  pulmonary function test
PFU — plaque-forming units
PG — phosphatidylglycerol
  plasma triglyceride

PG *(continued)*
  prostaglandin
  pyoderma gangrenosum
pg — picogram
PGA — pteroylglutamic acid
PGD — phosphogluconate dehydrogenase
  phosphoglyceraldehyde dehydrogenase
PGDH — phosphogluconate dehydrogenase
PGDR — plasma-glucose disappearance rate
PGH — pituitary growth hormone
PGI — phosphoglucoisomerase
  potassium, glucose and insulin
PGK — phosphoglycerate kinase
PGM — phosphoglucomutase
PGO — ponto-geniculo-occipital
PGP — postgamma proteinuria
PgR — progesterone receptor
PGTR — plasma glucose tolerance rate
PH — pharmacopeia
  prostatic hypertrophy
  pulmonary hypertension
Ph — phenyl
pH — hydrogen ion concentration
PHA — passive hemagglutination
  phytohemagglutinin
  pulse height analyzer
phacomalacia
phacomatosis
phacosclerosis
Phaenicia
phaeohyphomycosis

phage
phagocyte
    alveolar p's
    endothelial p.
    globuliferous p.
    melaniferous p.
    mononuclear p.
    sessile p.
phagocytic
phagocytoblast
phagocytolysis
phagocytosis
    vacuole alteration p.
phagolysosome
phagosome
phako-anaphylactic-endophthalmitis
phakomatosis
phalangeal
phalanx (phalanges)
phalloidin
pH alteration
phaneroplasm
phanerosis
phantom
    p. bar
    p. four-quadrant bar
    Hine-Duley p.
    p. limb
    p. spike and wave
pharmacodynamics
pharmacogenetics
pharmacokinetics
pharmacology
pharmacopeia
pharyngeal
    p. artery
    p. auditory tube ostium
    p. branch
    p. cavity
    p. fornix
    p. mucous gland

pharyngeal *(continued)*
    p. mucous membrane
    p. mucus
    p. muscle
    p. pouch
    p. recess
    p. submucosa
    p. tonsil
    p. tubal ostium
pharyngitis
Pharyngobdellida
pharyngoconjunctival fever
pharyngoesophageal
pharyngolaryngitis
pharyngopalatine
pharyngotympanic tube
pharynx
phase
    continuous p.
    disperse p.
    exponential p.
    inductive p.
    lag p.
    logarithmic p.
    M p.
    meiotic p.
    mobile p.
    moving p.
    S p.
    stationary p.
phasmid
Phasmidia
PHBB — propylhydroxybenzyl benzimidazole
Phe — phenylalanine
phenacaine hydrochloride
phenacemide
phenacetin
phenaceturic acid
phenaglycodol
phenanthrene
phenazocine

phenazopyridine hydrochloride
phencyclidine
phendimetrazine
phene
phenelzine sulfate
phenethylamine
phenformin hydrochloride
phenindamine tartrate
phenindione
pheniramine maleate
phenmetrazine hydrochloride
phenobarbital
phenocopy
phenogenetics
phenol
    p. liquefactum
    p. red
    p. salicylate
    p. sulfatase
phenolic esterase
phenolphthalein
phenolsulfonphthalein
phenom
phenomenon (phenomena)
    Felton p.
    Huebener-Thomsen-
      Friedenreich p.
    Jod-Basedow p.
    Kanagawa p.
    Pfeiffer's p.
    prozone p.
    Raynaud's p.
    Sanarelli-Shwartzman p.
    Shwartzman's p.
phenothiazine
phenothioxin
phenotype
    Bombay p.
    McLeod p.
phenotypic
    p. variance

phenoxybenzamine hydro-
    chloride
phenoxyethanol
phenprocoumon
phensuximide
phentermine
phentolamine
    p. hydrochloride
    p. mesylate
phenyl
    p. *p*-aminosalicylate
    p. cyclohexanol
    p. dimethyl urea
    p. mercuric acetate
    p. mercuric chloride
    p. mercuric salt
    p. salicylate
N-phenylacetamide
phenylacetic acid
phenylacetylglutamine
phenylalanine
    p. hydroxylase
    p. mustard
phenylalanyl
phenylaminopropane
phenylbutazone
phenylcarbinol
phenyldiphenyloxadiazole
p-phenylenediamine
phenylephrine
    p. bitartrate
    p. hydrobromide
    p. hydrochloride
    p. tannate
phenylethanolamine-*N*-methyl
    transferase
phenylhydrazine
phenylketonuria
phenyllactic acid
phenylmercuric
    p. nitrate

phenylmercuric *(continued)*
   p. triethanol ammonium lactate
o-phenylphenol
phenylpropanolamine
phenylpropylmethylamine
phenylpyruvate tautomerase
phenylpyruvic
   p. acid
   p. oligophrenia
phenylpyruvicaciduria
phenylthiocarbamide
phenylthiocarbamoyl
phenylthiourea
phenyltoloxamine
phenyramidol hydrochloride
phenytoin
pheochrome
pheochromoblastoma
pheochromocyte
pheochromocytoma
pheomelanin
pheresis
pheromone
PHI — phosphohexoisomerase
Phialophora
   P. compactum
   P. dermatitidis
   P. gougerotii
   P. jeanselmei
   P. mutabilis
   P. parasitica
   P. repens
   P. richardsiae
   P. spinifera
   P. verrucosa
phialophore
phialospore
Philadelphia chromosome
phimosis
pH indicator

PHK — platelet phosphohexokinase
PHLA — postheparin lipolytic activity
phlebarteriectasia
phlebectasia
phlebitis
phlebogram
phlebography
phlebolith
phleborheography
phlebosclerosis
phlebothrombosis
Phlebotomus
   P. argentipes
   P. chinensis
   P. intermedius
   P. macedonicum
   P. noguchi
   P. papatasii
   P. sergenti
   P. verrucarum
   P. vexator
phlebotomus
   p. fever
   p. fever virus
phlegm
phlegmasia
   p. alba dolens
   p. cerulea dolens
phlegmon
phlorhizin
phloroglucin
phloroglucinol
phloxine
phlyctenular conjunctivitis
phlyctenule
phlyctenulosis
phobic
   p. neurosis
   p. personality

phobic *(continued)*
   p. psychoneurosis
phocomelia
pholcodine
Phoma
   P. hibernica
phonation
phonendoscope
phonoangiography
phonoauscultation
phonocardiography
phonocatheterization
phonogram
Phoridae
phorocytosis
phosgene
phosphagen
phosphatase
   acid p.
   alkaline p.
   serum p.
phosphate
   acid p.
   ammonium magnesium p.
   calcium p.
   carbamyl p.
phosphatemia
phosphatid
   p. histiocytosis
phosphatidate phosphatase
phosphatidylcholine
   p.-cholesterol acyltransferase
phosphatidylethanolamine
phosphatidylglycerol
phosphatidylinositide
phosphatidylinositol
phosphatidylserine
phosphaturia
phosphide
phosphine

phosphoadenosine diphosphosulfate
phosphoadenosine phosphosulfate
phosphoadenylate 3-nucleotidase
phosphoamidase
phosphocholine
phosphocreatine
phosphodiesterase
phosphoenolpyruvate
phosphoethanolamine
phosphofructokinase
phosphoglucokinase
phosphoglucomutase
phosphogluconate dehydrogenase
phosphogluconic acid
phosphoglyceraldehyde
phosphoglycerate
   p. kinase
   p. phosphomutase
phosphoglycerides
phosphoglyceromutase
phosphoguanidine
phosphohexoisomerase
phosphohexokinase
phosphoketolase
phosphokinase
phospholipase
phospholipid
   p. methylation
phosphomevalonate kinase
phosphomevalonic acid
phosphomolybdic acid
phosphomonoesterase
phosphonoacetic acid
phosphopantetheine
phosphopantothenoylcysteine synthetase
phosphoprotein

phosphopyridoxal
phosphopyruvate
    p. carboxylase
    p. hydratase (enolase)
phosphoribokinase
phosphoribosyl
    p.-formylglycineamidine synthetase
    p.-glycineamide formyltransferase
    p.-glycineamide synthetase
    p.-pyrophosphate amidotransferase
phosphoribosyl-aminoimidazole
    p.-a. carboxamide formyltransferase
    p.-a. carboxylase
    p.-a. succinocarboxamide synthetase
    p.-a. synthetase
phosphoribosylpyrophosphate
phosphoric
    p. acid
    p. diester hydrolase
    p. monoester hydrolase
phosphorus
    p. isotope
phosphorylase
    p. kinase
    p. phosphatase
phosphorylation
phosphoserine phosphatase
phosphotransferase
phosphotungstic acid
    p. a. hematoxylin
phostex
photic
    p. stimulation
photoallergy
photoautotroph
photocatalysis
photocell
photochemical
photochemistry
photochromogen
photochromogenic
    p. mycobacterium
photocoagulation
photoconductive cell
photoconvulsive response
photodermatitis
photodiode
photodynamic
photoelectric
photoelectron
photofluorography
photographic effect
photoheterotroph
photoheterotrophic
photolithotroph
photoluminescence
photolysis
photolytic
photometer
photometrazol threshold
photometric
photomicrograph
photomicrography
photomicroscope
photomultiplier tube
photomyoclonic response
photomyogenic response
photon
    Compton p.
photoophthalmia
photoorganotroph
photoparoxysmal
photophobia
photopic
photoptometer
photoreaction
photoreceptor
photoretinitis

photoscan
photosensitive
    p. porphyria
photosensitivity
photosensitization
photostable
photosynthesis
phototaxis
phototoxic
phototoxicity
phototransistor
phototrophic
phototropism
photovoltaic cell
PHP — primary hyperparathyroidism
        pseudohypoparathyroidism
phrenic
    p. artery
    p. vein
phrenicocolic
phrenoplegia
phrenosin
phrygian cap
phthalic acid
phthalocyanine dye
phthalylsulfacetamide
phthalylsulfathiazole
phthiriasis
Phthirus
    P. pubis
phthisis bulbi
Phycomycetes
phycomycosis
phylactic
phylaxis
phyllodes
phylloquinone
phylogeny
phylum (phyla)
physaliphorous

Physaloptera
    P. caucasica
    P. mordens
physalopteriasis
Physalopteridae
physicochemical
physiologic
    p. chemistry
    p. dead space
    p. hypogammaglobulinemia
physiology
physis
physisorption
physostigmine
    p. salicylate
    p. sulfate
phytanic acid
phytin
Phytobdella
phytobezoar
phytohemagglutinin
phytol
phytomitogen
phytonadione
phytophotodermatitis
PI — phosphatidylinositol
    protamine insulin
    pulmonary incompetence
    pulmonary infarction
PIA — plasma insulin activity
pia-arachnitis
pia-arachnoid
pia-glia
pia mater
    p. m. encephali
    p. m. spinalis
Piazza's test
PICA — posterior inferior cerebellar artery
pica
Pichia
    P. membranaefaciens

Pick's
- bodies
- cells
- disease
- tubular adenoma

pickwickian disease
picocurie
picofarad
picogram
picometer
picornavirus
picosecond
picrate
picric acid
picrotoxin
PID — pelvic inflammatory disease
- plasma iron disappearance

PIDT — plasma-iron disappearance time
PIE — pulmonary infiltration and eosinophilia
- pulmonary interstitial emphysema

piedra
- black p.
- white p.

Piedraia
- *P. hortae*

Pierre Robin syndrome
piezoelectric effect
PIF — peak inspiratory flow
- prolactin-inhibiting factor
- proliferation inhibitory factor

PIFR — peak inspiratory flow rate
pigeon breast
pigment
- calculous p.

pigment *(continued)*
- ceroid p.
- cirrhosis p.
- deposition p., bilharzial
- deposition p., malarial
- endogenous p.
- epithelial p.
- exogenous p.
- melanotic p.

pigmentary
- p. cirrhosis
- p. degeneration
- p. dermatosis

pigmentation
- arsenic p.
- bismuth p.
- hematin p.
- hematoidin p.
- hemofuscin p.
- hemoglobin p.
- lead p.
- lipochrome p.
- melanin p.
- porphyrin p.
- wear-and-tear p.

pigmented
- p. pilocytic astrocytoma
- p. purpuric lichenoid dermatitis
- p. villonodular synovitis
- p. villonodular tenosynovitis

PII — plasma inorganic iodine
Pila
pilocarpine
piloid astrocytoma
pilomatrixoma
pilonidal
- p. cyst
- p. sinus

pilus (pili)
piminodine esylate

pineal
  p. body
  p. corpora arenacea
  p. gland
  p. recess
  p. secretory rate
pinealocyte
pinealoma
pinene
pineoblastoma
pinguecula
pinocytoma
pinocytosis
pinocytotic
pinosome
pinta
pinworm
pion
PIP — proximal interphalangeal
pipamazine
pipazethate hydrochloride
pipenzolate bromide
piperacetazine
piperacillin sodium
piperazine
piperidolate hydrochloride
piperocaine hydrochloride
piperoxan hydrochloride
pipestem cirrhosis
pipet
pipethanate
pipette
PIPJ — proximal interphalangeal joint
pipobroman
pipradrol hydrochloride
Pirenella
piriform
  p. muscle
  p. recess
Pirquet's reaction
pisiform bone

PIT — plasma iron turnover
PITR — plasma iron turnover rate
Pittsburgh pneumonia agent
pituicyte
pituitary
  p. acidophil cell
  p. adrenocorticotropic cell
  p. alpha cell
  p. amphophil cell
  anterior lobe of p.
  p. basophil cell
  p. beta cell
  p. capsule
  p. cell
  p. chromophobe cell
  p. dwarfism
  p. endocrine disorder
  p. extract
  p. failure
  p. fossa
  p. gland
  p. gonadotropic failure
  p. growth hormone
  p. hormone
  p. hypertrophic amphophil cell
  p. mammotropic cell
  p. myxedema
  p. pars intermedia
  p. pars tuberalis
  posterior lobe of p.
  p. reserve
  p. stalk
  p. thyrotropic cell
  p. tumor
pit viper
pityriasis
  p. alba
  p. capitis
  p. lichenoides et varioliformis acuta

pityriasis *(continued)*
   p. linguae
   p. pilaris
   p. rosea
   p. rubra pilaris
   p. versicolor
Pityrosporon
   P. orbiculare
   P. ovale
   P. versicolor
2-pivalyl-1,3-indandione
Pizzolato's peroxide-silver method
PK — Prausnitz-Küstner (reaction)
   psychokinesis
   pyruvate kinase
PKU — phenylketonuria
PKV — killed poliomyelitis vaccine
pkV, kVp — peak kilovoltage
PL — phospholipid
   placebo
   placental lactogen
   pulpolingual
PLA — pulpolinguoaxial
   pulpolabial
placebo
placenta (placentas, placentae)
   p. accreta
   battledore p.
   bilobate p.
   p. circummarginata
   circumvallate p.
   duplex p.
   p. fenestrata
   p. increta
   p. membranacea
   multilobate p.
   p. multipartita
   p. percreta
   p. previa

placenta *(continued)*
   p. spuria
   p. succenturiata
   p. trilobate
   p. tripartita
   twin p., dichorionic
   twin p., monoamniotic
   twin p., monochorionic
   twin p., monochorionic diamniotic
placental
   p. cotyledon
   p. fetal surface
   p. fluids
   p. fragment
   p. lactogen
   p. maternal surface
   p. membrane
   p. polyp
   p. spaces
   p. sulfatase
   p. villi
placentitis
placentography
placode
plagiocephaly
plague
   p. bacillus
   black p.
   bubonic p.
   cellulocutaneous p.
   hemorrhagic p.
   pneumonic p.
   septicemic p.
   sylvatic p.
   urban p.
Planck's
   constant
   radiation law
plane
   auriculoinfraorbital p.
   axiobuccolingual p.

plane *(continued)*
- axiomesiodistal p.
- coronal p.
- frontal p.
- horizontal p.
- interparietal p.
- intertubercular p.
- labiolingual p.
- mediodistal p.
- midsagittal p.
- occipital p.
- orbital p.
- parasagittal p.
- popliteal p.
- sagittal p.
- sternal p.
- sternoxiphoid p.
- transpyloric p.
- vertical p.

planigraphy
planimeter
planimetry
Planorbis
Plantago
plantar
- p. aponeurosis
- p. artery
- p. fibromatosis
- p. reflex
- p. vein
- p. wart

plantaris muscle
plantodorsal
plaque
- atheromatous p.
- Hollenhorst p's
- McCallum's p.
- senile p.

plasma
- p. alteration
- p. cell
- p. clotting time

plasma *(continued)*
- p. dyscrasia
- p. exchange
- p. hemoglobin
- p. iron turnover rate
- p. level
- p. membrane
- p. protein fraction
- p. recalcification
- p. renin activity
- p.-thrombin clot method
- p. thromboplastin antecedent deficiency
- p. thromboplastin component
- p. triglyceride
- p. volume

plasmablast
plasmacrit
plasmacyte
plasmacytic
- p. cells
- p. leukemia
- p. myeloma
- p. tissue

plasmacytoma
plasmacytosis
plasmagene
plasmahaut
plasmalemma
plasmalogen
plasmapheresis
plasmarrhexis
plasmid
- conjugative p.
- p. integration
- oligomeric p.
- p. transfer

plasmin
- p. coagulation

plasminogen
plasmocyte

Plasmodiidae
Plasmodium
    P. *falciparum*
    P. *malariae*
    P. *ovale*
    P. *pleurodyniae*
    P. *vivax*
    P. *vivax minuta*
plasmodium
    exoerythrocytic p.
plasmolysis
plasmon
plasmoptysis
plasmotype
plate
    alar p.
    axial p.
    chorionic p.
    cribriform p.
    epiphyseal p.
    ethmovomerine p.
    Fresnel zone p.
    subgerminal p.
    tarsal p.
    tympanic p.
    ventrolateral p.
platelet
    p. activating factor
    p. adhesiveness test
    p. aggregation test
    p. autoantibodies
    p. concentrate
    p. count
    p. defect
    p.-derived growth factor
    p.-free plasma
    p. isoantibodies
    p.-poor plasma
    p. retention test
    p.-rich plasma
    p. survival test
    p. thrombus

plateletpheresis
platinosis
platinum
platybasia
Platyhelminthes
platypnea
platysma muscle
PLD – platelet defect
pleiotropy
pleocytosis
pleokaryocyte
pleomorphic
    p. carcinoma
    p. lipoma
pleomorphism
Pleospora
plerocercoid
Plesiomonas shigelloides
plethora
plethysmogram
plethysmograph
plethysmography
pleura (pleurae)
pleural
    p. cavities
    p. effusion
    p. fibroma
    p. fluids
    p. friction rub
pleuralgia
Pleur. Fl. – pleural fluid
pleurisy
    fibrinous p.
pleuritis
    acute fibrinous p.
    fibrinous p.
    obliterative p.
Pleuroceridae
pleurodesis
pleurodynia
pleurography
pleurohepatitis

pleuropneumonia
   p.-like organism
pleuroscopy
PLEVA — pityriasis lichenoides et varioliformis acuta
plexiform
   p. neurofibroma
   p. neuroma
plexitis
plexus
   Auerbach's p.
   Bonnet's p.
   brachial p.
   cavernous p.
   enteric p.
   Meissner's nerve p.
   myenteric p.
   submucosal p.
   subserosal p.
plica (plicae)
   p. interureterica
   p. palmata
plication
ploidy
PLS — prostaglandin-like substance
PLT — psittacosis–lymphogranuloma venereum–trachoma
plumbism
Plummer's disease
Plummer-Vinson syndrome
pluripotent myeloid stem cell
plutonium
PLV — live poliomyelitis vaccine
   panleukopenia virus
   phenylalanine-lysine-vasopressin
PM — photomultiplier tube

PM *(continued)*
   polymorph
   postmortem
   pulpomesial
Pm — promethium
pm — picometer
PMA — prevalence of gingivitis (papillary, marginal, attached)
   progressive muscular atrophy
PMB — para-hydroxymercuribenzoate
   polymorphonuclear basophil
PMC — pseudomembranous colitis
PMD — primary myocardial disease
   progressive muscular dystrophy
PME — polymorphonuclear eosinophil
PMF — progressive massive fibrosis
PMI — point of maximal impulse
   point of maximal intensity
PML — progressive multifocal leukoencephalopathy
PMN — polymorphonuclear neutrophil
PMR — perinatal mortality rate
   proportionate morbidity ratio
   proportionate mortality ratio
PMS — phenazine methosulfate
   postmitochondrial supernatant

PMS *(continued)*
    pregnant mare serum
PMSG — pregnant mare serum
    gonadotropin
PMT — Porteus maze test
PN — periarteritis nodosa
    peripheral neuropathy
    pneumonia
    positional nystagmus
    pyelonephritis
P_{NA} — plasma sodium
PND — paroxysmal nocturnal
    dyspnea
pneumarthrosis
pneumatocele
pneumatosis
    p. cystoides intestinalis
    p. intestinalis cystica
pneumoarthrography
pneumobacillus
    Friedländer's p.
pneumococcal
pneumococcus (pneumococci)
pneumoconiosis
Pneumocystis
    P. carinii
pneumocystography
pneumocystosis
pneumoencephalography
pneumograph
pneumography
pneumolithiasis
pneumomediastinum
pneumonectomy
pneumonia
    acute gelatinous p.
    aspiration p.
    atypical p.
    chemical p.
    confluent p.
    desquamative interstitial p.

pneumonia *(continued)*
    diffuse p.
    focal p.
    Friedländer's p.
    fungal p.
    giant cell p.
    Hemophilus influenzae p.
    hemorrhagic p.
    hypostatic p.
    inhalation p.
    interstitial p.
    Klebsiella p.
    lipid p.
    lipoid p.
    lobar p.
    lobular p.
    mycoplasmal p.
    organized p.
    paratuberculous p.
    Pittsburgh p. agent
    plasma cell p.
    pneumococcal p.
    primary atypical p.
    primary influenza virus p.
    rheumatic p.
    staphylococcal p.
    streptococcal p.
    unresolved p.
    uremic p.
    viral p.
pneumonic plague
pneumonitis
    desquamative interstitial p.
    interstitial p.
    rheumatic p.
    uremic p.
pneumonocyte
pneumoperitoneum
pneumopyelography
pneumoretroperitoneum
pneumotachogram

pneumothorax
    spontaneous p.
    therapeutic p.
pneumoventriculography
pneumovirus
PNH – paroxysmal nocturnal hemoglobinuria
PNP – para-nitrophenol
PNPP – para-nitrophenylphosphate
PNS – peripheral nervous system
PNU – protein nitrogen unit
PO – parieto-occipital
    polonium
    posterior
PO_2 or pO_2 – oxygen partial pressure (tension)
POB – phenoxybenzamine
podocyte
podophyllin resin
poetin
pOH – hydroxyl concentration
poik – poikilocyte
poikiloblast
poikilocyte
poikilocytosis
poikiloderma
    p. atrophicans vasculare
    Civatte's p.
poikilodermatomyositis
point
    alveolar p.
    apophysiary p.
    auricular p.
    conjugate p.
    craniometric p.
    Erb's p.
    isobestic p.
    isoionic p.
    jugomaxillary p.
    p. mutation

point *(continued)*
    occipital p.
    refraction p.
    supraclavicular p.
    thermal death p.
Poiseuille's law
Poison Control Center
poisoning
    antimony p.
    arsenic p.
    blood p.
    carbon disulfide p.
    carbon monoxide p.
    carbon tetrachloride p.
    chloroform p.
    cyanide p.
    desquamative interstitial p.
    ethyl alcohol p.
    heavy metal p.
    lead p.
    manganese p.
    mercury p.
    methyl alcohol p.
    naphthol p.
    nitroanilene p.
    oxygen p.
    paraldehyde p.
    salmonellal p.
    scombroid p.
    tetrachlorethane p.
    thallium p.
Poisson distribution
pokeweed mitogen
polar
    p. body
    p. compound
polarimeter
polarimetry
polarity
polarization
polarize
polarized light

polarography
poldine methylsulfate
pole
    animal p.
    vitelline p.
polio — poliomyelitis
polioencephalitis
poliomyelitis
    acute anterior p.
    immunization reaction p.
    virus p.
poliovirus, types I, II, III
pollex (pollices)
pollicis artery
polonium
poloxalkol
poly — polymorphonuclear leukocyte
polyacrylamide
polyadenylate
polyadenylic acid
polyagglutination
polyamide
polyamine-methylene resin
polyangiitis
polyarteritis nodosa
polyarthritis
polybrominated biphenyl
polycarbophil
polychlorinated biphenyl
polychromasia
polychromatic
    p. normoblast
polychromatocyte
polychromatocytosis
polychromatophilia
polychromatophilic
    p. normoblast
    p. rubricyte
polychromatosis
polychromemia
polyclave

polyclonal
polycyclic aromatic hydrocarbon
polycystic
    p. change
    p. kidney
    p. ovary
    p. ovary syndrome
polycyte
polycythemia
    p. hypertonica
    myelopathic p.
    p. rubra
    splenomegalic p.
    p. vera
polycytosis
polydactyly
polydeoxyribonucleotide synthetase
polyelectrolyte
polyembryony
polyemia
    p. aquosa
    p. hyperalbuminosa
    p. polycythaemica
    p. serosa
polyendocrine
    p. adenomatosis
polyene
polyenoic acid
polyester
polyether
polyethylene glycol alkyl ester
polygalacturonase
polygenic
polygon
polygraphic
polygyny
polyhedral
polyhedron
polyhelminthism
polyhydramnios

polyhydric alcohol
polykaryocyte
polymastia
polymer
polymerase
polymerization
polymetaphosphate
polymethine dye
polymicrobial
polymorphic
polymorphism
polymorphocyte
polymorphonuclear
    p. basophil
    p. eosinophil
    p. leukocyte
    p. leukocytic infiltrate
    p. neutrophil
polymyalgia rheumatica
polymyositis
polymyxin
    p. sulfate
polyneuritic-type hypertrophic muscular atrophy
polyneuritis
polyneuropathy
polynuclear
polynucleate
polynucleolar
polynucleotide
    p. ligase
    p. nucleotidyltransferase
    p. phosphorylase
polyomavirus
polyostotic fibrous dysplasia
polyp
    adenomatous p.
    aural p.
    cervical p.
    choanal p.
    cholesterol p.
    cockscomb p.

polyp *(continued)*
    colorectal p.
    endometrial p.
    fibroepithelial p.
    gastric p.
    granulomatous p.
    inflammatory p.
    laryngeal p.
    lymphoid p.
    nasal p.
    papillary adenomatous p.
    placental p.
    retention p.
    umbilical p.
polyparasitism
polypeptide
polyphagia
polyphase
polyphenism
polyphosphoric acid
polyploid
polyploidy
polypnea
polypoid
    p. adenoma
    p. hyperplasia
polyposis
polypropylene glycol
polypyrrylmethane
polyradiculoneuritis
polyribosome
polysaccharide
polyserositis
polysomaty
polysome
polysomnogram
polysomnography
polysomy
polysorbate
polyspermy
polyspike complex
polystyrene

polysulfide
polytene chromosome
polytetrafluoroethylene
polythelia
polythiazide
polyunsaturated
polyuria
polyuridylic acid
polyvinyl
    p. alcohol fixative method
    p. chloride
polyvinylpyrrolidone
POMP — prednisone, Oncovin, methotrexate, 6-mercaptopurine
Pompe's disease
ponceau B
pons (pontes)
    basilar p.
    decussation p.
    p. longitudinal fasciculi
    p. nucleus
    p. reticular formation nucleus
    spinothalamic p.
    p. superficial transverse fibers
    p. superior central nucleus
    tegmental p.
    transverse p.
Pontiac fever
pontine artery
ponto-geniculo-occipital spike
poorly differentiated lymphocytic lymphoma
POP — plasma oncotic pressure
popliteal
    p. artery
    p. vein
POPOP — 1,4-bis-α-(5-phenyloxazolyl)-benzene

population
pore
    alveolar p.
    gustatory p.
    p's of Kohn
    nuclear p.
porencephaly
Porges-Meier test
Porges-Salomon test
pork tapeworm
Porocephalus
    P. armillatus
    P. clavatus
    P. constrictus
    P. denticulatus
porokeratosis
    Mibelli's p.
poroma
    eccrine p.
porosity
porphin
porphobilinogen
    p. deaminase
    p. synthase
porphyria
    acute intermittent p.
    congenital p.
    p. cutanea tarda
    p. erythropoietica
    hepatic p.
    latent p.
    photosensitive p.
porphyrin
porphyrinuria
porta hepatis
portal
    p. cirrhosis
    p. hypertension
    p. lymph node
    p. tract
    p. vein

Porter-Silber
   chromogens
   reaction
Porteus maze test
portocaval shunt
pos. — positive
position
   anatomic p.
   decubitus p.
   occipitoanterior p.
   occipitoposterior p.
   occipitotransverse p.
positive
   p. pressure
   p. pressure breathing
positron
   p. beta decay
   p.-emission tomography
pos. pr. — positive pressure
post — posterior
     postmortem
postauricular
postbrachial
postcentral
   p. fissure
   p. gyrus
   p. sulcus
postchromation
posterior
   p. abdominal wall
   p. auricular artery
   p. auricular nerve
   p. cerebral artery
   p. chamber
   p. circumflex humeral artery
   p. column
   p. commissure
   p. communicating artery
   p. cusp
   p. dislocation

posterior *(continued)*
   p. displacement
   p. facial vein
   p. femoral cutaneous nerve
   p. forceps
   p. fornix
   p. fossa
   p. gray column
   p. horn
   p. inferior cerebellar artery
   p. intercostal artery
   p. lateral nucleus of thalamus
   p. leaflet
   p. limb
   p. limb bud
   p. lobe of pituitary
   p. lobe of prostate
   p. lunate lobule
   p. mediastinum
   p. meningeal artery
   p. papillary muscle
   p. parietal artery
   p. parietal gyrus
   p. parolfactory area
   p. pituitary
   p. quadrangular lobule
   p. quadrigeminal body
   p. retromandibular vein
   p. segment
   p. semilunar lobule
   p. sinus of Valsalva
   p. spinal artery
   p. superior alveolar nerve
   p. superior ansiform lobule
   p. synechia
   p. temporal artery
   p. terminal vein
   p. thalamic capsule
   p. tibial artery
   p. tibial tendon

posterior *(continued)*
    p. tibial vein
    p. tubercle
    p. ventral nucleus
    p. wall of oropharynx
    p. wall of stomach
posteroanterior
posterointermediate
    p. ventral nucleus
posterolateral
    p. artery
    p. fissure of cerebellum
    p. ventral nucleus
posteromedial
posteroventralis nucleus
postganglionic sympathetic fiber
posthemorrhagic anemia
postheparin lipolytic activity
posthepatic cirrhosis
postinfectious
    p. encephalomyelitis
    p. glomerulonephritis
postlingual fissure
postlunate fissure
postmature labor
postmaturity
postmenarcheal
postmenopausal
    p. endometrium
postmenstrual endometrium
postmordant
postmortem
postnecrotic cirrhosis
postnodular fissure
post-op — postoperative
postoperative shock
postpartum
postprandial
postpubertal
    p. hyperpituitarism
    p. panhypopituitarism
postpubescence
postreceptor
poststenotic dilatation
poststreptococcal
posttransfusion hepatitis
postulate
    Ehrlich's p.
    Koch's p's
postural
potable
potassium
    p. acetate
    p. *p*-aminosalicylate
    p. bicarbonate
    p. chlorate
    p. chloride
    p. chromate
    p. citrate
    p. cyanate
    p. cyanide
    p. dichromate
    p. enteropathy
    p. ferrocyanide
    p. guaiacolsulfonate
    p. hydroxide
    p. hydroxide (KOH) test
    p. imbalance
    p. iodide
    p. isotope
    p. oxalate
    p. perchlorate
    p. permanganate
    p. phosphate
    p. salt
    p. tartrate
    p. thiocyanate
    p. thiosulfate
    p. warfarin
potency
potential
    corneoretinal p.
    Donnan's p.

potential *(continued)*
  resting membrane p.
potentiometry
Potter-Bucky
  diaphragm
  grid
Pott's aneurysm
pouch
  branchial p.
  craniobuccal p.
  Douglas's p.
  first pharyngeal p.
  fourth pharyngeal p.
  Pavlov's p.
  pharyngeal p.
  Rathke's p.
  rectouterine p.
  rectovaginal p.
  rectovesical p.
  second pharyngeal p.
  third pharyngeal p.
  vesicouterine p.
povidone
  p.-iodine
Powassan virus
poxvirus
PP – pancreatic polypeptide
  partial pressure
  pellagra preventive
  permanent partial
  pink puffers (emphysema)
  postpartum
  postprandial
  prothrombin-proconvertin
  protoporphyrin
  proximal phalanx
  pulse pressure
  pyrophosphate
PPA – phenylpyruvic acid
PPB – platelet-poor blood

PPB *(continued)*
  positive-pressure breathing
ppb – parts per billion
PPBS – postprandial blood sugar
PPD – paraphenylenediamine
  phenyldiphenyloxadiazole *(indurated)*
  purified protein derivative
PPD-S – purified protein derivative–standard
PPF – plasma protein fraction
ppg – picopicogram
PPH – postpartum hemorrhage
  primary pulmonary hypertension
  protocollagen proline hydroxylase
PPHP – pseudopseudohypoparathyroidism
PPLO – pleuropneumonia-like organism
ppm – parts per million
PPP – pentose phosphate pathway
  platelet-poor plasma
PPR – Price precipitation reaction
PPS – pepsin
  postpump syndrome
PPT – plant protease test
Ppt or ppt – precipitate
  prepared
PPV – positive-pressure ventilation
PQ – permeability quotient
  pyrimethamine-quinine
PR – partial remission
  peripheral resistance

PR *(continued)*
   prosthion
   protein
   pulse rate
Pr — praseodymium
   presbyopia
   prism
PRA — plasma renin activity
Prader-Willi syndrome
pralidoxime
   p. chloride
pramoxine hydrochloride
praseodymium
Prausnitz-Küstner reaction
prazepam
prazosin hydrochloride
PRBV — placental residual blood volume
PRC — packed red cells
PRCA — pure red cell agenesis
   pure red cell aplasia
PRD — partial reaction of degeneration
   postradiation dysplasia
prealbumin
preamplifier
preauricular
prebetalipoprotein
prebiventral fissure
precancerous
   p. dysplasia
precentral
   p. fissure
   p. gyrus
   p. sulcus
precipitant
precipitate
   keratotic p.
precipitation
precipitin
precision

precocious
   p. adrenarche
   p. pseudopuberty
   p. puberty
precocity
preculminate fissure
precuneus
precursor
predator
predecidual
prediabetes
prednisolone
prednisone
preeclampsia
preejection period
preexcitation syndrome
prefibrinolysin
preganglionic sympathetic fiber
pregnancy
   aborted ectopic p.
   corpus luteum of p.
   ectopic p.
   extrauterine p.
   first trimester p.
   ovarian p.
   parasitic ectopic p.
   ruptured ectopic p.
   second trimester p.
   third trimester p.
   toxemia of p.
   tubal p.
pregnanediol
pregnanetriol
pregnenolone
preictal
preinvasive
Preiser's disease
Preisz-Nocard bacillus
prelaryngeal lymph node
preleukemia
prelytic sphere

Prevotella bivia

premature
- p. abnormal placenta
- p. atrial contraction
- p. climacteric
- p. contraction
- p. ejaculation
- p. infant
- p. labor
- p. menopause
- p. rupture
- p. separation of the placenta
- p. ventricular contraction

prematurely
- p. closed foramen ovale
- p. separated placenta

prematurity
premenarcheal
premenopausal
premenstrual
- p. endometrium
- p. tension

premolar
premorbid
premotor cortex
premyeloblast
premyelocyte
prenatal
prenyltransferase
preoccipital notch
preoptic
preovulatory
preparation
- allergenic protein p's
- biomechanical p.
- heart-lung p.
- impression p.

preproprotein
prepubertal
- p. hyperpituitarism
- p. panhypopituitarism

prepubescence
prepuce
- p. of clitoris
- p. of penis
- redundant p.

preputial
prepyramidal fissure
pre-rolandic artery
presbycardia
presbycusis
presbyopia
prescription
presenile dementia
presentation
- abnormal obstetrical p.
- arm p.
- breech p.
- compound p.
- face p.
- transverse p.
- umbilical cord p.

prespermatogonia
pressure
- atrophy p.
- cone p.
- p. crescent
- diverticulum p.
- groove p.
- p.-volume curve

presumptive heterophile test
presymphysial lymph node
presystolic gallop
pretracheal lymph node
prevalence
PRFM — prolonged rupture of fetal membranes
PRI — phosphoribose isomerase
priapism
Price-Jones curve
Price precipitation reaction
prickling sensation

prilocaine hydrochloride
primaquine
    p. phosphate
    p. sensitivity
primary
    p. adrenal insufficiency
    p. amenorrhea
    p. fibrinolysis
    p. fissure
    p. ovarian follicle
    p. spermatocyte
primate
primed lymphocyte typing
primidone
primigravida
primipara
primitive
    p. erythroblast
    p. mesoblast
    p. neuroblastic cell
primordial
    p. dwarf
    p. germ cell
    p. ovum
    p. sex cell
primordium (primordia)
principle
    antianemia p.
    Fick's p.
    follicle-stimulating p.
    hematinic p.
    immediate p.
    luteinizing p.
    prothrombin-converting p.
    proximate p.
    ultimate p.
printed circuit
P-R interval
Prinzmetal's angina
prism
    adamantine p's
    Nicol p.

prismatic
pristanic acid
PRL — prolactin
PRM — phosphoribomutase
        preventive medicine
Pro — proline
pro — prothrombin
proaccelerin
probability
    p. distribution
proband
probe
    p. of patent foramen ovale
probenecid
probit transformation
proboscis
probucol
procainamide
procaine
    p. amide hydrochloride
    p. hydrochloride
    p. penicillin G
procallus
procarbazine
procaryote
procedure
procentriole
proceptivity
process
    acromion p.
    alveolar p.
    articular p.
    caudate p.
    ciliary p.
    clinoid p.
    coracoid p.
    coronoid p.
    costal p.
    dendritic p.
    falciform p.
    mastoid p.
    odontoid p.

414 PROCESS – PROJECTION

process *(continued)*
    olecranon p.
    pterygoid p.
    spinous p.
    styloid p.
    Tomes' p.
    transverse p.
    uncinate p. of pancreas
    xiphoid p.
processor
processus
    p. vaginalis peritonei
prochlorperazine
    p. edisylate
    p. maleate
procidentia
procoagulant
procollagen
proconvertin
proctatresia
proctitis
proctocele
proctoptosis
proctoscopy
proctosigmoidoscopy
procyclidine
    p. hydrochloride
product
    cleavage p.
    contact activation p.
    fibrinolytic split p's
    fission p.
    gene p.
    spallation p's
    substitution p.
production-defect anemia
proenzyme
proerythroblast
proerythrocyte
Professional Standards Review Organization
profibrinolysin
profile
    liver p.
profunda femoris
    p. f. artery
    p. f. vein
progenitor
progeny
progeria
progestational
    p. endometrium
    p. hormones
progesteroid
progesterone
    p. receptor
progestin
progestogen
proglottid
prognathism
prognosis
progonoma
    melanotic p.
program evaluation and review technique
progranulocytic leukemia
progravid
progressive
    p. bulbar palsy
    p. cerebellar dyssynergia
    p. massive fibrosis
    p. multifocal leukoencephalopathy
    p. muscular atrophy
    p. muscular dystrophy
    p. pigmentary dermatosis
    p. spinal muscular atrophy
    p. systemic sclerosis
prohormone
proinsulin
projection
    Caldwell p.
    Fischer p.
    Towne p.

Prokaryotae
prokaryote
prokaryotic
Proketazine
prolactin
    p.-inhibiting factor
    p.-releasing factor
prolactinoma
prolan
prolapse
prolapsed umbilical cord
prolidase
proliferate
proliferation
    p. inhibitory factor
proliferative
    p. chronic arthritis
    p. endometrium
    p. glomerulonephritis
    p. inflammation
    p. myositis
    p. synovitis
proline
    p. dehydrogenase
    p. hydroxylase
    p. oxidase
    p. oxoglutarate dioxygenase
prolinemia
prolinuria
prolonged
    p. bleeding time
    p. coagulation time
    p. P-R interval
    p. QRS complex
prolyl
prolymphocyte
PROM — premature rupture of membranes
    prolonged rupture of membranes
promastigote

promazine hydrochloride
promegakaryoblast
promegakaryocyte
promegaloblast
prometaphase
promethazine hydrochloride
promethestrol dipropionate
promethium
promoblast
promonocyte
promoxolane
promyelocyte
    basophilic p.
    eosinophilic p.
    neutrophilic p.
pronation
pronator quadratus muscle
pronator teres muscle
pronephros
pronormoblast
pronucleus
propagating thrombosis
propagation
propane
propanediolphosphate dehydrogenase
propanenitrile
propanoic acid
propantheline bromide
proparacaine
propenyl
propepsin
properdin
proper fasciculus
prophage
prophase
prophylactic
prophylaxis
propiomazine hydrochloride
propionate
    p. carboxylase
    p. metabolism

Propionibacteriaceae
Propionibacterium
   P. acnes
   P. avidum
   P. granulosum
   P. lymphophilum
propionic acid
propionitrile
propionyl–coenzyme A carboxylase
proplasmacyte
proportional counter
propositus (propositi)
propoxycaine
propoxyphene
propranolol
   p. hydrochloride
proprioceptive
proprioceptor
proprotein
proptometer
proptosis
propyl
   p. alcohol
   p. diethyl succinamate
   p. gallate
propylene
   p. dichloride
   p. glycol
propylhexedrine
propyliodone
propylthiouracil
prorubricyte
prosection
prosencephalon
prosodemic
prosopagnosia
prosopalgia
prosoplasia
prosostomate trematodes
prostacyclin

prostaglandin
   p. endoperoxide
prostanoic acid
prostate
prostatic
   p. acid phosphatase
   p. duct
   p. gland
   p. muscle
   p. secretion
   p. tumor
   p. utricle
prostatitis
prostatocystitis
prostatography
prostatolith
prosthesis
   Starr-Edwards p.
prosthetic
prosthion
prostration
   heat p.
prot — protein
protactinium
protaminase
protamine
   p. insulin
   p. sulfate
   p. titration test
   p. zinc
protan
protanomaly
protanopia
protease
Proteeae
proteidin
   pyocyanase p.
protein
   Bence Jones p.
   C-reactive p.
   p. denaturation

protein *(continued)*
    p. electrophoresis
    p. hormone
    p. hydrolysate
    p. kinase
    Lathyrus p.
    M p.
    nonhistone chromosomal p.
    p. plasma
    p. synthesis
proteinase
    Bothrops atrox serine p.
protein-bound iodine
proteinemia
proteinosis
    alveolar p.
    lipoid p.
proteinuria
    Bence Jones p.
proteoclastic
proteoglycan
proteolipid
proteolysis
proteolytic
Proteomyces
proteose
proteosuria
Proteus
    P. inconstans
    P. mirabilis
    P. morganii
    P. OX-K, OX-2, OX-19
    P. rettgeri
    P. stuartii
    P. vulgaris
prothipendyl hydrochloride
prothrombin
    p. consumption time
prothrombinase
prothrombinogen
prothrombinokinase
prothrombinopenia

protirelin
protist
Protista
protium
protoanemonin
Protobacterieae
protocatechuate oxygenase
protocol
protocoproporphyria
protodiastolic
    p. gallop
protohemin
protokylol hydrochloride
proton
protoplasm
protoplasmic
    p. astrocyte
    p. astrocytoma
protoplast
protoporphyria
protoporphyrin
protoporphyrinogen oxidase
protoporphyrinuria
Prototheca
    P. ciferrii
    P. filamenta
    P. portoricensin
    P. segbwema
    P. wickerhamii
    P. zopfi
prototype
protoveratrine A or B
Protozoa
protozoan
    p. parasite
protozoon (protozoa)
protozoophage
protransglutaminase
protriptyline
protrusion
protuberance
    external occipital p.

protuberance *(continued)*
    internal occipital p.
Providencia
    P. alcalifaciens
    P. providenciae
    P. stuartii
provitamin
provocative chelation test
Prowazekia
Prower factor
prox — proximal
proximal
    p. convoluted renal tubule
    p. radioulnar joint
    p. tibiofibular joint
prozone
    p. phenomenon
PRP — pityriasis rubra pilaris
    platelet-rich plasma
PRPP — phosphoribosylpyrophosphate
P-R segment
PRT — phosphoribosyltransferase
PRU — peripheral resistance unit
prurigo nodularis
pruritus
    p. ani
    p. vulvae
Prussian blue
prussic acid
PS — periodic syndrome
    phosphatidylserine
    population sample
    Porter-Silber (chromogen)
    prescription
    pulmonary stenosis
    pyloric stenosis
P/S — polyunsaturated-to-saturated fatty acids ratio
Ps. — *Pseudomonas*
ps — per second
    picosecond
PSA — polyethylene sulfonic acid
psammoma
psammomatous meningioma
PSC — Porter-Silber chromogen
    posterior subcapsular cataract
PSD — peptone-starch-dextrose
PSE — portal-systemic encephalopathy
Pseudamphistomum
    P. truncatum
pseudarthrosis
pseudoacini
pseudoaldosteronism
pseudoalleles
pseudoarthrosis
pseudobulbar palsy
pseudocholesteatoma
pseudocholinesterase
pseudochromhidrosis
pseudocirrhosis
pseudocyesis
pseudocylindroid
pseudocyst
pseudodecidual
pseudodiploid
pseudodiverticulum
pseudoephedrine hydrochloride
pseudoepitheliomatous hyperplasia
pseudohermaphrodism
pseudohermaphroditism
pseudohyperkalemia
pseudohyperplasia
pseudohypertrophy
pseudohypoparathyroidism
pseudoisochromatic
pseudolymphoma

pseudomelanosis coli
pseudomembrane
pseudomembranous
    p. acute inflammation
    p. colitis
    p. enterocolitis
pseudomonad
Pseudomonadaceae
Pseudomonadales
Pseudomonadineae
Pseudomonas
    P. acidovorans
    P. aeruginosa
    P. alcaligenes
    P. cepacia
    P. diminuta
    P. eisenbergii
    P. fluorescens
    P. fragi
    P. kingii
    P. mallei
    P. maltophilia
    P. multivorans
    P. nonliquefaciens
    P. paucimobilis
    P. pseudoalcaligenes
    P. pseudomallei
    P. putida
    P. putrefaciens
    P. pyocyanea
    P. stutzeri
    P. syncyanea
    P. testosteroni
    P. viscosa
Pseudomonilia
pseudomucinous
    p. cystadenocarcinoma
    p. cystadenoma
    p. degeneration
pseudomyiasis
pseudomyxoma peritonei
pseudoneurotic schizophrenia

pseudoparakeratosis
pseudopodium (pseudopodia)
pseudopolycythemia
pseudopolyp
pseudopolyposis
pseudopseudohypoparathyroidism
pseudopuberty
pseudosarcoma
pseudosarcomatous fasciitis
pseudosclerosis
    Jakob-Creutzfeldt p.
    Westphal-Strümpell p.
pseudotumor
pseudouridine
pseudoxanthoma elasticum
PSG — peak systolic gradient
       polysomnogram
       presystolic gallop
PSGN — poststreptococcal
        glomerulonephritis
p.s.i. — pounds per square inch
psilocin
psilocybin
psittacosis
psoas
    p. abscess
    p. muscle
psoriasiform dermatitis
psoriasis
    exfoliative p.
    pustular p.
    p. vulgaris
psoriatic
Psorophora
PSP — periodic short pulse
       phenolsulfonphthalein
       positive spike pattern
       progressive supranuclear
         palsy
PSRO — Professional Standards
        Review Organization

PSS — physiological saline solution
progressive systemic sclerosis
PST — penicillin, streptomycin and tetracycline
psychalgia
psychataxia
psychiatry
psychoendocrinology
psychology
psychomotor
    p. epilepsy
    p. variant
psychoneurosis
    anxiety p.
    obsessive-compulsive p.
    phobic p.
psychoneurotic
psychopathic
    p. inferiority
    p. personality
psychosexual
psychosin
psychosis (psychoses)
    affective p.
    involutional p.
    Korsakoff's p.
    manic-depressive p.
    puerperal p.
    schizophrenic p.
psychosomatic
psychrophile
psyllium
    p. hydrophilic mucilloid
PT — parathyroid
paroxysmal tachycardia
pneumothorax
prothrombin time
PTA — persistent truncus arteriosus
phosphotungstic acid

PTA *(continued)*
plasma thromboplastin antecedent
post-traumatic amnesia
PTAH — phosphotungstic acid hematoxylin
PTB — patellar tendon–bearing
PTC — phenylthiocarbamide
phenylthiocarbamoyl
plasma thromboplastin component
PTE — parathyroid extract
pulmonary thromboembolism
PTED — pulmonary thromboembolic disease
pteridine
pterin
pterion
pteroic acid
pteroylglutamic acid
pteroylpolyglutamate
pterygium
    p. coli
    congenital p.
pterygoid
    p. muscle
pterygopalatine nerve
PTFE — polytetrafluoroethylene
PTH — parathormone
parathyroid hormone
post-transfusion hepatitis
PTHS — parathyroid hormone secretion (rate)
PTI — persistent tolerant infection
PTM — post-transfusion mononucleosis
PTMA — phenyltrimethylammonium

ptosis
PTP — post-tetanic potentiation
PTR — peripheral total resistance
PTS — para-toluenesulfonic acid
PTT — partial thromboplastin time
    particle transport time
PTU — propylthiouracil
PTX — parathyroidectomy
ptyalin
ptyalism
PU — peptic ulcer
    pregnancy urine
Pu — plutonium
pubarche
puberty
pubic symphysis
pubis
public antigen
Puchtler's
    alkaline Congo red method
    Sirius red method
PUD — pulmonary disease
pudendal
    p. artery
    p. nerve
    p. plexus
    p. vein
    p. venous plexus
pudendum (pudenda)
    p. femininum
    p. muliebre
PUE — pyrexia of unknown etiology
puerpera
puerperal
puerperium
PUFA — polyunsaturated fatty acid

pul — pulmonary
Pulex
    P. irritans
Pulicidae
pullorin
Pullularia
    P. pullulans
pullulate
pulmonary
    p. adenomatosis
    p. alveolar macrophage
    p. alveolar microlithiasis
    p. alveolar proteinosis
    p. alveoli
    p. artery
    p. blastoma
    p. capillary blood volume
    p. circulation
    p. congestion
    p. distomiasis
    p. edema
    p. embolism
    p. emphysema
    p. eosinophilia
    p. fibrosis
    p. hemosiderosis
    p. hypertension
    p. infarct
    p. interstitial emphysema
    p. lymph node
    p. osteoarthropathy
    p. perfusion
    p. perfusion scan
    p. plexus
    p. pneumonitis
    p. sarcoidosis
    p. surfactant
    p. tissue resistance
    p. trunk
    p. vein
    p. ventilation scan
    p. wedge pressure

pulmonic
    p. ring
    p. valve
pulmonic valve
    p. v. anterior cusp
    p. v. commissure
    p. v. cusp
pulmonology
pulp
    putrescent p.
    vertebral p.
pulpefaction
pulpitis
    putrescent p.
pulse
    alternating p.
    anacrotic p.
    bigeminal p.
    bisferiens p.
    carotid p.
    Corrigan's p.
    p. deficit
    dicrotic p.
    p. height analyzer
    irregular p.
    jugular venous p.
    paradoxical p.
    Quincke's p.
pulsion diverticulum
pulsus (pulsus)
    p. parvus
    p. tardus
pulvinar
    p. nucleus
    p. thalami
pump
    calcium p.
    cardiac balloon p.
    infusion p.
    perfusion p.
    peristaltic p.
    sodium-potassium p.

punctate
puncture
PUO — pyrexia of unknown origin
pupil
    Adie's p.
    Argyll Robertson p.
    bounding p.
    tonic p.
pupillary
    p. membrane
pure red cell aplasia
purified protein derivative
purinase
purine
    p. nucleoside phosphorylase
Purkinje's
    cells
    fibers
purpura
    allergic p.
    anaphylactoid p.
    p. annularis telangiectodes
    fibrinolytic p.
    Henoch's p.
    Schönlein's p.
    thrombocytopenic p.
    thrombotic thrombocytopenic p.
purulent
pus
    p. bonum et laudabile
    ichorous p.
    sanious p.
pustular
    p. psoriasis
pustule
putamen
putrefaction
putrescent pulpitis
PV — peripheral vascular
    peripheral vein

PV *(continued)*
    peripheral vessels
    plasma volume
    polycythemia vera
    portal vein
P & V — pyloroplasty and vagotomy
PVA — polyvinyl alcohol
PVA fixative method
PVA lacto-phenol medium
PVC — polyvinyl chloride
    postvoiding cystogram
    premature ventricular contraction
    pulmonary venous congestion
PVD — peripheral vascular disease
PVF — portal venous flow
PVM — pneumonia virus of mice
PVP — penicillin V potassium
    peripheral vein plasma
    polyvinylpyrrolidone
    portal venous pressure
PVR — peripheral vascular resistance
    pulmonary vascular resistance
PVS — premature ventricular systole
PVT — paroxysmal ventricular tachycardia
    portal vein thrombosis
PW — posterior wall
P wave
PWB — partial weight-bearing
PWI — posterior wall infarct
PWM — pokeweed mitogen
Px — pneumothorax
PXE — pseudoxanthoma elasticum

pycno-. *See* pykno-
pyelitis
    p. cystica
    p. glandularis
pyelogram
pyelography
pyelonephritis
Pyemotes
pygomelus
pygopagus
pyknodysostosis
pyknosis
pyknotic
pylephlebitis
pyloric
    p. antrum
    p. Brunner's glands
    p. gland, gastric
    p. lymph node
    p. sphincter
    p. stenosis
pylorospasm
pylorus
pyocolpos
pyocyanea
pyocyanin
pyoderma
    p. gangrenosum
pyogenic
pyometra
pyonephrosis
pyorrhea
pyosalpinx
pyoureter
pyramid
pyramidal
    p. cell
    p. decussation
    p. lobe, thyroid gland
    p. tract
pyramidalis muscle
pyran

pyranose
pyranoside
pyrathiazine
pyrazinamide
Pyrenochaeta
   P. romeroi
pyrethrin
pyrethrum
pyrexia
pyridine
   p. aldoxime methiodide
   p. nucleotide
pyridostigmine bromide
pyridoxal
   p. kinase
   p. phosphate
pyridoxamine
pyridoxic acid
pyridoxine
pyriform
pyrilamine maleate
pyrimethamine
pyrimidine
pyrithione zinc
pyrocatechol
pyrogallic acid
pyrogallol
pyrogen
pyrogenic
pyroglobulin
pyroglobulinemia
pyroglutamase
pyroglutamate
   p. hydroxylase
pyroglutamicaciduria
pyrolysis
pyronin

pyrophosphatase
   inorganic p.
   nucleotide p.
pyrophosphate
pyrophosphokinase
pyrophosphomevalonate decarboxylase
pyrophosphoric acid
pyrophosphorylase
pyrophosphotransferase
pyroracemic acid
pyrrobutamine phosphate
pyrrole
pyrrolia
pyrrolidone carboxylate
pyrroline
   p.-5-carboxylate dehydrogenase
   p.-2-carboxylate reductase
   p.-5-carboxylate reductase
pyruvate
   p. carboxylase
   p. decarboxylase
   p. dehydrogenase
   p. kinase
   p. phosphokinase
pyruvic acid
pyrvinium
   p. chloride
   p. pamoate
pyuria
PZ – pancreozymin
PZA – pyrazinamide
PZ-CCK – pancreozymin-cholecystokinin
PZI – protamine zinc insulin

Q

Q — coulomb (electric quantity)
Q_B — total body clearance
Q_{10} — temperature coefficient
QC — quinine-colchicine
Q fever
QNS — quantity not sufficient
QO_2 or qO_2 — oxygen quotient
QP — quanti-Pirquet reaction
QRS complex
QRZ — wheal reaction time
quadrat
quadrate
quadratus
    q. femoris muscle
    q. lumborum muscle
    q. plantae muscle
quadribasic
quadriceps
    q. femoris muscle
    q. tendon
quadriceptor
quadricuspid
quadrigeminal
quadriplegia
quadripolar
quadrivalent
qualitative
quantasome
quantatrope
quantimeter
quantitative
quantum (quanta)
quarantine
quartile
quartz
quasidominance
quassation
quaternary

quazodine
Queckenstedt's test
quercetin
Quervain's disease
Queyrat's erythroplasia
QUICHA — quantitative inhalation challenge apparatus
quicksilver
Quick's test
quinacrine
quinaldinic acid
quinate
    q. dehydrogenase
Quincke's
    disease
    pulse
quinestrol
quinethazone
quingestanol acetate
quinic acid
quinidine
quinine
    q.-colchicine
    q. hydrochloride
    q. sulfate
quinoid
quinoline
quinology
quinone
    q. oxime benzoyl hydrazine
    q. reductase
quinovose
quinquecuspid
quinquevalent
quintisternal
quotient
    albumin q.
    caloric q.

quotient *(continued)*
    protein q.
    rachidean q.

quotient *(continued)*
    respiratory q.
Q wave

R

R — Behnken's unit
    organic radical
    Rankine (scale)
    Réaumur (scale)
    rectal
    regression coefficient
    respiration
    Rinne test
    rotengen
    rough colony
R. — *Rickettsia*
R_A — airway resistance
R_x — prescription
RA — renal artery
    rheumatoid arthritis
    right atrial
Ra — radium
rabies
    r. virus
RA cell
racemase
racemate
racemization
racemose aneurysm
racephedrine
rachianesthesia
rachidial
rachigraph
rachiometer
rachis
rachischisis
rachitic
rachitis
RAD — right axis deviation

rad — radial
    radiation absorbed dose
radar
Radford nomogram
radial
    r. artery
    r. immunodiffusion
    r. nerve
    r. vein
radian
radiant
radiation
    cosmic r.
    r. damage
    r. dermatitis
    electromagnetic r.
    gamma r.
    infrared r.
    r. injury
    ionizing r.
    r. necrosis
    r. reaction
    r. response
    ultraviolet r.
radiative capture
radical
    acid r.
    alcohol r.
    free r.
radicular
radiculitis
radiculoganglionitis
radiculomedullary
radiculomeningomyelitis

radiculomyelopathy
radiculoneuropathy
radiculopathy
radioactive
   r. gold
   r. iodine uptake
radioactivity
radioallergosorbent test
radioassay
radioautography
radiobiology
radiocarpal
   r. joint
   r. ligament
radiochemical
radiochromatogram
radiodense
radiodermatitis
radioencephalography
radioenzymatic assay
radiogold colloid
radiograph
radiographic
radiography
radioimmunoassay
radioimmunoelectrophoresis
radioiodine
radioisotope
radiolabeled
radiologic
radiologist
radiology
radiolucency
radiolucent
radiolysis
radiometer
radionecrosis
radionuclide
radiopacity
radiopaque
radiopharmaceutical
radiophosphorus

radiopulmonography
radioreceptor
radiorenography
radioresistant
radioscopic
radioscopy
radiosensitivity
radioulnar
radio waves
radium
   r. isotope
radius (radii)
radix (radices)
radon
RADTS — rabbit antidog thymus serum
RAE — right atrial enlargement
RAF — rheumatoid arthritis factor
raffinose
ragocyte
RAH — right atrial hypertrophy
RAI — radioactive iodine
RAI scan
   RAI s. uptake
Raillietina
   R. celebensis
   R. demerariensis
RAIU — radioactive iodine uptake
RA latex fixation test
rale
RAM — random-access memory
Raman spectroscopy
Ramon flocculation
Ramsden's eyepiece
RAMT — rabbit antimouse thymocyte
ramus (rami)
   r. communicans
   dorsal r.
   ventral r.

random
- r. access
- r.-access memory
- r. coil
- r. error
- r. sample
- r. variable

randomization

Rankine temperature scale

ranula

ranular

Ranvier's node

RAO — right anterior oblique

Raoult's law

RAP — right atrial pressure

raphe

rapid eye movement

rapid plasma reagin test

rarefaction

RARLS — rabbit antirat lymphocyte serum

RAS — renal artery stenosis

Rasmussen's aneurysm

RAST — radioallergosorbent test

rat bite fever

rate
- age-specific r.
- case fatality r.
- cause-specific death r.
- circulation r.
- incidence r.
- morbidity r.
- mortality r.
- prevalence r.
- Rourke-Ernstein sedimentation r.
- sedimentation r.
- standardized r.

RATHAS — rat thymus antiserum

Rathke's
- pouch
- pouch tumor

ratio
- De Ritis r.
- myeloid-erythroid r.
- proportionate mortality r.
- standard morbidity r.
- standard mortality r.

Rattus

RATx — radiation therapy

rauwolfia
- r. serpentina

ray
- alpha r.
- beta r.
- cathode r.
- cosmic r.
- delta r.
- gamma r.
- grenz r's
- infrared r.
- monochromatic r.
- necrobiotic r.
- positive r.
- refracted r.
- roentgen r.
- titanium r.
- ultraviolet r.
- W r's
- x r's

Raynaud's
- disease
- phenomenon

RB — respiratory bronchiole

Rb — rubidium

RBA — rose bengal antigen

RBB — right bundle branch

RBBB — right bundle branch block

RBC — red blood cell

RBC *(continued)*
   red blood count
RBC/hpf — red blood cells per high power field
RBCM — red blood cell mass
RBCV — red blood cell volume
RBE — relative biological effectiveness
RBF — renal blood flow
RBL — Reid's base line
RBP — retinol-binding protein
RC — red cell
   red cell casts
   retrograde cystogram
RCA — right coronary artery
RCBV — regional cerebral blood volume
RCC — red cell count
RC circuit
RCD — relative cardiac dullness
RCF — red cell folate
   relative centrifugal force
RCM — red cell mass
   right costal margin
R colony
RCR — respiratory control ratio
RCS — reticulum cell sarcoma
RCV — red cell volume
RD — Raynaud's disease
   reaction of (to) degenertion
   resistance determinant
   respiratory disease
   right deltoid
   right dorsoanterior
rd — rutherford
RDE — receptor-destroying enzyme
RDI — rupture-delivery interval
RDP — right dorsoposterior
RDS — respiratory distress syndrome
RE — radium emanation
   regional enteritis
   reticuloendothelial
Re — rhenium
REA — radioenzymatic assay
reabsorption
reactance
   capacitive r.
   inductive r.
reactant
reaction
   alloxan-Schiff r.
   Arthus r.
   Bauer r.
   Bence Jones r.
   Berthelot's r.
   chemical r.
   Christeller r.
   Dold's r.
   Edman r.
   Ehrlich's r.
   false-negative r.
   false-positive r.
   Feulgen's r.
   foreign body r.
   Fujiwara r.
   giant cell r.
   glycine-arginine r.
   Gruber-Widal r.
   inflammatory r.
   Jarisch-Herxheimer r.
   Jones-Mote r.
   Langhans' type of giant cell r.
   Liebermann-Burchardt r.
   Meinicke turbidity r.
   Nagler's r.
   Nessler r.
   Nickerson-Kveim test r.
   Ninhydrin-Schiff r.

reaction *(continued)*
   performic acid–Schiff r.
   Perls' r.
   Pirquet's r.
   Porter-Silber r.
   Prausnitz-Küstner r.
   Price precipitation r.
   r. quotient
   reagin r.
   Schmorl's r.
   sigma r.
   Szent-Györgyi r.
   Wassermann r.
   Weil-Felix r.
   Widal r.
   Zimmermann's r.
reactive
reactivity
readout
readthrough
read-write memory
reagent
   Bial's r.
   chlorous acid r.
   Cleland's r.
   Coleman-Schiff r.
   diazo r.
   Drabkin's r.
   Ehrlich's diazo r.
   Folin-Ciocalteu r.
   gold chloride r.
   Hanker-Yates r.
   Mandelin's r.
   Marquis r.
   Millon's r.
   Schiff's r.
   Selivanoff's (Seliwanow's) r.
   Sickledex r.
reagin
reaginic antibody
real number
Réaumur scale
recalcification
recanalization
receiver operating characteristic
receptor
   acetylcholine r's
   adrenergic r's
   cholinergic r.
   complement r.
   contiguous r.
   dominant r.
   gustatory r.
   sessile r.
   visual r.
   volume r's
recess
   duodenojejunal r.
recessive
   r. gene
recessus (recessi)
recipient
reciprocal
recombinant
   r. DNA
recon
recovery
rectal
   r. ampulla
   r. artery
   r. crypt of Lieberkühn
   r. lumen
   r. mucous membrane
   r. mucus
   r. muscularis propria
   solitary, lymphoid r. nodule
   r. submucosa
   r. vein
rectification
rectifier
   bridge r.

rectifier *(continued)*
    full-wave r.
    half-wave r.
rectilinear
    r. scanner
rectocele
rectosigmoid colon
rectouterine
rectovaginal
    r. fistula
    r. septum
rectovesical
    r. pouch
    r. septum
rectum
rectus
    r. abdominis muscle
    r. capitis muscle
    r. femoris muscle
    r. inferior branch, oculomotor nerve
    r. medialis branch, oculomotor nerve
    r. muscle
    r. superior branch, oculomotor nerve
recurrence
recurrent
    r. artery
    r. laryngeal nerve
recursion
red
    r. blood cells
    r. cell aplasia
    Congo r.
    r. infarct
    r. mite
    r. nucleus
    Sirius r.
redox
    r. potential
    r. reaction

reduced nicotinamide-adenine dinucleotide
reductant
reductase
reduction
reduviid
Reduviidae
Reduvius
Reed-Sternberg cell
reentry
Reese-Ecker method
Rees's culture medium
REF — renal erythropoietic factor
reflection
    Bragg r.
    diffuse r.
    specular r.
    total internal r.
reflex
    accommodation r.
    Achilles r.
    audiocular r.
    autonomic r.
    axon r.
    Babinski's r.
    Bainbridge r.
    baroreceptor r.
    Bezold-Jarisch r.
    carotid sinus r.
    ciliospinal r.
    cochleopupillary r.
    conditioned r.
    corneal r.
    cough r.
    cremasteric r.
    Cushing's r.
    enterogastric r.
    extensor plantar r.
    flexion r.
    flexor plantar r.
    gag r.

reflex *(continued)*
    H r.
    Hering-Breuer r.
    Hoffmann's r.
    increased flexion r.
    increased stretch r.
    ischemic r.
    light r.
    mass r.
    monosynaptic r.
    oculocephalic r.
    oculovestibular r.
    patellar tendon r.
    polysynaptic r.
    pupillary r.
    spinal r.
    stretch r.
    suckling r.
    withdrawal r.
reflux
    hepatojugular r.
    vesicoureteral r.
refract
refraction
refractive
refractometer
refractory
Refsum's disease
REG — radioencephalogram
Regan isoenzyme
regeneration
    epimorphic r.
    morphallactic r.
regenerative endometrium
region
    C r.
regional
    r. colitis
    r. enteritis
    r. enterocolitis
    r. ileitis

register
registry
regression
regulation
regurgitation
    cardiac valvular r.
rehydration
Reid's
    base line
    index
Reifenstein's syndrome
Reil's limiting sulcus
reinfection
Reinke crystals
reinnervation
Reinsch's test
Reissner's
    fiber
    membrane
Reiter protein complement-fixation test
Reiter's syndrome
Reitland-Franklin unit
rejection
    homograft r.
    hyperacute r.
relapse
relapsing fever
relation
    Duane-Hunt r.
relative
    r. biological effectiveness
    r. cardiac volume
    r. centrifugal force
    r. standard deviation
relaxin
relay
releasing hormone
REM — rapid eye movement
    roentgen-equivalent — man

remission
remnants
    Cloquet's canal r.
    sinus venosus r.
REMP — roentgen-equivalent — man period
ren (renes)
    r. mobilis
    r. unguliformis
renal
    r. adenoma
    r.-adrenal axis
    r. amyloidosis
    r. area cribrosa
    r. artery
    r. calculi
    r. calyx
    r. cell carcinoma
    r. colic
    r. columns
    r. corpuscle
    r. cortex
    r. cortical interstitial tissue
    r. cortical necrosis
    r. dysplasia
    r. edema
    r. failure
    r. glycosuria
    r. hypertension
    r. infarct
    r. medullary interstitial tissue
    r. osteodystrophy
    r. papilla
    r. pelvic cavity
    r. pelvis
    r. pyramid
    r. rickets
    r. sinus
    r. stones
    r. tubular acidosis

renal *(continued)*
    r. tubular basement membrane
    r. tubular neck
    r. tubules
    r. vein
    r. vein thrombosis
    r. vessels
Rendu-Osler disease
Rendu-Weber-Osler disease
renin
    r.-angiotensin-aldosterone system
    r.-sodium profiling
rennin
renogram
Renshaw cell
reovirus, types 1, 2 and 3
REP — roentgen equivalent — physical
repair
    density-dependent r.
    fibrous r.
    postoperative r.
    primary r.
    secondary r.
reparative
    r. giant cell granuloma
repeated DNA sequences
replacement
    fibrous r.
replication
replicon
repolarization
repression
    catabolite r.
    end-product r.
    negative control r.
    positive control r.
reproduction
reproductive

reptilase
RER — rough endoplasmic reticulum
RES — reticuloendothelial system
rescinnamine
resection
resectoscopy
reserpine
reserve
   r. cell carcinoma
   r. cell hyperplasia
reservoir
   chromatin r.
   r. of virus
residual
residue
resin
resistance
   electrode r.
   r. plasmid
   total peripheral r.
   total pulmonary r.
   r. transfer factor
resistivity
resistor
resolution
resonance
   r. fluorescence
resorcinol
   r. monoacetate
resorption
   bone r.
   lacunar r.
   osteoclastic r.
resp — respiratory
respiration
   aerobic r.
   anaerobic r.
   artificial r.
   Cheyne-Stokes r.
   cogwheel r.

respiration *(continued)*
   interrupted r.
   Kussmaul r.
respirator
   Drinker r.
respiratory
   r. acidosis
   r. alkalosis
   r. bronchiole
   r. disorder
   r. distress syndrome
   r. epithelium
   r. exanthematous virus
   r. exchange ratio
   r. failure
   r. fluids
   r. infection virus
   r. protein
   r. quotient
   r. rate disorder
   r. rhythm disorder
   r. sound
   r. spaces
   r. syncytial virus
   r. syndrome
   r. system
   r. tract
respirometer
   Wright r.
response
   immune r.
rest
   cartilaginous r.
   congenital r.
   embryonal r.
   epithelial r.
   Erdheim r.
   mesonephric r.
   müllerian r.
   paramesonephric r.
   Walthard's cell r's
   wolffian r.

restiform
restriction endonuclease
restrictive
retained
    r. placental fragment
    r. products of conception
retardation
    growth r.
    mental r.
    psychomotor r.
rete (retia)
    acromial r.
    articular r.
    calcaneal r.
    r. cell tumor
    r. ovarii
    r. of patella
    r. testis
    r. vasculosum
    r. venosum
retention
    r. content
    r. cyst
    r. fluid
    r. gas
    r. meconium
    r. mucus
    r. polyp
    urinary r.
retic — reticulocyte
reticular
    r. activating system
    r. colliquation
    r. formation
    r. lamina
    r. layer
    r. membrane of cochlear duct
    r. nucleus of thalamus
    r. tissue
reticulin
    r. fibril alteration

reticulin *(continued)*
    r. M
reticulocyte
    r. production index
reticulocytopenia
reticulocytosis
reticuloendothelial
    r. cell hyperplasia
    r. cells
    r. sarcoma
    r. system
reticuloendotheliosis
    systemic r.
reticulohistiocytic granuloma
reticulohistiocytoma
reticulosis
    medullary histiocytic r.
reticulospinal
reticulum (reticula)
    endoplasmic r.
    granular r.
    sarcoplasmic r.
    stellate r.
reticulum cell
    r. c. hyperplasia
    r. c. lymphosarcoma
    r. c. sarcoma
    thymic r. c.
retina
retinaculum (retinacula)
    retinacula cutis
    r. extensorum
    r. flexorum
retinal
    r. anlage tumor
    r. artery
    r. detachment
    r. microaneurysm
    r. vein
retinene isomerase
retinitis
    r. pigmentosa

retinitis *(continued)*
    r. proliferans
retinoblastoma
retinoic acid
retinol-binding protein
retinopathy
    diabetic r.
retinoscopy
retinotopic
Retortamonas
    R. intestinalis
retraction
retroflexion
retrograde
retrohyoid bursa
retrolental fibroplasia
retrolenticular
retromammary
retromandibular
retroperitoneal
    r. fibromatosis
retroperitoneum
retroperitonitis
retropharyngeal
retrospective study
retroversion
retrovirus
Rettgerella rettgeri
reverse
    r. agglutination
    r. banding
    r. peristalsis
    r. transcriptase
    r. triiodothyronine
reversed albumin-globulin ratio
reversible
revivescence
Reye's syndrome
Reynold's number
RF — Reitland-Franklin (unit)
    relative fluorescence
    releasing factor

RF *(continued)*
    rheumatic fever
    rheumatoid factor
RFA — right femoral artery
    right frontoanterior
R factor
RFB — retained foreign body
RFLA — rheumatoid factor–like activity
RFP — right frontoposterior
RFS — renal function study
RFT — right frontotransverse
RG — right gluteal
RH — reactive hyperemia
    relative humidity
    releasing hormone
Rh — Rhesus (factor)
    rhodium
rh — rheumatic
Rhabditis
    R. hominis
rhabdocyte
Rhabdomonas
rhabdomyolysis
rhabdomyoma
rhabdomyosarcoma
    alveolar r.
    embryonal r.
rhabdovirus
Rh agglutinin
rhamnulokinase
Rh antigen
RHBF — reactive hyperemia blood flow
Rh blood group
RHD — relative hepatic dullness
    rheumatic heart disease
rhenium
rheobase
Rhesus factor
rheum — rheumatic

rheumatic
    r. arteritis
    r. arthralgia
    r. endocarditis
    r. fever
    r. heart disease
    r. myocarditis
    r. nodule
    r. pneumonia
    r. valvulitis
rheumatid
rheumatism
rheumatoid
    r. agglutinator
    r. ankylosing spondylitis
    r. aortitis
    r. arteritis
    r. arthritis
    r. episcleritis
    r. factor reaction
    r. heart disease
    r. nodule
    r. scleritis
rhinal
Rh incompatibility
rhinencephalon
rhinitis
    allergic r.
    atrophic r.
    fetid r.
    r. sicca
    vasomotor r.
Rhinocladium
rhinocleisis
rhinoentomophthoromycosis
rhinonasopharyngitis
rhinopharyngitis
rhinophycomycosis
rhinophyma
rhinorrhea
rhinoscleroma
rhinosporidiosis

Rhinosporidium seeberi
rhinovirus
Rhipicentor
Rhipicephalus
    R. sanguineus
Rh isoimmunization syndrome
Rhizobiaceae
Rhizobium
Rhizoglyphus
    R. parasiticus
Rhizopoda
Rhizopus
    R. equinus
    R. niger
    R. nigricans
    R. rhizopodoformis
RHL — right hepatic lobe
RHLN — right hilar lymph node
rhm — roentgen (per) hour (at one) meter
Rh neg — Rhesus factor negative
rhodamine
Rhodesian trypanosomiasis
rhodium
Rhodnius prolixus
Rhodophyllus sinuatus
rhodopsin
Rhodotorula
    R. mucilaginosa
    R. rubra
rhodotorulosis
RhoGAM vaccine
rhombencephalon
rhomboid
    r. fossa
    r. muscle
    r. nucleus
rhombomere
rhonchus (rhonchi)
rhopheocytosis

Rhus

Rh pos — Rhesus factor positive
rhythm
- Berger's r.
- bigeminal r.
- cardiac r.
- gallop r.
- respiratory r.

RI — refractive index
- regional ileitis
- respiratory illness

RIA — radioimmunoassay
ribavirin
riboflavin
- r. deficiency
- r. kinase
- r. loading test
- r. phosphate

ribokinase
ribonuclease
ribonucleic acid
ribonucleoprotein
ribonucleoside
ribonucleotide
ribose
ribosephosphate
- r. isomerase
- r. pyrophosphokinase

ribosomal
ribosome
ribosuria
ribosylnicotinamide kinase
ribothymidylic acid
ribulokinase
ribulose
- r. phosphate epimerase

Richet's aneurysm
Richter's
- hernia
- syndrome

ricin
ricinoleic acid

rickets
Rickettsia
- *R. akamushi*
- *R. akari*
- *R. australis*
- *R. burnetii*
- *R. canada*
- *R. conorii*
- *R. diaporica*
- *R. mooseri*
- *R. muricola*
- *R. nipponica*
- *R. orientalis*
- *R. pavlovskii*
- *R. pediculi*
- *R. prowazekii*
- *R. quintana*
- *R. rickettsii*
- *R. sibiricus*
- *R. tsutsugamushi*
- *R. typhi*
- *R. wolhynica*

rickettsia (rickettsiae)
Rickettsiaceae
rickettsial
rickettsialpox
Rickett's organism
RID — radial immunodiffusion
ridge
- truncus arteriosus r.
- urogenital r.

Riedel's
- lobe
- struma
- thyroiditis

Riehl's melanosis
RIF — right iliac fossa
RIFA — radioiodinated fatty acid
rifamide
rifampicin
rifampin

rifamycin
Rift Valley fever
Rift Valley fever virus
right
    r. anterior oblique
    r. axis deviation
    r. bundle branch block
    r. posterior oblique
    r.-sided aortic arch
    r.-sided ductus arteriosus
rigidity
    decerebrate r.
    lead-pipe r.
    muscular r.
    nuchal r.
rigor mortis
RIHSA — radioactive iodinated human serum albumin
Riley-Day syndrome
ring
    Balbiani's r's
    Bandl's r.
    Kayser-Fleischer r.
    Schatzki's r.
    vascular r.
    Waldeyer's tonsillar r.
Ringer's lactate solution
ringworm
Rinne's test
ripple factor
RISA — radioactive iodinated serum albumin
risk factor
ristocetin
RITC — rhodamine isothiocyanate
Ritter-Oleson technique
Ritter's disease
RIU — radioactive iodine uptake
RK — rabbit kidney
    right kidney

RKY — roentgen kymography
RLC — residual lung capacity
RLF — retrolental fibroplasia
RLL — right lower lobe
RLN — recurrent laryngeal nerve
RLP — radiation-leukemia-protection
RLQ — right lower quadrant
RLS — Ringer's lactate solution
RM — radical mastectomy
    respiratory movement
RMA — right mentoanterior
RMK — rhesus monkey kidney
RML — right middle lobe
RMP — rapidly miscible pool
    right mentoposterior
RMS — root-mean-square
RMSF — Rocky Mountain spotted fever
RMT — retromolar trigone
    right mentotransverse
RMV — respiratory minute volume
Rn — radon
RNA — ribonucleic acid
RNA
    messenger RNA
    RNA nucleotidyltransferase
    RNA polymerase
    ribosomal RNA
    soluble RNA
    transfer RNA
RNase — ribonuclease
RND — radical neck dissection
RNP — ribonucleoprotein
RO — Ritter-Oleson (technique)
ROA — right occipitoanterior
robertsonian translocation
Robin's syndrome
ROC — receiver operating characteristic

Rochalimaea
   henselae (per S Rite)
   R. quintana
Rocky Mountain spotted fever
rodenticide
Rodrigues' aneurysm
rod-shaped
roentgenkymography
roentgenogram
roentgenography
roentgenology
roentgen rays
Roger
   maladie de R.
ROH — rat ovarian hyperemia (test)
Rokitansky-Aschoff sinus
rolandic epilepsy
Rolando's fissure
Roller's nucleus
ROM — range of motion
        rupture of membranes
Romaña's sign
Romanowsky's stain
ronnel
root
   belladonna r.
   bitter r.
   cochlear r.
   facial r.
   r.-mean-square
   motor r.
   sensory r.
ROP — right occipitoposterior
Ropes test
rosacea-like tuberculid
rosaniline
rose bengal sodium
Rosenmüller's
   fossa
   lymph node
Rosenthal's
   syndrome

Rosenthal's *(continued)*
   vein
roseola
   r. infantum
   r. infantum virus
   r. vaccination
Rose's test
rosette
   malarial r.
Rose-Waaler test
rostral
   r. displacement
   r. lamina, corpus callosum
rostrum (rostra)
   r. corpus callosi
   r. sphenoidale
ROT — right occipitotransverse
rotavirus
rotenone
Rothera's test
Roth's spot
Rotor's syndrome
rotoxamine
Rotter's
   syndrome
   test
Rouget's
   cell
   pericyte
rough endoplasmic reticulum
rouleau (rouleaux)
roundworm See pg. 232
Rourke-Ernstein sedimentation rate
Rous
   sarcoma virus
   test
Rowntree and Geraghty's test
RP — reactive protein
       refractory period
       resting pressure
       retrograde pyelogram

Ascaris (l type

Rp — pulmonary resistance
RPA — right pulmonary artery
RPCF — Reiter protein complement-fixation
RPCFT — Reiter protein complement-fixation test
RPE — retinal pigment epithelium
RPF — renal plasma flow
RPG — retrograde pyelogram
RPGN — rapidly progressive glomerulonephritis
RPI — reticulocytic production index
rpm — revolutions per minute
RPO — right posterior oblique
RPR — rapid plasma reagin
RPS — renal pressor substance
RPV — right pulmonary veins
RQ — respiratory quotient
RR — radiation response
    renin release
    respiratory rate
    response rate
RRA — radioreceptor assay
RR-HPO — rapid recompression — high pressure oxygen
RRP — relative refractory period
RRR — renin-release rate
RS — Reed-Sternberg cell
    respiratory syncytial
RSA — relative specific activity
    reticulum cell sarcoma
    right sacroanterior
RSB — right sternal border
RSC — rested-state contraction
RScA — right scapuloanterior
RScP — right scapuloposterior
RSD — relative standard deviation
RSP — right sacroposterior
RSR — regular sinus rhythm
RST — radiosensitivity test
    right sacrotransverse
RSV — respiratory syncytial virus
    right subclavian vein
    Rous sarcoma virus
R-S variation
RS virus
RT — reaction time
    room temperature
RTA — renal tubular acidosis
RTD — routine test dilution
RTF — replication and transfer
    resistance transfer factor
    respiratory tract fluid
RU — rat unit
    resistance unit
    retrograde urogram
Ru — ruthenium
rub
    pericardial friction r.
    pleural-pericardial friction r.
rubella
    r. virus
rubeola
    r. virus
rubidium
Rubin's test
rubivirus
rubriblast
rubricyte
rubrospinal
rubrum
    r. Congo
    r. scarlatinum

rudimentary
    r. finger
    r. lung
    r. structure
    r. testis syndrome
    r. uterus, male
Ruffini's corpuscle
ruga (rugae)
RUL — right upper lobe
rule
    Clark's r.
Rumpel-Leede test
runt disease
Runyon's classification
rupture
    inflammatory r.
    premature r.
ruptured
    r. aneurysm
    r. ectopic pregnancy
    r. myocardial infarct
    r. umbilical cord
RUQ — right upper quadrant
RUR — resin-uptake ratio
RURTI — recurrent upper respiratory tract infection
Rusconi's anus
Russell-Crooke cell
Russell's
    body
    unit
    viper venom
Russell-Silver syndrome

Russian spring-summer encephalitis virus
Russula emetica
ruthenium
rutherford
RV — rat virus
    residual volume
    respiratory volume
    right ventricle
    rubella virus
RVB — red venous blood
RVD — relative vertebral density
RVE — right ventricular enlargement
RVEDP — right ventricular end-diastolic pressure
RVH — right ventricular hypertrophy
RVI — relative value index
RVR — renal vascular resistance
    resistance to venous return
RVRA — renal vein renin activity
    renal venous renin assay
RVRC — renal vein renin concentration
RVT — renal vein thrombosis
R wave
ryania

S

S — sacral
    serum
    smooth (colony)
    soluble
    spherical lens

S *(continued)*
    sulfur
    supravergence
    Svedberg unit of sedimentation coefficient

S. — *Salmonella*
   Schistosoma
   Spirillum
   Staphylococcus
   Streptococcus
s — second, seconds
SA — salicylic acid
   sarcoma
   secondary amenorrhea
   secondary anemia
   serum albumin
   sinoatrial
   Stokes-Adams
   surface area
SAB — significant asymptomatic bacteriuria
sabadilla
Sabethes
Sabhi agar
Sabin-Feldman dye test
Sabin vaccine
Sabouraud's dextrose agar
sac
   endolymphatic s.
   lacrimal s.
saccharase
saccharic acid
saccharoid
Saccharomyces
   S. albicans
   S. anginae
   S. apiculatus
   S. cantliei
   S. capillitii
   S. carlsbergensis
   S. cerevisiae
   S. coprogenus
   S. epidermica
   S. galacticolus
   S. glutinis
   S. hominis
   S. lemonnieri

Saccharomyces (continued)
   S. mellis
   S. mycoderma
   S. neoformans
   S. pastorianus
saccharomyces
   Busse's s.
saccharomycosis
saccharopine
   s. dehydrogenase
saccharopinuria
Saccomanno's fixative
saccular
   s. aneurysm
   s. bronchiectasis
saccule
saccus
SACD — subacute combined degeneration
Sachs-Georgi test
sacral
   s. artery
   s. bursa
   s. lymph node
   s. myotome
   s. nerve
   s. plexus
   s. region
   s. spinal cord
   s. vein, lateral
   s. vertebra of intervertebral disc
sacralization
   lumbar vertebra s.
sacrococcygeal
sacroiliac joint
sacrum
safflower oil
saffron
safrol
SAG — Swiss-type agammaglobulinemia

sagittal
    s. sinus
    s. suture
sago spleen
SAH — subarachnoid hemorrhage
Saint Anthony's fire
St. Louis encephalitis
St. Louis encephalitis virus
Saksenaea
sal — saline
    saliva
salicylamide
salicylanilide
salicylate
    s. isoamyl
    s. phenyl
salicylic acid
salicylsalicylic acid
saline
    s. agglutinin
    s. infusion
    physiologic s.
Salisbury common cold virus
saliva
salivary
    s. gland
    s. virus
Salk vaccine
Salmonella
    S. arizonae
    S. choleraesuis
    S. derby
    S. enteritidis
    S. gallinarum
    S. hirschfeldii
    S. indiana
    S. minnesota
    S. montevideo
    S. muenchen
    S. newington
    S. oranienburg

Salmonella (continued)
    S. paratyphi, A, B, C
    S. schottmülleri
    S. sendai
    S. thompson
    S. typhi
    S. typhimurium
    S. typhisuis
    S. typhosa
    S. virginia
salmonella (salmonellae)
    s. agglutinins
Salmonella-Shigella agar
salmonellosis
salpingitis
    follicular s.
    s. isthmica nodosa
salpingo-oophorectomy
salpingo-oophoritis
salpingopharyngeus muscle
salpinx
    s. auditiva
    s. uterina
salsalate
Saltatoria
saltatory
    s. conduction
salt-losing crisis
Salvia
    S. horminium
    S. sclarea
Salzman method
SAM — sulfated acid mucopolysaccharide
samarium
Sanarelli-Shwartzman phenomenon
sandalwood oil
Sandhoff's disease
Sanfilippo's syndrome
sanguivorous
San Joaquin fever

SA node
santonin
Santorini's
    cartilage
    duct
SAP — serum alkaline phosphatase
        systemic arterial pressure
saphenous
    s. nerve
    s. vein
saponification
saponin
    steroid s.
    triterpenoid s.
Sappinia diploidea
saprol
sapronosis
saprophyte
Saprospira
saramycetin
Sarcina
sarcina (sarcinae)
sarcocyst
sarcocystin
Sarcocystis
sarcocyte
Sarcodina
sarcoid
    Boeck's s.
    granuloma s.
    Spiegler-Fendt s.
sarcoidosis
sarcolemma
sarcoma (sarcomas, sarcomata)
    alveolar s.
    ameloblastic s.
    botryoid s.
    s. botryoides
    cerebellar s.
    endometrial stromal s.

sarcoma *(continued)*
    endothelial s.
    Ewing's s.
    giant cell s.
    hemangioendothelial s.
    Hodgkin's s.
    Kaposi's s.
    Kupffer's cell s.
    lymphangioendothelial s.
    mast cell s.
    meningeal s.
    mesothelial s.
    multiple hemorrhagic s.
    neurogenic s.
    osteogenic s.
    periosteal s.
    reticuloendothelial s.
    reticulum cell s.
    small cell s.
    spindle cell s.
    stromal s.
    synovial s.
    undifferentiated s.
Sarcomastigophora
sarcomatosis
    meningeal s.
sarcomere
Sarcophaga
    S. carnaria
    S. dux
    S. fuscicauda
    S. haemorrhoidalis
    S. nificornis
    S. rubicornis
Sarcophagidae
sarcoplasm
sarcoplasmic
Sarcoptes
    S. scabiei
sarcoptidosis
sarcosine
    s. dehydrogenase

sarcosine *(continued)*
    s. oxidase
sarcosinemia
Sarcosporidia
sarcosporidiosis
sartorius muscle
    s. m. bursa
SAS — supravalvular aortic stenosis
sat — saturated
satellite
    s. cell
    s. colony
    s. DNA
    nucleolar s.
satellitosis
saturated
    s. fatty acid
    s. phosphatidylcholine
saturation
satyriasis
SB — serum bilirubin
    sternal border
Sb — antimony (stibium)
$SbCl_3$ — antimony trichloride
SBE — subacute bacterial endocarditis
SBF — splanchnic blood flow
SBN — single-breath nitrogen (test)
Sb_2O_3 — antimony trioxide
Sb_2O_5 — antimony pentoxide
Sb_4O_6 — antimony trioxide
SBP — systemic blood pressure
    systolic blood pressure
SBTI — soybean trypsin inhibitor
SC — closure of the semilunar valves
    sacrococcygeal
    sickle cell
    sternoclavicular

SC *(continued)*
    subcutaneous
    succinylcholine
Sc — scandium
scabies
scala (scalae)
    s. tympani
    s. vestibuli
scalded skin syndrome
scale
    absolute s.
    Baumé's s.
    Benoist' s.
    Celsius s.
    centigrade s.
    Fahrenheit temperature s.
    hydrometer s.
    Kelvin temperature s.
    Rankine temperature s.
    Réaumur s.
scalene
    s. lymph node
    s. muscles
    s. region
scalenus anticus syndrome
scalp
    gyrate s.
scan
    bilirubin s.
    brain s.
    CAT (computed axial tomography) s.
    gallium s.
    kidney s.
    krypton s.
    liver s.
    RAI s.
    RISA s.
    spleen s.
    technetium s.
scandium
scanner

scanning
    s. electron microscope
    fluorescent s.
scanography
scaphocephaly
scaphoid
    s. bone
    s. facies
scapula (scapulae)
scapular
scarabiasis
scarlet
    Biebrich s.
    s. fever
    s. G
    s. R
    water-soluble s.
Scarpa's ganglion
SCAT — sheep cell agglutination test
Scatchard equation
scatter
    s. diagram
scattergram
scattering
Scaurus
SCC — squamous cell carcinoma
SCD — subacute combined degeneration (of spinal cord)
    sudden cardiac death
    sudden coronary death
ScDA — scapulodextra anterior
ScDP — scapulodextra posterior
Scedosporium apiospermum
SCG — serum chemistry graft
SCH — succinylcholine
Schaedler blood agar
Schales and Schales method for chloride
Schamberg's disease

Schatzki's ring
Schaumann's bodies
Scheie's syndrome
Scheloribates
Schick test
Schiff's
    base
    biliary cycle
    reagent
Schilder's disease
Schiller's test
Schilling
    blood count
    test
Schilling-type monocytic leukemia
Schimmelbusch's disease
Schirmer's test
schistocyte
Schistosoma
    S. haematobium
    S. intercalatum
    S. japonicum
    S. mansoni
Schistosomatidae
Schistosomatoidea
schistosome
schistosomiasis
schistosomicide
schizoaffective schizophrenia
Schizoblastosporion
schizogony
schizoid
schizomycete
schizont
Schizophora
schizophrenia
    acute undifferentiated s.
    catatonic s.
    chronic undifferentiated s.
    hebephrenic s.
    paranoid s.

schizophrenia *(continued)*
   pseudoneurotic s.
   schizoaffective s.
   simple s.
schizophrenic psychosis
Schizophyllum commune
Schizosaccharomyces
Schlemm's canal
Schmidt-Lantermann segment
Schmidt's syndrome
Schmitz's bacillus
Schmorl's
   bacillus
   nodule
   reaction
Schönlein's purpura
Schottmüller's disease
Schüffner's dots
Schultz-Dale test
Schumm's test
schwannoma
   malignant s.
Schwann's
   cell
   sheath
   white substance
Schweninger-Buzzi disease
sciatica
sciatic nerve
scillaren
scilliroside
scintigram
scintigraphy
scintillation
   s. camera
   s. counter
   s. crystal
scintillator
scintiphotograph
scintiscanning
scirrhous carcinoma

SCJ — squamocolumnar junction
SCK — serum creatine kinase
ScLA — scapulolaeva anterior
sclera (sclerae)
   lamina cribrosa sclerae
scleredema
   s. adultorum
sclerema
   s. neonatorum
scleritis
   rheumatoid s.
sclerodactyly
scleroderma
scleromyxedema
sclerosing
   s. adenosis
   s. hemangioma
   s. osteitis
   s. sinusitis
sclerosis
   amyotrophic lateral s.
   disseminated s.
   endocardial s.
   endomyocardial s.
   lobar s.
   multiple s.
   primary endocardial s.
   progressive systemic s.
   subacute combined s.
   tuberous s.
sclerotium
ScLP — scapulolaeva posterior
SCM — Society of Computer Medicine
scolecoid
scolex (scoleces)
scoliosis
S colony
Scolopendra
scop — scopolamine

scopolamine
Scopularaiopsis
   S. americana
   S. aureus
   S. blochi
   S. brevicaulis
   S. cinereus
   S. koningi
   S. minimus
scopulariopsosis
Scorpiones
scotochromogen
scotochromogenic
   s. mycobacterium
scotoma (scotomata)
scotopic
SCP – single-celled protein
SCPK – serum creatine phosphokinase
SCR – silicon-controlled rectifier
scratch test
scrofuloderma
scrotal
   s. raphe
   s. septum
scrotum
scrub typhus
SCS – silicon-controlled switch
SCT – sex chromatin test
      staphylococcal clumping test
scurvy
Scutigera
scybalum (scybala)
SD – septal defect
      serologically defined
      serum defect
      spontaneous delivery
      standard deviation
      streptodornase

S/D – systolic to diastolic
SDA – sacrodextra anterior
      specific dynamic action
SD antigen
S-D curve – strength-duration curve
SDE – specific dynamic effect
SDH – serine dehydrase
      sorbitol dehydrogenase
      succinate dehydrogenase
SDM – standard deviation of the mean
SDP – sacrodextra posterior
SDS – sodium dodecyl sulfate
      sudden death syndrome
SDT – sacrodextra transversa
SE – standard error
     Starr-Edwards (prosthesis)
Se – selenium
seatworm
sebaceous
   s. adenocarcinoma
   s. adenoma
   s. carcinoma
   s. cyst
   s. gland
seborrhea
seborrheic
   s. dermatitis
   s. keratosis
sebum
Seckel's syndrome
secobarbital
secondary
   s. active transport
   s. amenorrhea
   s. coil
   s. constriction
   s. culture

secondary *(continued)*
    s. granule
    s. lysosome
    s. sex character
    s. structure
    s. x-rays
second cranial nerve
second degree
    s. d. burn
    s. d. frostbite
    s. d. heart block
    s. d. radiation injury
secretin
secretinase
secretion
secretor
    s. factor
    s. gene
    s. phenotype
secretory
    s. alteration
    s. component
    s. endometrium
    s. granule
    s. IgA
section
    s. cutting
    s. freeze substitution technique
SED — skin erythema dose
    spondyloepiphyseal dysplasia
sedation
sedative
sediment
    urinary s.
sedimentation
    s. coefficient
    s. equilibrium
    erythrocyte s.
    s. techniques
    velocity-diffusion s.

sedimentation rate
    Rourke-Ernstein s. r.
    Westergren's s. r.
    Wintrobe's s. r.
    zeta s. r.
sedoheptulokinase
sed rate — sedimentation rate
SEE — standard error of the estimate
SEG — sonoencephalogram
seg — segmented (leukocyte)
segment
    bronchopulmonary s.
    cranial s's
    frontal s.
    hepatic s's
    interannular s.
    medullary s.
    mesoblastic s.
    neural s.
    occipital s.
    Okazaki's s's
    P-R s.
    protovertebral s.
    pubic s.
    renal s's
    rivinian s.
    sacral s.
    Schmidt-Lantermann s.
    spinal s.
    S-T s.
    uterine s.
Segmentina
Segmentininae
segs — segmented neutrophils
Seitz filter
seizure
Selas filter
Seldinger technique
selection
    s. against dominant mutations

selection *(continued)*
    s. against heterozygotes
    s. against homozygotes
    s. against recessive mutations
    coefficient of s.
    directional s.
    natural s.
    s. pressure
selenium
    s. isotope
    s. sulfide
selenocyte
selenoid body
selenomethionine
Selivanoff's (Seliwanow's) reagent
sellar
sella turcica
SEM — scanning electron microscope
        standard error of the mean
semeiography
semen
semicarbazide hydrochloride
semicircular
    s. canal
    s. duct
semiconductor
semiinterquartile range
semilunar
    s. cartilage
seminal
    s. colliculus
    s. duct
    s. fluid
seminal vesicle
    s. v. adventitia
    s. v. mucosa
    s. v. muscularis

seminiferous
    s. epithelium
    s. tubule
seminoma
semipermeable
semipronation
semiquantitative
semiquinone
semisupination
semitendinosus muscle
Semliki Forest virus
Sendai virus
Senear-Usher disease
senescence
Sengstaken-Blakemore tube
senile
    s. amyloidosis
    s. atrophy
    s. dementia
    s. elastosis
    s. endometrium
    s. involution
    s. keratosis
    s. plaque
senility
senna
sensation
    burning s.
    prickling s.
    tingling s.
sensibility
    epicritic s.
    protopathic s.
sensitivity
sensitization
sensor
sensory
    s. afferent system
    s. aphasia
    s. epithelium
    s. ganglion

sensory *(continued)*
    s. radicular neuropathy
    s. receptor
    s. root
    s. structure
sentinel node
SEP — sensory evoked potential
        somatosensory evoked potential
        systolic ejection period
Sepsidae
sepsis
septal
    s. cartilage
    s. fibrosis of liver
    s. hypertrophy
    s. leaflet of tricuspid valve
    s. papillary muscle
septal defect
    atrial s. d.
    interatrial s. d.
    interventricular s. d.
    ventricular s. d.
septate
    s. cervix
    s. uterus
    s. vagina
septation
septic
    s. embolus
    s. infarct
    s. shock
septicemia
Septra
septum (septa)
    alveolar s.
    atrial s.
    atrioventricular s.
    deviated s.
    interatrial s.
    intermuscular s.

septum (septa) *(continued)*
    interventricular s.
    nasal s.
    s. pellucidum
    s. primum
    rectovaginal s.
    rectovesical s.
    scrotal s.
    s. secundum
    s. spurium
    tracheoesophageal s.
    s. transversum
    urorectal s.
    ventricular s.
seq — sequela
        sequestrum
sequela (sequelae)
sequence
sequential
    s. access
    s. analysis
sequestered antigen
sequestration
    bronchopulmonary s.
sequestrum
SER — smooth endoplasmic reticulum
        systolic ejection rate
Sereny test
serial
    s. data transmission
Sericopelma
    S. communis
serine
    s. deaminase
    L-s. dehydratase
    s. hydroxymethyltransferase
seroconversion
serodiagnosis
serofibrinous
    s. effusion

serologic
  s. reaction
  s. test for syphilis
serological
serologically defined antigen
serology
seroma
seromucous
seronegative
serophilic
seropositive
serosa
  appendiceal s.
  colonic s.
  duodenal s.
  gallbladder s.
  gastric s.
  small intestinal s.
  tubal s.
  urinary bladder s.
  uterine s.
serosanguineous
serotonergic
serotonin
serotype
serous
  s. acute inflammation
  s. acute synovitis
  s. atrophy
  s. cyst
  s. cystadenocarcinoma, papillary
  s. cystadenoma, papillary
  s. cystoma
  s. effusion
  s. gland
  s. inflammation
serpiginous
serrate
Serratia
  S. indica
  S. kiliensis

Serratia (continued)
  S. liquefaciens
  S. marcescens
  S. piscatorum
  S. plymuthica
  S. rubidaea
Serratieae
serratus
  s. anterior muscle
  s. posterior muscle
Sertoli-Leydig cell tumor
Sertoli's cell
serum (sera)
  s. albumin
  anallergenic s.
  anticholera s.
  anticomplementary s.
  antidiphtheric s.
  antihepatic s.
  antilymphocyte s.
  antimeningococcus s.
  antipertussis s.
  antiplague s.
  antiplatelet s.
  antipneumococcus s.
  antirabies s.
  antiscarlatinal s.
  antistaphylococcus s.
  antistreptococcus s.
  antitetanic s.
  antityphoid s.
  antivenomous s.
  s. creatinine
  cytotrophic s.
  endotheliolytic s.
  s. equinum
  s. glutamate oxaloacetate transaminase
  s. glutamate pyruvate transaminase
  s. hepatitis
  s. hepatitis virus

serum (sera) *(continued)*
- heterologous s.
- hog cholera s.
- homologous s.
- hyperimmune s.
- immune s.
- inactivated s.
- leukocytolytic s.
- motile s.
- nephrotoxic s.
- s. osmolality
- pericardial s.
- plague s.
- polyvalent s.
- prophylactic s.
- s. protein electrophoresis
- s. prothrombin conversion accelerator deficiency
- s. prothrombin time
- salvarsanized s.
- s. sickness
- streptococcus s.
- thyrotoxic s.

serumal
servomechanism
servomotor
seryl-RNA-synthetase
sesame oil
sesamoid bone
sesquiterpene
sessile
SET — systolic ejection time
seventh cranial nerve
Severinghaus electrode
Sever's disease
sex
- s. chromatin
- s. chromosome
- s. determination
- s. differentiation
- s. reversal
- s. steroid

sex cell
- primordial s. c.

sexduction
sexivalent
sexual
- s. deviation
- s. exhibitionism
- s. impotence
- s. perversion

sexually transmitted disease
Sézary syndrome
SF — scarlet fever
  spinal fluid
Sf — Svedberg flotation units
SFD — skin-film distance
SFEMG — single-fiber electromyography
SFP — screen filtration pressure
  spinal fluid pressure
SFS — split function study
SG — serum globulin
  skin graft
  specific gravity
S-G — Sachs-Georgi (test)
SGA — small for gestational age
SGOT — serum glutamic-oxaloacetic transaminase
SGP — serine glycerophosphatide
SGPT — serum glutamic-pyruvic transaminase
SGV — salivary gland virus
SH — serum hepatitis
  sex hormone
  sinus histiocytosis
  sulfhydryl
shadow
Sharpey's perforating fibers
SHB — sulfhemoglobin
SHBD — serum hydroxybutyrate dehydrogenase
Shea-Anthony antral balloon

sheath
- carotid s.
- rectus s.
- Schwann's s.
- tendon s.

Sheehan's syndrome
sheep cell agglutination test
SHG — synthetic human gastrin
shield
- gonadal s.
- syringe s.

shift
- chloride s.
- s. to the left
- regenerative blood s.
- s. register
- s. to the right

Shiga's bacillus
Shigella
- *S. alkalescens*
- *S. ambigua*
- *S. arabinotarda Type A, B*
- *S. boydii*
- *S. ceylonensis*
- *S. dispar*
- *S. dysenteriae*
- *S. etousae*
- *S. flexneri*
- *S. madampensis*
- *S. newcastle*
- *S. paradysenteriae*
- *S. parashigae*
- *S. schmitzii*
- *S. shigae*
- *S. sonnei*
- *S. wakefield*

shigellosis
shikimate dehydrogenase
shin
- saber s.

shingles
Shinowara-Jones-Reinhard unit

SHO — secondary hypertrophic osteoarthropathy
shock
- anaphylactic s.
- anaphylactoid s.
- s. artifact
- cardiogenic s.
- colloid s.
- endotoxic s.
- endotoxin s.
- faradic s.
- hemoclastic s.
- hemorrhagic s.
- histamine s.
- hypoglycemic s.
- hypovolemic s.
- insulin s.
- micro s.
- neurogenic s.
- osmotic s.
- peptone s.
- protein s.
- septic s.
- serum s.
- thyrotoxin s.
- toxic s.
- vasogenic s.

Shope papilloma
shortened
- s. bleeding time
- s. coagulation time

shortening
- abnormal s.

shoulder
Shrapnell's membrane
shuffling gait
shunt
- anatomic s.
- arteriovenous s.
- Israels' s.
- physiologic s.
- venous-to-arterial s.

Shwartzman's phenomenon
SI — International System
   sacroiliac
   saturation index
   serum iron
   soluble insulin
   stroke index
SIADH — syndrome of inappropriate antidiuretic hormone
sialadenitis
sialic acid
sialidase
sialography
sialolithiasis
sialomucin
sialorrhea
Siamese twins
Sia test
Sibine
Sibley-Lehninger unit
sibling
Sicariidae
sicca syndrome
SICD — serum isocitric dehydrogenase
sickle cell
   s. c. anemia
   s. c. disease
   s. c. thalassemia
   s. c. trait
Sickledex reagent
sickling
   s. test
SID — sudden infant death
side effect
sideramine
sideroachrestic anemia
Siderobacter
sideroblast
sideroblastic anemia
Siderocapsa

Siderocapsaceae
siderochrome
Siderococcus
siderocyte
siderocytic
sideroderma
siderofibrosis
sideromycin
sideropenia
sideropenic dysphagia
siderophagocytosis
siderophilin
siderophore
siderosilicosis
siderosis
siderosome
siderotic
SIDS — sudden infant death syndrome
Siggaard-Andersen alignment nomogram
sigma
   s. rhythm
sigmavirus
sigmoid
   s. artery
   s. colon
   s. sinus
sigmoiditis
sigmoidoscopy
sign
   Babinski's s.
   Blumberg's s.
   Brudzinski's s.
   Chaddock's s.
   Chvostek's s.
   Cullen's s.
   Goodell's s.
   Hegar's s.
   Kernig's s.
   Nikolsky's s.
   Pemberton's s.

sign *(continued)*
    Romaña's s.
    Trousseau's s.
    Unschuld's s.
signal
    s. averaging
    s. level
    s. node
signal-to-noise ratio
signature
signet ring
    s. r. adenocarcinoma
    s. r. carcinoma
    s. r. cell
significance
    s. level
    s. probability
significant
    s. digits
SIJ — sacroiliac joint
silane
silanization
silica
silicate
silicic acid
silicofluoride salt
silicon
    s.-controlled rectifier
    s.-controlled switch
    s. dioxide
silicone
silicosis
silver
    mild s. protein
    s. sulfadiazine
silver nitrate
    Barnett-Bourne acetic alcohol s. n.
silyation
Simbu virus
simethicone
simian sarcoma virus

Simmonds' disease
Simmons' citrate agar
Sims-Huhner test
simulation
Simuliidae
Simulium
Sindbis virus
singer's node
single-blind
single-breath nitrogen test
single diffusion test
sinistrocardia
    isolated s.
sinoatrial
    s. block
    s. node
sinus
    accessory s.
    Aschoff-Rokitansky s.
    s. bradycardia
    branchial cleft s.
    cavernous s.
    circular s.
    s. confluens
    draining s.
    dural s.
    ethmoid s.
    frontal s.
    s. histiocytosis
    inferior petrosal s.
    inferior sagittal s.
    inflammatory s.
    lactiferous s.
    maxillary s.
    occipital s.
    paranasal s.
    pilonidal s.
    s. rectus
    renal s.
    Rokitansky-Aschoff s.
    sigmoid s.
    sphenoid s.

sinus *(continued)*
    sphenoparietal s.
    straight s.
    superior petrosal s.
    superior sagittal s.
    s. tract, inflammatory
    transverse s.
    urogenital s.
    Valsalva's posterior s.
    s. venosus
sinusitis
    sclerosing s.
sinusoid lymph node
Siphonaptera
Siphunculina
Sipple's syndrome
sirenomelia
Sirius red
SIRS — soluble immune response suppressor
SISI — short-increment sensitivity index
Sisyrosea
sitosterols
situs inversus
sixth cranial nerve
Sjögren's syndrome
SJR — Shinowara-Jones-Reinhard (unit)
SK — streptokinase
skatole
skatoxyl
skeletal
    s. age
    s. dysplasia
    s. muscle
skeleton
    appendicular s.
    axial s.
    cardiac s.
    gill arch s.

skeleton *(continued)*
    visceral s.
Skene's gland
skew
skewed distribution
skiagraph
skiametry
skin
    s.-film distance
    s.-reactive factor
    shagreen s.
    s. tag
    s. test
SKSD — streptokinase-streptodornase
skull
    natiform s.
SL — sensation level
       Sibley-Lehninger (unit)
       streptolysin
SLA — sacrolaeva anterior
        slide latex agglutination
SLD or SLDH — serum lactic dehydrogenase
SLE — St. Louis encephalitis
        systemic lupus erythematosus
sleep
    s. apnea
    s. deprivation
    drug-induced s.
    NREM s.
    s. spindle
sleeping sickness
sleepwalking
SLEV — St. Louis encephalitis virus
SLI — splenic localization index
slide
SLKC — superior limbic keratoconjunctivitis

SLN — superior laryngeal nerve
SLO — streptolysin-O
slow-reacting substance of
    anaphylaxis
SLP — sacrolaeva posterior
SLR — *Streptococcus lactis* R
SLS — segment long-spacing
    (collagen)
SLT — sacrolaeva transversa
slurring
Sly disease
SM — streptomycin
    submucous
    suction method
    systolic mean
    systolic murmur
Sm — samarium
SMA — superior mesenteric
    artery
SMA-12 profile test
SMAF — specific macrophage-
    arming factor
small cell
    s. c. carcinoma
    s. c. sarcoma
smaller occipital nerve
small intestine
smallpox
    coherent s.
    confluent s.
    discrete s.
    hemorrhagic s.
    s. immunization
    inoculation s.
    malignant s.
    modified s.
    s. virus
smear
    Breed s.
    fungi s.
    Papanicolaou's s.

smear *(continued)*
    peripheral blood s.
    TB s.
smegma
    s. clitoridis
    s. embryonum
    s. preputii
Smith-Strang disease
SMON — subacute myelo-
    optical neuropathy
smooth
    s. endoplasmic reticulum
    s. muscle
SMP — slow-moving protease
SMR — somnolent metabolic
        rate
    standard mortality
        ratio
    submucous resection
SMRR — submucous resection
    and rhinoplasty
SN — serum-neutralizing
    suprasternal notch
Sn — tin
snakebite
snapback DNA
SNB — scalene node biopsy
Snellen chart
Snell's law
SNM — Society of Nuclear
    Medicine
SNOP — Systematized Nomen-
    clature of Pathology
SNR — signal-to-noise ratio
SO — salpingo-oophorectomy
SOB — short(ness) of breath
SOC — sequential-type oral
        contraceptive
Society of Computer Medicine
Society of Nuclear Medicine
sodium

sodium
- s. acetrizoate
- s. alginate
- s. aminosalicylate
- s. arsanilate
- s. arsenate
- s. arsenite
- s. ascorbate
- s. bicarbonate
- s. biphosphate
- s. bitartrate
- s. cacodylate
- s. caprylate
- s. caustic alkali
- s. chloride and dextrose injection
- s. chloride and fructose injection
- s. chloride, isotonic
- s. chloride injection
- s. chromate
- s. citrate
- s. cyanide
- s. dehydrocholate
- s. diatrizoate
- s. 2,4-dichlorophenoxyethyl sulfate
- s. dihydrogen phosphate
- s. dinitro-ortho-cresylate
- s. diprotrizoate
- s. diuresis
- s. dodecyl sulfate
- s. endothal
- s. escape
- s. estrone sulfate
- s. ethyl xanthate
- etidronate s.
- s. fluoride
- s. fluoroacetate
- s. fluosilicate
- s. glutamate
- s. hexafluorosilicate

sodium *(continued)*
- s. hyposulfate
- s. indigotindisulfonate
- s. iodide
- s. iodipamide
- s. iodomethamate
- s. ion
- s. isopropyl xanthate
- s. isotope
- s. lactate injection
- s. levothyroxine
- s. liothyronine
- s. mercaptomerin
- s. metaborate
- s. *N*-methyl dithiocarbamate
- s. monofluoroacetate
- s. morrhuate
- s. nitrite
- s. nitroprusside
- s. oxalate
- s. pentachlorophenate
- s. perborate
- s. pertechnetate
- s. phosphate
- s. phytate
- s. polyanetholsulfonate
- s. polystyrene sulfonate
- s. propionate
- s. psylliate
- s. rhodanide
- s. ricinoleate
- s. salicylate
- s. selenate
- s. silicate
- s. silicofluoride
- s. succinate
- s. sulfate
- s. sulfide
- s. sulfite
- s. sulfocyanate
- s. tartrate

sodium *(continued)*
   s. tetraborate
   s. tetradecyl
   s. thiocyanate
   s. thioglycollate
   s. thiosulfate
   s. trichloroacetate
   s. warfarin
soft
   s. chancre
   s. palate
   s. tissue
   s. tubercle
software
SOL or Sol – solution
          space-occupying lesion
sol
   metal s.
   solid s.
solanine
solanocyte
solanoid
Solanum
solar keratosis
sole
   convex s.
solenoid
Solenopsis
soleus muscle
solid
   s. carcinoma
   s.-phase radioimmunoassay
   s.-state radiation detector
   s. teratoma
solitary
   s. cyst
   s. lymphoid nodule
   s. plasmacytoma
solubility
   s. coefficient

soluble
   s. immune response suppressor
solute
solution
   Balamuth's buffer s.
   Burow's s.
   Cajal's formol ammonium bromide s.
   Dakin's s.
   Dragendorff's s.
   Fehling's s.
   formaldehyde s.
   formol ammonium bromide s.
   Fowler's s.
   Hucker-Conn crystal violet s.
   Lugol's s.
   Ringer's lactate s.
solvate
solvent
solvolysis
SOM – secretory otitis media
        serous otitis media
soma
somasthenia
somatesthesia
somatic
somatomammotropin
somatomedin A, B, C
somatosensory
   s. evoked potential
somatostatin
somatostatinoma
somatotrope
somatotrophic
somatotropic
somatotropin
somesthesia
somite

somnambulism
somnolence
Somogyi unit
sonar
sonication
Sonne-Duval bacillus
Sonne dysentery
sonogram
sonolucent
sorbefacient
sorbitol
    s. dehydrogenase
Sotos' syndrome
SOTT — synthetic medium old tuberculin trichloroacetic acid (precipitated)
sound
    alteration s., cardiac
    alteration s., heart
    respiratory s., abnormal
    s. waves
source
    s. language
    s. program
    s. statement
South American blastomycosis
Southern blot technique
SP — shunt procedure
    skin potential
    status post
    steady potential
    summating potential
    suprapubic
    symphysis pubis
    systolic pressure
2-S P — transport medium used for mycoplasma isolation
sp. (spp.) — species
SPA — suprapubic aspiration
space (spaces)
    apical s.
    capsular s.

space (spaces) *(continued)*
    Disse's s's
    female genital s.
    fetal s.
    Fontana's s.
    gastrointestinal s.
    Held's s.
    His's s.
    iliocostal s.
    intervillous s.
    male genital s.
    medullary s.
    meningeal s.
    periaxial s.
    phrenocostal s.
    placental s.
    respiratory s.
    retrobulbar s.
    urinary tract s.
    Virchow-Robin s.
SPAI — steroid protein activity index
sparganosis
Sparganum proliferum
sparteine
spasm
    torsion s.
spastic
    s. bulbar palsy
    s. colitis
    s. gait
spasticity
spatial
    s. distortion
    s. frequency
    s. resolution
SPBI — serum protein-bound iodine
SPCA — serum prothrombin conversion accelerator

SPE — serum protein electrophoresis
Spearman's rank correlation coefficient
speciation
species
specific
    s. coagulation factor deficiency
    s. etiologic agent not identified
    s. gravity
    s. macrophage-arming factor
    s. rotation
specificity
    neuronal s.
    organ s.
    species s.
    spill-over s.
specimen
spectinomycin
spectral
    s. interference
    s. resolution
    s. response
spectrin
spectrofluorometer
spectrograph
spectrometer
spectrometry
spectrophotometry
    infrared s.
    ultraviolet/visible s.
spectroscopy
    Raman s.
spectrum (spectra)
speculum (specula)
speech
    s. disorder
    s. impediment
    slurred s.

Spelotrema
sperm
    s. count
    muzzled s.
spermatic
    s. cord
    s. vein
spermatid
spermatocele
spermatocyte
spermatogenesis
spermatogenic
    s. arrest
    s. epithelium
    s. granuloma
    s. maturation arrest
spermatogonium (spermatogonia)
spermatozoon (spermatozoa)
spermia
spermidine
spermine
spermiogenesis
SPF — specific pathogen-free
    split products of fibrin
sp. gr. — specific gravity
SPH — secondary pulmonary hemosiderosis
sph — spherical
    spherical lens
sphaceloderma
Sphaerophorus
    S. necrophorus
S phase
sphenoid
    s. bone
    s. sinus
    s. suture
spheno-occipital synchondrosis
sphenopalatine ganglion
sphenoparietal sinus
sphenopetrosal synchondrosis

sphere
    attraction s.
    embryonic s.
    segmentation s.
    vitelline s.
spherical
    s. aberration
spherocyte
spherocytic
spherocytosis
spheroid
spheroplast
spherule
spherulin
sphincter
    s. of ampulla
    anal s.
    s. ani externus muscle
    cardiac s.
    cardioesophageal s.
    inguinal s.
    s. of Oddi
    palatopharyngeal s.
    s. pupillae muscle
    pupillary s.
    pyloric s.
    rectal s.
    s. urethrae muscle
sphinganine
sphingenine
sphingoin
sphingolipid
sphingolipidosis
sphingolipodystrophy
sphingomyelin
    s. phosphodiesterase
sphingomyelinase
sphingomyelinosis
sphingophospholipid
sphingosine
sphygmic

SPI — serum precipitable iodine
spiculated
spicule
spider
    s. angioma
    black widow s.
    s. nevus
Spiegler-Fendt sarcoid
Spielmeyer-Vogt disease
spike
    s. and dome complex
    H s.
    s. and slow-wave complex
    s. and slow-wave rhythm
spina bifida
    s. b. cystica
    s. b. occulta
    open s. b.
spinal
    s. accessory nerve
    s. arachnoid
    s. artery
    s. cord
    s. dura mater
    s. epidural space
    s. ganglion
    s. nerve
    s. pia mater
    s. puncture
    s. region of subdural space
    s. sensory afferent system
    s. somatosensory evoked potential
    s. subarachnoid space
    s. tap
    s. tract nucleus
    s. tract of trigeminal nerve
spinal fluid
    s. f. culture
    s. f. leukocyte count
    s. f. pressure

spinalis muscle
spindle
    s. alteration
    barbiturate s.
    bipolar s.
    multipolar s.
    s. muscle
    s. tendon
spindle cell
    s. c. carcinoma
    s. c. lipoma
    s. c. melanoma
    s. c. nevus
    s. c. sarcoma
spine
    anterior inferior iliac s.
    anterior superior iliac s.
    ischial s.
    posterior inferior iliac s.
    posterior superior iliac s.
spinocerebellar
spino-olivary tract
spinorubral
spinotectal
spinothalamic
spiradenoma
    eccrine s.
spiral
    s. canal, cochlea
    Curschmann's s's
    s. fracture
    s. ganglion
    Herxheimer's s.
    s. lamina
    s. membrane
    s. plica
spiramycin
spirilla
Spirillaceae
Spirillum
    S. minor
    S. minus

spirillum
    Obermeier's s.
Spirochaeta
    S. daxensis
    S. eurystrepta
    S. marina
    S. plicatilis
    S. stenostrepta
spirochetal
spirochete
spirochetemia
spirochetosis
spirogram
Spirometra
spirometric
spirometry
spironolactone
Spiruroidea
Spitz nevus
SPL — sound pressure level
        spontaneous lesion
splanchnic
    s. nerve
spleen
    accessory s.
    Banti's s.
    lardaceous s.
splenectomy
splenic
    s. anemia of infants
    s. artery
    s. capsule
    s. cords
    s. corpuscle
    s. flexure
    s. hilus
    s. lymphatic follicle
    s. neutropenia
    s. red pulp
    s. sinusoids
    s. trabeculae
    s. tumor

splenic *(continued)*
   s. vein
   s. white pulp
splenitis
   spodogenous s.
splenium
   s. corporis callosi
splenius muscle
splenogonadal fusion
splenohepatomegaly
splenomegaly
   fibrocongestive s.
splenoportography
splenosis
spondylitis
   ankylosing s.
   tuberculous s.
spondylolisthesis
spondylosis
   cervical s.
   lumbar s.
spongioblast
spongioblastoma
   s. multiforme
   s. polare
   s. unipolare
spongiosis
spongy
   s. degenerative-type leukodystrophy
   s. nevus
spont — spontaneous (delivery)
spontaneous
   s. abortion
   s. pneumothorax
sporangiophore
sporangiospore
sporangium (sporangia)
spore
   bacterial s.
   fungal s.
sporoblast

sporocyst
sporogony
Sporothrix
   S. schenckii
sporotrichosis
Sporotrichum
   S. beurmanni
   S. schenckii
sporozoan
sporozoite
sporozoon (sporozoa)
spot
   Bitot's s's
   Koplik's s's
   mongolian s.
   Roth's s.
spotted fever
Sprinz Nelson syndrome
sprue
   celiac s.
   nontropical s.
   tropical s.
SPS — sodium polyanetholsulfonate
   sulfite polymyxin sulfadiazine
Spumavirinae
sputum
   s. coctum
   s. crudum
   s. cruentum
   globular s.
   nummular s.
SQ — subcutaneous
squalene cyclohydroxylase
squama (squamae)
squamocolumnar junction
squamous
   s. epithelium
   s. metaplasia
   s. papilloma
   s. suture

SS-A antigens
SS-B

SQUAMOUS CELL — STAGE 467

squamous cell
   s. c. carcinoma
   s. c. carcinoma and adeno-carcinoma, mixed
   s. c. carcinoma-in-situ
   s. c. papilloma
squamous cell index
   crowded s. c. i.
   eosinophilic s. c. i.
   karyopyknotic s. c. i.
   maturation s. c. i.
SQUID — superconducting quantum-interference device
squill
SR — sarcoplasmic reticulum
   secretion rate
   sedimentation rate
   sensitization response
   sigma reaction
   sinus rhythm
   skin resistance
   superior rectus
   systemic resistance
Sr — strontium
sr — steradian
SRBC — sheep red blood cells
SRC — sedimented red cells
   sheep red cells
SRF — skin reactive factor
   somatotropin-releasing factor
   split renal function
   subretinal fluid
SRFS — split renal function study
SRNA — soluble ribonucleic acid
SRS — slow-reacting substance
SRSA — slow-reacting substance of anaphylaxis
S-R variation

SS — *Salmonella-Shigella*
   saturated solution
   statistically significant
   subaortic stenosis
   supersaturated
SSA — salicylsalicylic acid
   Ro skin-sensitizing antibody — see antigen
   sulfosalicylic acid (test)
SSD — source to skin distance
   sum of square deviations
SSKI — saturated solution of potassium iodide
SSN — severely subnormal
SSP — Sanarelli-Shwartzman phenomenon
   subacute sclerosing pan-encephalitis
SSPE — subacute sclerosing panencephalitis
SSS — scalded skin syndrome
   specific soluble substance
SSU — sterile supply unit
SSV — simian sarcoma virus
ST — esotropia
   sternothyroid
   subtalar
   subtotal
   surface tension
St — stoke
STA — serum thrombotic accelerator
stab — stab cell
   stab neutrophil
stabile
stability
stable
stachybotryotoxicosis
stage
   Tanner s.

? LA (leukocyte-activating) ? antigen

staging
Stagnicola
stain
    Achucárro's s.
    acid-Schiff s.
    alcian blue s.
    ATPase s.
    auramine-rhodamine s.
    azure-eosin s.
    Best's carmine s.
    Bethe's s.
    Bowie s.
    carbol fuchsin s.
    chlorazol black E. s.
    Ciaccio's s.
    Congo red s.
    cresyl violet s.
    Dorner s.
    eosin s.
    Feulgen's s.
    Giemsa s.
    Gimenez s.
    Gomori's trichrome s.
    Goodpasture's s.
    Gram's s.
    Gram-Weigert s.
    Gridley s.
    Heidenhain's azan s.
    Heidenhain's iron hematoxylin s.
    hematoxylin-eosin s.
    Jenner-Giemsa s.
    Kinyoun carbol fuchsin s.
    Leishman's s.
    Lendrum's inclusion body s.
    leukocyte acid phosphatase s.
    Macchiavello's s.
    Mallory's collagen s.
    Masson s.

stain *(continued)*
    Mayer's acid alum hematoxylin s.
    May-Grünwald-Giemsa s.
    methenamine silver s.
    pancreatic islet s.
    Papanicolaou's s.
    Pappenheim's s.
    polychrome methylene blue s.
    quinacrine s.
    Romanowsky's s.
    Taenzer-Unna s.
    Truant's s.
    van Gieson's s.
    Verhoeff's s.
    Wade-Fite-Faraco s.
    Wayson s.
    Weigert's s.
    Wright's s.
    Ziehl-Neelsen s.
staining
    bacterial s.
    bipolar s.
    H and E s.
    histologic s.
stalk
    abdominal s.
    allantoic s.
    cerebellar s.
    hypophyseal s.
    infundibular s.
    neural s.
    optic s.
    pituitary s.
    yolk s.
STA-MCA — superficial temporal artery to middle cerebral artery
standard
    s. curve

STANDARD – STEATORRHEA

standard *(continued)*
    s. deviation
    s. electrode potential
    s. enthalpy of formation
    s. error of the mean
    s. free energy
    s. reduction potential
    s. solution
    s. state
    s. temperature and pressure
standardize
standstill
    cardiac s.
stannic
    s. chloride
stannous
stanolone
stanozolol
stapes
Staph – Staphylococcus
staph – staphylococcus
staphylocoagulase
staphylococcal
    s. colitis
    s. enteritis
    s. folliculitis
    s. pharyngitis
    s. pneumonia
    s. sinusitis
    s. tonsillitis
staphylococcemia
staphylococcin
Staphylococcus
    S. albus
    S. aureus
    S. citreus
    S. epidermidis
    S. pyogenes aureus
    S. pyogenes var. *albus*
    S. saprophyticus
staphylococcus (staphylococci)
staphylokinase

staphylolysin
    α s., alpha s.
    β s., beta s.
    δ s., delta s.
    ϵ s., epsilon s.
    γ s., gamma s.
staphyloma
Starling's law
Starr-Edwards prosthesis
stasis
    bile s.
    dermatitis s.
    ulcer s.
Stasisia
stat – German unit of radium
        emanation
        immediately
static
statistic
statistical
    s. symbols
stat test
stature
status
    s. asthmaticus
    s. epilepticus
    s. marmoratus
    s. spongiosis
    s. thymicolymphaticus
STC – soft tissue calcification
STD – sexually transmitted
        disease
    skin test dose
    skin to tumor distance
std – saturated
steapsin
stearate
stearic acid
stearin
steatomatosis
steatopygia
steatorrhea

steatosis
Stefan-Boltzmann law
Stegobium
Steinert's disease
Stein-Leventhal syndrome
Stelangium
stellate
    s. fracture
    s. ganglion
stem cell
    s. c. leukemia
    s. c. lymphoma
Stender dish
stenosis
    aortic s.
    calcific s.
    congenital s.
    hypertrophic pyloric s.
    s. and incompetency
    mitral s.
    nodular calcific s.
    nodular calcific aortic s.
    pyloric s.
    subaortic s.
    valvular s.
Stensen's duct
stercradian
stercobilin
stercobilinogen
stercoraceous ulcer
Sterculia gum
stereocampimeter
stereochemistry
stereocilia
stereocinefluorography
stereognosis
stereoisomer
stereoisomerism
stereology
stereoscope
stereoscopic
stereotactic
stereotaxis
steric
sterigma (sterigmata)
sterile
sterility
sterilization
    chemical s.
    eugenic s.
    fractional s.
    intermittent s.
    mechanical s.
sterilizer
sternal
    s. notch
    s. puncture
    s. synchondrosis
Sternberg-Reed cell
sternoclavicular
sternocleidomastoid muscle
sternocostal
sternohyoid muscle
sternothyroid muscle
sternoxiphoid plane
sternum
steroid
    6-beta-hydroxylase s.
    11-alpha-hydroxylase s.
    11-beta-hydroxylase s.
    17-alpha-hydroxylase s.
    19-hydroxylase s.
    21-hydroxylase s.
    delta-isomerase s.
    s.-21-monooxygenase
steroid-binding
    s.-b. betaglobulin
steroidogenesis
sterol
    s. carrier proteins
Stevens-Johnson syndrome
Stewart-Treves syndrome
STH — somatotropic hormone
STI — systolic time interval

stibine
stibophen
stigma (stigmata)
stilbene dye
stilbestrol
stillbirth
   macerated s.
Still's disease
stimulus (stimuli)
   adequate s.
   maximal s.
   submaximal s.
   subthreshold s.
   supramaximal s.
   threshold s.
stipple cell
stippling
   basophilic s.
STK — streptokinase
STM — streptomycin
stoichiometry
stoke
Stokes-Adams syndrome
Stokes' law
Stoll's dilution egg count technique
stoma (stomas, stomata)
stomach
   bilocular s.
   dumping s.
   sclerotic s.
   thoracic s.
   trifid s.
stomal ulcer
stomatitis (stomatitides)
   aphthous s.
   gangrenous s.
   herpetic s.
   Vincent's s.
stomatocytosis
Stomoxys
   S. calcitrans

stool
   acholic s.
   tarry s.
storage disease
storiform
storm
   thyroid s.
Stormer viscosimeter
Stovall-Black method
STP — standard temperature and pressure
STPD — standard temperature and pressure, dry ($0°C$, 760 mm Hg)
strabismus
Strachan's syndrome
stramonium
strangulated hernia
strangulation
stratification
stratified
   s. epithelium
stratigraphy
stratum (strata)
   s. basale
   s. corneum
   s. granulosum
   s. lucidum
   s. spinosum
streak
   angioid s's
   germinal s.
   medullary s.
   meningeal s.
   primitive s.
Strengeria
strength-duration curve
strep — streptococcus
Streptobacillus
   S. moniliformis
   S. pseudotuberculosis
Streptococcaceae

streptococcal
- s. cellulitis
- s. erysipelas
- s. lymphangitis
- s. nasopharyngitis
- s. pharyngitis
- s. tonsillitis
- s. toxin immunization reaction

Streptococceae
Streptococcus
- *S. agalactiae*
- *S. anaerobius*
- *S. anginosus-constellatus*
- *S. bovis*
- *S. cremoris*
- *S. durans*
- *S. equi*
- *S. equisimilis*
- *S. evolutus*
- *S. faecalis*
- *S. faecium*
- *S. hemolyticus*
- *S. intermedius*
- *S. lactis*
- *S. liquefaciens*
- *S. MG*
- *S. MG-intermedius*
- *S. microaerophilic*
- *S. milleri*
- *S. mitis*
- *S. mutans*
- *S. pneumoniae*
- *S. pyogenes*
- *S. salivarius*
- *S. sanguis*
- *S. uberis*
- *S. viridans*
- *S. zooepidemicus*
- *S. zymogenes*

streptococcus (streptococci)
- alpha s.
- anhemolytic s.
- Bargen's s.
- beta s.
- Fehleisen's s.
- gamma s.
- group A s.
- group D s.
- group N s.
- hemolytic s.
- s. MG
- nonhemolytic s.
- s. of Ostertag

streptodornase
streptokinase
- s.-streptodornase

streptolysin
- s. O
- s. S

Streptomyces
- *S. madurae*
- *S. pelletieri*
- *S. somaliensis*

Streptomycetaceae
streptomycin
streptomycosis
Streptothrix
streptotrichosis
streptozocin
streptozotocin
streptozyme test

stress
- environmental s.
- s. reticulocyte

stretch
- receptor s.
- s. reflex

stria (striae)
- striae gravidarum
- s. medullaris
- s. terminalis
- Wickham's striae

striate
striation
    basal s.
striatonigral degeneration
striatostriatal fibers
stricture
stridor
    laryngeal s.
Strigeata
stripped nuclei
Strobane
strobe light
strobila (strobilae)
stroke
    heat s.
    sun s.
    s. volume
stroma (stromata)
stromal
    s. endometriosis
    s. hyperplasia
    s. sarcoma
stromatosis
    endometrial s.
Strong's bacillus
Strongylidae
Strongyloidea
Strongyloides
    S. fulleborni
    S. stercoralis
strongyloidiasis
strontium
    s. isotope
strophanthin
structural
    s. gene
    s. protein
structure
    s. collapse
    rudimentary s.
struma
    Hashimoto's s.
    aberrans

struma *(continued)*
    s. lymphomatosa
    s. ovarii
    Riedel's s.
Strümpell-Lorrain disease
strychnine
STS — serologic test for syphilis
    standard test for syphilis
S-T segment
STSG — split thickness skin graft
STT — serial thrombin time
STU — skin test unit
Stuart factor
study
    erythrokinetic s's
    fat absorption s's
stunted
    s. embryo
    s. fetus
stupor
    epileptic s.
    lethargic s.
    postconvulsive s.
Sturge-Weber disease
Sturge-Weber-Kalischer syndrome
stuttering
STVA — subtotal villose atrophy
stye
    meibomian s.
    zeisian s.
styloglossus muscle
stylohyoid muscle
styloid
    s. process
stylopharyngeus muscle
styptic
    chemical s.

styptic *(continued)*
  mechanical s.
  vascular s.
styramate
styrene
SUA — serum uric acid
      single umbilical artery
subacromial bursa
subacute
  s. bacterial endocarditis
  s. combined degeneration
  s. combined sclerosis
  s. glomerulonephritis
  s. inflammation
  s. necrotizing encephalopathy
  s. sclerosing panencephalitis
  s. spongiform encephalopathy
subaortic stenosis
  discrete s. s.
  idiopathic hypertrophic s. s.
subaponeurotic
subarachnoid
  s. cistern
  s. space
subbasal projection
subcallosal gyrus
subchorionic
subclavian
  s. artery
  s. lymphatic trunks
  s. vein
subclavicular
subclavius muscle
subcommissural
subcostal
  s. artery
  s. margin
  s. plane
  s. vein

subcu, subcut or subq — subcutaneous
subculture
subcutaneous
  s. bursa
  s. emphysema
  s. inguinal ring
  s. nodule
  s. tissue
  s. trochanteric bursa
subcutis
subdeltoid bursa
subdiaphragmatic
subdural
  s. empyema
  s. hematoma
  s. hygroma
  s. space
subependymal
  s. glioma
subepidermal
  s. fibrosis
subfascial bursa
subfornical
subfrontal sulcus
subhepatic fossa
subiculum
subinguinal lymph node
subinvolution
subjacent
sublenticular posterior limb
subleukemic leukemia
sublimation
sublingual
  s. caruncle
  s. duct
  s. gland
subluxation
submandibular
  s. gland
  s. lymph node

submaxillary
- s. duct
- s. ganglion
- s. gland
- s. glycoprotein

submental lymph node
submentovertical
submersion-immersion
submetacentric
submucosa
- adenoid s.
- anal canal s.
- appendiceal s.
- bronchial s.
- colonic s.
- duodenal s.
- esophageal s.
- gastric s.
- hypopharyngeal s.
- ileal s.
- jejunal s.
- laryngeal s.
- nasopharyngeal s.
- oropharyngeal s.
- pharyngeal s.
- rectal s.
- small intestinal s.
- tonsillar s.
- tracheal s.
- urinary bladder s.

submucosal
submuscular bursa
subparietal sulcus
subphrenic fossa
subpleural
subscapular
- s. artery
- s. lymph node
- s. nerve

subscapularis muscle
subseptate uterus
subserosa
- appendiceal s.
- colonic s.
- duodenal s.
- gallbladder s.
- gastric s.
- small intestinal s.
- tubal s.
- urinary bladder s.
- uterine s.

subspecies
substance
- agglutinable s.
- antidiuretic s.
- autacoid s.
- chromidial s.
- chromophil s.
- colloid s.
- cortical s.
- gelatinous s.
- glandular s.
- H s.
- hemolytic s.
- interfibrillar s.
- interspongioplastic s.
- medullary s.
- metachromatic s.
- periventricular s.
- reticular s.
- sarcous s.
- thromboplastic s.
- white s. of Schwann
- zymoplastic s.

substantia (substantiae)
- s. gelatinosa
- s. nigra

substernal goiter
substitution
- creeping s. of bone
- reaction s.

substrate

subsynchronous
subtelocentric
subtendinous bursa
subthalamic
    s. fasciculus
    s. nucleus
subthalamus
subtotal amputation
succinate dehydrogenase
succinchlorimide
succinic acid
Succinivibrio
    S. dextrinosolvens
succinylcholine chloride
succinyl-coenzyme A
    s.-c. A hydrolase
    s.-c. A synthetase
succinylsulfathiazole
Sucquet-Hoyer canal
sucrase
sucrose
    s. glucohydrolase
    s. hemolysis test
    s. intolerance
suction
    post-tussive s.
Suctoria
SUD — sudden unexpected death
        sudden unexplained death
sudamen (sudamina)
Sudan
    S. black
    S. G
    S. yellow G
    S. I, II, III, IV
sudanophil
sudanophilia
sudanophilic
    s. leukodystrophy

sudden
    s. cardiac death
    s. coronary death
    s. infant death syndrome
Sudeck's atrophy
sudoriferous gland
suffocation
suicidal
suicide
SUID — sudden unexplained infant death
sulci cutis
sulcomarginal fasciculus
sulcus (sulci)
    Campbell's cruciate s.
    central s.
    cingulate s.
    circular s.
    collateral s.
    dorsal s.
    fimbriodentate s.
    inferior frontomarginal s.
    inferior temporal s.
    intraparietal s.
    lateral occipital s.
    marginal s.
    middle frontal s.
    middle temporal s.
    olfactory s.
    orbital s.
    paracentral s.
    parieto-occipital s.
    postcentral s.
    precentral s.
    Reil's limiting s.
    subfrontal s.
    subparietal s.
    superior frontal s.
    superior temporal s.
    s. terminalis
    ventral lateral s.

sulfabenzamide
sulfacetamide
sulfachloropyridazine
sulfadiazine
sulfadimethoxine
sulfaethidole
sulfaguanidine
sulfamerazine
sulfameter
sulfamethazine
sulfamethizole
sulfamethoxazole
sulfamethoxypyridazine
sulfanilamide
sulfanilic acid
sulfaphenazole
sulfapyridine
sulfatase
sulfate
   acid s.
   adenylyltransferase s.
   chondroitin s.
   conjugated s.
   cupric s.
   ferrous s.
   neutral s.
   Nile blue s.
sulfatemia
sulfathiazole
sulfatidase
sulfatide
   s. lipidosis
   s. sulfatase
sulfation
sulfhemoglobin
sulfhemoglobinemia
sulfhemoglobinuria
sulfhydryl
sulfide
sulfinic acid
sulfinpyrazone

sulfinyl
sulfisomidine
sulfisoxazole
   acetyl s.
   s. diolamine
sulfite
   s. oxidase
   s. polymyxin sulfadiazine
   s. reductase
sulfmethemoglobin
sulfobromophthalein
sulfolipid
sulfolithocholylglycine
sulfomucin
sulfonamide
sulfonation
sulfone
sulfonethylmethane
sulfonic acid
sulfonmethane
sulfonyl
sulfonylurea
sulfoprotein
sulfoxide
sulfoxone sodium
sulfur
   s. dioxide
   s. dye
   s. isotope
   s. trioxide
sulfuric
   s. acid
   s. esterase
   s. ester hydrolase
sulfurous acid
sulfurtransferase
Sulkowitch's test
sulphenone
SUN — serum urea nitrogen
sunstroke
sup — superficial

sup *(continued)*
  superior
superconducting quantum-interference device
superficial
  s. cervical artery
  s. circumflex iliac vein
  s. dorsal nucleus
  s. epigastric artery
  s. lymphatics
  s. multicentric basal cell carcinoma
  s. palmar artery
  s. peroneal nerve
  s. sylvian vein
  s. temporal artery
  s. transverse fibers
  s. volar artery
  s. wound
superinfection
superior
  s. aperture
  s. brachium
  s. cardiac branch
  s. cardiac nerve
  s. central nucleus
  s. cerebellar artery
  s. cerebellar peduncle
  s. cerebral vein
  s. cervical ganglion
  s. colliculus
  s. colliculus of corpora quadrigemina
  s. commissure
  s. deep cervical lymph node
  s. displacement
  s. division, oculomotor nerve
  s. epigastric artery
  s. frontal gyrus
  s. frontal sulcus

superior *(continued)*
  s. fronto-occipital fasciculus
  s. ganglion
  s. genicular artery
  s. gluteal nerve
  s. hemorrhoidal artery
  s. hemorrhoidal vein
  s. intercostal artery
  s. laryngeal aperture
  s. laryngeal nerve
  s. left pulmonary vein
  s. lingular bronchus
  s. longitudinal fasciculus
  s. mediastinum
  s. medullary velum
  s. mesenteric artery
  s. mesenteric ganglion
  s. mesenteric plexus
  s. mesenteric vein
  s. nasal turbinate
  s. oblique muscle
  s. oblique nerve
  s. occipital gyrus
  s. olivary nucleus
  s. ophthalmic vein
  s. pancreaticoduodenal artery
  s. parietal lobe
  s. petrosal sinus
  s. phrenic artery
  s. phrenic vein
  s. posterior fissure
  s. principal preoptic nucleus
  s. rectal artery
  s. rectal vein
  s. rectus muscle
  s. right pulmonary vein
  s. sagittal sinus
  s. segment

superior *(continued)*
- s. sensory nucleus
- s. striate vein
- s. temporal gyrus
- s. temporal sulcus
- s. thalamic radiation
- s. thoracic artery
- s. thyroid artery
- s. trunk, brachial plexus
- s. vena cava
- s. vena cava syndrome

supernatant
supernumerary
superoinferior
superoxide
- s. dismutase

supersaturated
supersecretion
supersonic
Superstitionia
supervoltage
supination
supinator muscle
supine
support
supporting structure
suppressibility
suppression
suppressor
- s. gene
- s. lymphocyte

suppuration
suppurative
- s. acute appendicitis
- s. acute inflammation
- s. appendicitis
- s. chronic inflammation
- s. chronic otitis media
- s. granulomatous inflammation
- s. inflammation

supracallosal gyrus

suprachiasmatic nucleus
supraclavicular
- s. lymph node
- s. nerve
- s. region

suprageniculate nucleus
suprahyoid muscle
supramammillary
- s. decussation
- s. nucleus

supramarginal
- s. artery
- s. gyrus

supranuclear
supraoptic nucleus
supraorbital
- s. artery
- s. nerve

suprapatellar
- s. bursa

suprapubic
- s. needle aspiration

suprarenal
suprascapular
supraspinatus muscle
suprasternal
supratentorial
supratrochlear
- s. artery
- s. nerve

supravital
- s. staining

supreme genicular artery
sural
- s. artery
- s. nerve

suramin sodium
surface
- s.-active agent
- s. alteration
- s.-barrier detector
- s. epithelium

surfactant
surgical
    s. amputation
    s. defect
    s. dissection
    s. incision
    s. instrument
    s. pathology
    s. scar
    s. wound
suroplantar
survival
    red blood cell s.
SUS — stained urinary sediment
susceptibility
suspension
suspensory ligament
suspicious cytologic alteration
suture
    coronal s.
    ethmoidomaxillary s.
    frontal s.
    intermaxillary s.
    lacrimal s.
    lambdoid s.
    nasal s.
    palatal s.
    parietomastoid s.
    sagittal s.
    sphenoid s.
    squamous s.
    temporozygomatic s.
    zygomaticomaxillary s.
SUUD — sudden unexpected, unexplained death
SV — severe
    simian virus
    snake venom
    stroke volume
    subclavian vein
    supravital

SVAS — supravalvular aortic stenosis
SVC — slow vital capacity
    superior vena cava
SVCG — spatial vectorcardiogram
SVD — spontaneous vaginal delivery
    spontaneous vertex delivery
Svedberg flotation unit
SVI — stroke volume index
SVM — syncytiovascular membrane
SVR — systemic vascular resistance
SW — spiral wound
    stroke work
Swan-Ganz catheter
S wave
sweat gland
    s. g. adenocarcinoma
    s. g. adenoma
    s. g. carcinoma
    s. g. tumor
sweating
    excessive s.
Sweet method
swelling
    cloudy s.
SWI — stroke work index
Swift's disease
Swiss cheese hyperplasia
Swiss-type agammaglobulinemia
Swiss-type hypogammaglobulinemia
Sx — signs
    symptoms
sycosis
Sydenham's chorea

Sylvest's disease
Sylvius
    aqueduct of S.
    fissure of S.
    iter of S.
sym — symmetrical
    symptoms
symbiont
symbiosis
symblepharon
symbol, symbols. *See* Symbols and Prefixes, Appendix 8.
symmetric
    s. distribution
symmetry
    bilateral s.
    s. element
    radial s.
sympathectomy
sympathetic
    s. fiber
    s. ganglion
    s. nervous system
    s. ophthalmitis
    s. trunk
sympathicoblastoma
sympathicogonioma
sympathomimetic
symphysis
    s. menti
    s. pubis
    s. sacrococcygea
sympodia
symport
symptom
symptomatic
symptomatology
symptomatolytic
synapse
synapsis
synaptic
    s. cleft

synaptic *(continued)*
    s. transmission
    s. vesicles
synaptonemal complex
synaptosome
synarthrosis
Syncephalastrum
syncephalus
synchondrosis
    costochondral s.
    petroso-occipital s.
    spheno-occipital s.
    sphenopetrosal s.
    sternal s.
synchronized
    s. culture
synchronous
    s. data transmission
syncopal
syncope
    cardiac s.
    carotid sinus s.
    exertional s.
    micturition s.
    postural s.
    vasovagal s.
syncytial
    s. alteration
    s. endometritis
    s. trophoblast
syncytiotrophoblast
syncytium
syndactyly
syndesis
syndesmitis
syndrome, syndromes. *See* Eponymic Diseases and Syndromes, Appendix 2.
syndrome of inappropriate antidiuretic hormone
synechia (synechiae)
syneresis

synergism
synergist
synergy
Syn. Fl. — synovial fluid
Syngamidae
Syngamus
    S. laryngeus
    S. trachea
syngamy
syngeneic
syngraft
synkaryon
synophthalmia
synorchism
Synosternus
    S. pallidus
synostosis
synotus
synovia
synovial
    s. fluid
    s. layer of articular capsule
    s. membrane
    s. plica
    s. sarcoma
    s. tendon sheath
    s. tissue
    s. villus
synovioma
synovitis
    acute serous s.
    pigmented villonodular s.
    proliferative s.
syntenic
synteny
syntexis
synthase
synthetase
synthetic
syntrophism
syntropic

Syphacia
    S. obvelata
syphilid
syphilis
syphilitic
    s. aneurysm
    s. aortitis
syringadenoma
    papillary s.
syringe
    fountain s.
    hypodermic s.
    probe s.
syringobulbia
syringocystadenoma
    s. papilliferum
syringoencephalomyelia
syringoma
    chondroid s.
syringomyelia
syringomyelocele
syrosingopine
system
    Bactec s.
    Kell blood s.
systematic
Systematized Nomenclature of Pathology
systemic
    s. familial primary amyloidosis
    s. lupus erythematosus
    s. primary amyloidosis
    s. reticuloendotheliosis
    s. sclerosis
systemoid
systole
systolic
    s. hypertension
    s. murmur
    s. pressure

systolic *(continued)*
   s. time interval

Sz — schizophrenia
Szent-Györgyi reaction

T

T — temperature
  tension (intraocular)
  tesla
  thoracic
  thorax
  thymidine
  torque
  tritium
T+ — increased tension
T− — decreased tension
T½ — terminal half-life
T_3 — triiodothyronine
T_4 — thyroxine
T. — *Taenia*
  Treponema
  Trichophyton
  Trypanosoma
t — temporal
  tertiary
  test of significance
TA — alkaline tuberculin
  therapeutic abortion
  titratable acid
  toxin-antitoxin
  tube agglutination
Ta — tantalum
TAB — typhoid, paratyphoid A
      and paratyphoid B
tabanid
Tabanidae
Tabanus
tabes dorsalis
table
  periodic t.
taboparesis

tache
tachogram
tachometer
tachyarrhythmia
tachycardia
  atrial t.
  junctional t.
  nodal t.
  paroxysmal auricular t.
  paroxysmal ventricular t.
  ventricular t.
tachyphylaxis
tachypnea
tactile
  t. anesthesia
  t. disc
  t. hypesthesia
TAD — thoracic asphyxiant
      dystrophy
Taenia
  T. africana
  T. bremneri
  T. canina
  T. confusa
  T. diminuta
  T. echinococcus
  T. lata
  T. murina
  T. nana
  T. philippina
  T. saginata
  T. solium
  T. taeniaeformis
Taeniarhynchus
taeniasis

Taeniidae
Taenzer-Unna stain
TAF — albumose-free tuberculin
toxoid-antitoxin floccules
trypsin-aldehyde-fuchsin
tag
    anal t.
    hymenal t.
    skin t.
T agglutination
TAH — total abdominal hysterectomy
tail
    t. of caudate nucleus
    t. of epididymis
    t. of pancreas
    t. poikilocyte
Takata-Ara test
Takayasu's syndrome
TAL — thymic alymphoplasia
talbutal
talipes
    t. calcaneovalgus
    t. calcaneovarus
    t. calcaneus
    t. cavus
    t. equinovalgus
    t. equinovarus
    t. equinus
    t. planovalgus
    t. valgus
talocalcaneonavicular
talocrural
talus (tali)
TAM — toxoid-antitoxin mixture
TAME — toluene-sulfo-trypsin arginine methyl ester

tamoxifen
tamponade
    cardiac t.
tangent
tangential projection
Tangier disease
tannase
tanned red cell hemagglutination inhibition test
Tanner stage
tannic acid
tantalum
    t. isotope
T antigen (tumor antigen)
TAO — thromboangiitis obliterans
triacetyloleandomycin
tapetum
tapeworm
    beef t.
    dwarf t.
    fish t.
    pork t.
TAPVD — total anomalous pulmonary venous drainage
TAR — thrombocytopenia with absence of the radius
TARA — tumor-associated rejection antigen
tare
target cell
tarry
tarsal
    t. artery
    t. bone
    t. gland
    t. joint
    t. plate
    t. tunnel syndrome
tarsometatarsal
tarsus

tartaric acid
tart cell
tartrate
tartrazine
taste
    t. bud
    color t.
    franklinic t.
TAT — tetanus antitoxin
    thromboplastin activation test
    total antitryptic activity
    toxin-antitoxin
    turn-around time
    tyrosine aminotransferase
tattoo
taurine
taurochenodeoxycholate
taurocholemia
taurocholic acid
taurodeoxycholic acid
taurolithocholic acid
Taussig-Bing syndrome
tautomer
tautomeral
tautomerase
    phenylpyruvate t.
tautomerism
    keto-enol t.
    proton t.
    ring chain t.
    valence t.
taxis
taxon (taxa)
taxonomy
Tay-Sachs disease
TB — terminal bronchiole
    toluidine blue
    tracheobronchitis
    tubercle bacillus

TB *(continued)*
    tuberculosis
Tb — terbium
TBA — tertiary butylacetate
    testosterone-binding affinity
    thiobarbituric acid
T banding
TBC — tuberculosis
TBD — total body density
TBF — total body fat
TBG — thyroxine-binding globulin
TBGP — total blood granulocyte pool
TBH — total body hematocrit
TBI — thyroxine-binding index
    total body irradiation
TBII — TSH-binding inhibitory immunoglobulin
TBK — total body potassium
TBM — tuberculous meningitis
    tubular basement membrane
TBN — bacillus emulsions
TBP — thyroxine-binding protein
TBPA — thyroxine-binding prealbumin
TB-RD — tuberculosis–respiratory disease
TBS — total body solute
    tribromosalicylanilide
    triethanolamine-buffered saline
TB smear
TBT — tolbutamide test
    tracheobronchial toilet
TBV — total blood volume
TBW — total body water
    total body weight

TBX — whole body irradiation
TC — taurocholate
    temperature compensation
    tetracycline
    thermal conductivity
    tissue culture
    total cholesterol
    tubocurarine
Tc — technetium
TCA — tricarboxylic acid
    trichloroacetate
    trichloroacetic acid
    tricyclic antidepressant
TCAP — trimethylcetylammonium pentachlorophenate
TCBS — thiosulfate citrate bile salts sucrose
TCC — trichlorocarbanilide
TCD — tissue culture dose
TCD_{50} — median tissue culture dose
TC detector
TCE — trichloroethylene
T cell
    T c.-replacing factor
TCF — total coronary flow
TCH — total circulating hemoglobin
TCI — transient cerebral ischemia
TCID — tissue culture infective dose
$TCID_{50}$ — median tissue culture infective dose
TCIE — transient cerebral ischemic episode
TCM — tissue culture medium
TCP — tricresyl phosphate
tcRNA — translation control RNA
TCSA — tetrachlorosalicylanilide
TCT — thrombin-clotting time
    thyrocalcitonin
TD — tetanus-diphtheria
    thoracic duct
    thymus-dependent
    torsion dystonia
    transverse diameter
TDA — TSH-displacing antibody
TDF — thoracic duct fistula
    thoracic duct flow
TDI — toluene-diisocyanate
    total-dose infusion
TDL — thoracic duct lymph
TDP — thoracic duct pressure
    thymidine diphosphate
TDT — terminal deoxynucleotidyl transferase
TE — threshold energy
    tissue-equivalent
    total estrogen (excretion)
    tracheoesophageal
Te — tellurium
    tetanus
TEA — tetraethylammonium
TEAC — tetraethylammonium chloride
tearing
TeBG — testosterone-estradiol–binding globulin
technetium
    t.-99m aggregated albumin
    t.-99m albumin microspheres
    t.-99m dihydrothiotic acid
    t.-99m dimercaptosuccinic acid
    t.-99m diphosphonate
    t.-99m etidronate sodium
    t.-99m glucoheptonate

technetium *(continued)*
    t.-99m iron ascorbate complex
    t.-99m medronate sodium
    t.-99m pentetic acid
    t.-99m pertechnetate
    t.-99m polyphosphate
    t.-99m pyrophosphate
    t.-99m red blood cells
    t.-99m serum albumin
    t.-99m sulfur colloid
technician
technique
    Brecher's new methylene blue t.
    Brown-Brenn t.
    Carey's Ranvier t.
    Corbin t.
    Dennis t.
    dilution-filtration t.
    Ficoll-Hypaque t.
    fluorescent antibody t.
    Highman's Congo red t.
    Hotchkiss-McManus PAS t.
    Knott's t.
    Kohn's one-step staining t.
    Laurell t.
    McMaster t.
    plaque t.
    Ritter-Oleson t.
    scintillation counting t.
    Seldinger t.
    Southern blot t.
    Stoll's dilution egg count t.
    time diffusion t.
    zinc sulfate centrifugal flotation t.
technologist
technology
tectobulbar tract
tectorial membrane
tectospinal tract
tectum
    t. of mesencephalon
TED — threshold erythema dose
    thromboembolic disease
Tedion
TEE — tyrosine ethyl ester
TEF — tracheoesophageal fistula
tegmen (tegmina)
    t. tympani
tegmental pons
tegmentum (tegmenta)
TEIB — triethyleneiminobenzoquinone
teichoic acid
TEL — tetraethyl acid
tela (telae)
    t. choroidea
    t. conjunctiva
    t. subcutanea
    t. submucosa
    t. subserosa
telangiectasia
    hereditary hemorrhagic t.
telangiectasis
telecardiography
telemetry
telencephalon
teleomorph
teleroentgenography
tellurate
tellurite
tellurium
    t. dioxide
telocentric
telodendron
telomere
telophase
TEM — transmission electron microscope

TEM *(continued)*
    triethylenemelamine
temperature
  absolute t.
  body t.
  t. coefficient
  critical t.
  optimum t.
  subnormal t.
template
temporal
  t. artery
  t. bone
  t. branch
  t. dispersion
  t. epilepsy
  t. fascia
  t. gyrus
  t. horn
  t. lobe
  t. muscle
  t. operculum
  t. pole
  t. radiation
  t. region
  t. sulcus
temporomandibular
temporo-occipital fasciculus
temporopontile
temporopontine
temporozygomatic
TEN — toxic epidermal necrolysis
tenac — tenaculum
tenaculum
tenderness
tendinitis
tendo (tendines)
  t. Achillis
  t. calcaneus
  t. conjunctivus
  t. cordiformis

tendo (tendines) *(continued)*
  t. cricoesophageus
  t. oculi
tendon
  Achilles t.
  ankle t.
  anterior tibial muscle of t.
  biceps t.
  calcaneal t.
  central t.
  digital t.
  elbow t.
  patellar t.
  posterior tibial muscle of t.
  t. quadriceps
  t. sheath
  shoulder t.
  spindle t.
  superior oblique muscle of t.
  triceps t.
  wrist t.
Tenebrio
tenesmus
tenia (teniae)
  t. choroidea
  teniae coli
  t. libera
  t. mesocolica
  t. omentalis
  t. plexus
  t. telae
  t. thalami
  t. ventriculi quarti
  t. ventriculi tertii
Tenney changes
tenosynovitis
  t. crepitans
  pigmented villonodular t.
  villous t.
tension
  premenstrual t.

tensor veli palatini muscle
tenth cranial nerve
tentorial branch, ophthalmic nerve
tentorium (tentoria)
    t. cerebelli
    t. of hypophysis
TEP — thromboendophlebectomy
TEPP — tetraethyl pyrophosphate
teracurie
terahertz
teratocarcinoma
teratogen
teratogenesis
teratogenic
teratology
teratoma
    adult cystic t.
    benign t.
    embryonal t.
    malignant t.
    monodermal t.
    solid t.
terbium
terbutaline sulfate
terebene
teres major muscle
teres minor muscle
terminal
    t. airway unit
    amino t.
    t. bar alteration
    t. bronchiole
    carboxyl t.
    t. cisterna
    t. deletion
    t. deoxynucleotidyl transferase
    t. deoxyribonucleotidyl transferase

terminal *(continued)*
    t. vein
termination
    t. codon
    t. factor
    t. sequence
Ternidens
    T. diminutus
terpene
terpin
terpineol
terpin hydrate
tertiary
    t. syphilis
TES — trimethylaminoethanesulfonic acid
Teschen virus
tesla
test
    Abrams' t.
    acetic acid and potassium ferrocyanide t.
    acetic acid t.
    acetoacetic acid t.
    acetoin t.
    acetone t.
    acid elution t.
    acidified serum t.
    acidity reduction t.
    acid-lability t.
    acidosis t.
    acid perfusion t.
    acid phosphatase t.
    ACTH t.
    Adamkiewicz's t.
    Adler's t.
    adrenalin t.
    adrenocortical inhibition t.
    adrenocorticotropic hormone stimulation t.
    agglutination t.
    A/G ratio t.

test *(continued)*
- albumin t.
- aldolase t.
- aldosterone stimulation t.
- aldosterone suppression t.
- alizarin t.
- alkali denaturation t.
- alkaline phosphatase t.
- alkali t.
- alkali tolerance t.
- alkaloid t.
- alpha amino nitrogen t.
- Ames t.
- amylase t.
- antiglobulin t.
- antitoxoplasma antibody t.
- Anton t.
- Apt t.
- arginine t.
- Argo corn starch t.
- arylsulfatase t.
- Aschheim-Zondek t.
- ascorbate cyanide t.
- ascorbic acid t.
- automated reagin t.
- A-Z t.
- Bachman t.
- bacitracin disk t.
- Baker's acid hematein t.
- Baker's pyridine extraction t.
- barium t.
- Beard t.
- Bence Jones protein t.
- Benedict's t.
- bentonite flocculation t.
- Bernstein t.
- Betke-Kleihauer t.
- bile acid t.
- bile pigment t.
- bile solubility t.
- bilirubin t., direct, indirect

test *(continued)*
- bilirubin tolerance t.
- biuret t.
- blood urea nitrogen t.
- Bloor's t.
- Bloxam's t.
- Boas' t.
- Bonanno's t.
- Bradshaw's t.
- bromocriptine suppression t.
- bromosulfalein t.
- brucella agglutination t.
- butanol extractable iodine t.
- calcium t.
- calcium oxalate t.
- CAMP t.
- candida precipitin t.
- capillary fragility t.
- carbohydrate identification t.
- carbon dioxide combining power t.
- Casoni's intradermal t.
- Castellani's t.
- catalase t.
- catecholamine t.
- cephalin-cholesterol flocculation t.
- cephalin flocculation t.
- cetylpyridium chloride t.
- Chediak's t.
- chi-squared t.
- cholesterol t.
- cholesterol-lecithin flocculation t.
- cholinesterase t.
- chromogenic cephalosporin t.
- cis-trans t.
- citrate t.

test *(continued)*
- Clark's t.
- clomiphene t.
- coagulase t.
- coagulation t.
- coagulation time t.
- colloidal gold t.
- compatibility t.
- complement-fixation (C-F) t.
- complement lysis sensitivity t.
- Congo red t.
- Coombs' t., direct, indirect
- coproporphyrin t.
- cortisone-glucose tolerance t.
- C-reactive protein t.
- creatine t.
- creatinine clearance t.
- cyanide-ascorbate t.
- cyanide-nitroprusside t.
- Davidsohn's differential t.
- deoxyribonuclease (DNase) t.
- deoxyuridine suppression t.
- dexamethasone suppression t.
- dextrose t.
- Diagnex Blue t.
- Dick t.
- dilution t.
- dinitrophenylhydrazine t.
- direct antiglobulin t.
- disaccharide tolerance t.
- disk diffusion t.
- dithionite t.
- Dixon's t.
- Dold's t.
- Donath-Landsteiner t.
- Donné's t.
- double diffusion t.

test *(continued)*
- Dragendorff's t.
- dye excretion t's
- edrophonium chloride t.
- Ehrlich's t.
- electrophoresis t.
- Elek t.
- Ellsworth-Howard t.
- enzyme-linked antibody t.
- euglobulin clot t.
- fat absorption t.
- febrile agglutination t.
- Fehling's t.
- ferric chloride t.
- ferric ferricyanide reduction t.
- Feulgen's t.
- fibrinogen t.
- fibrin titer t.
- Fishberg's concentration t.
- flocculation t.
- fluorescent treponemal antibody absorption t.
- foam stability t.
- formol-gel t.
- fragility t.
- Francis' skin t.
- Frei t.
- Friedman's t.
- frog t.
- galactose tolerance t.
- gastrin-calcium infusion stimulation t.
- gastrin-protein meal stimulation t.
- gastrin-secretin stimulation t.
- gastrointestinal blood loss t.
- gastrointestinal protein loss t.
- Gerhardt's t.

test *(continued)*
    glucagon t.
    glucose tolerance t.
    glutathione stability t.
    glycogen storage t.
    Gordon's t.
    Graham-Cole t.
    Gravindex t.
    Guthrie's t.
    Ham t.
    Hanger's t.
    Harrison's t.
    heat precipitation t.
    Heinz body t.
    hemagglutination t.
    heterophile antibody t.
    Hicks-Pitney thromboplastin generation t.
    Hinton t.
    hippuric acid t.
    Histalog t.
    histamine t.
    Hogben t.
    Hollander t.
    homogentisic acid t.
    Howard t.
    17-hydroxycorticosteroid t.
    5-hydroxyindoleacetic acid t.
    icterus index t.
    Ide t.
    IMViC t's
    indican t.
    indigo-carmine t.
    indole t.
    indophenol t.
    insulin clearance t.
    insulin tolerance t.
    interference t.
    intradermal t.

test *(continued)*
    iodine-131 uptake t.
    iron-binding capacity t.
    isoiodeikon t.
    isoniazid phenotype t.
    isopropanol precipitation t.
    ^{131}I (radioactive iodine) uptake t.
    Jones-Cantarow t.
    Kahn t.
    Katayama's t.
    17-ketosteroid t.
    Kolmer's t.
    Kunkel's t.
    Kveim t.
    lactic acid t.
    lactic dehydrogenase t.
    lactose tolerance t.
    Ladendorff's t.
    Lange's colloidal gold t.
    latex fixation t.
    latex slide agglutination t.
    LE t.
    leucine aminopeptidase t.
    Levinson t.
    levulose tolerance t.
    limulus lysate t.
    lipase t.
    lipid t.
    lymphocyte transfer t.
    Machado-Guerreiro t.
    magnesium t.
    malaria film t.
    mallein t.
    Malmejde's t.
    Mantoux skin t.
    Master two-step t.
    mastic t.
    Mazzotti t.
    melanin t.
    methylene blue t.

test *(continued)*
    Metopirone t.
    Middlebrook-Dubos hemagglutination t.
    monocyte function t.
    Monospot t.
    Mosenthal's t.
    Motulsky dye reduction t.
    mucoprotein t.
    Murphy-Pattee t.
    Napier formol-gel t.
    nitrate utilization t.
    nitroblue tetrazolium t.
    nitroprusside t.
    nonprotein nitrogen t.
    Obermayer's t.
    Obermüller's t.
    occult blood t.
    oleic acid uptake t.
    Optochin susceptibility t.
    osazone t.
    osmotic fragility t.
    oxidation-fermentation t.
    pancreatic islet cell antibody t.
    Pandy's t.
    Papanicolaou's t.
    partial thromboplastin time t.
    patch t.
    Paul-Bunnell-Barrett t.
    Paul-Bunnell t.
    perchlorate discharge t.
    Petri's t.
    phenolphthalein t.
    phenolsulfonphthalein t.
    phentolamine t.
    phenylketonuria t.
    phosphatase t.
    phospholipid t.
    phosphoric acid t.
    Piazza's t.

test *(continued)*
    plasma hemoglobin t.
    platelet aggregation t.
    Porges-Meier t.
    Porges-Salomon t.
    porphobilinogen t.
    porphyrin t.
    Porteus maze t.
    potassium t.
    potassium hydroxide (KOH) t.
    precipitin t.
    presumptive heterophile t.
    prolactin t.
    protamine titration t.
    protein t.
    protein-bound iodine t.
    prothrombin t.
    provocative chelation t.
    purine bodies t.
    quantitation t.
    Queckenstedt's t.
    Quick's t.
    radioactive iodine t.
    radioallergosorbent t.
    RA latex fixation t.
    rapid plasma reagin t.
    reactone red t.
    Reinsch's t.
    Reiter protein complement-fixation t.
    resorcinol t.
    riboflavin loading t.
    Rinne's t.
    Ropes t.
    rose bengal t.
    Rose's t.
    Rose-Waaler t.
    Rothera's t.
    Rotter's t.
    Rous t.
    Rowntree and Geraghty's t.

Schober's

494 TEST – TEST

test *(continued)*
- Rubin's t.
- Rumpel-Leede t.
- Sabin-Feldman dye t.
- Sachs-Georgi t.
- Schick t.
- Schiller's t.
- Schilling t.
- Schirmer's t.
- Schultz-Dale t.
- Schumm's t.
- scratch t.
- secretin t.
- sedimentation t.
- Sereny t.
- serology t.
- serum alkaline phosphatase t.
- serum globulin t.
- sheep cell agglutination t.
- Sia t.
- sickle cell t.
- sickling t.
- silver nitroprusside t.
- Sims-Huhner t.
- single-breath nitrogen t.
- single diffusion t.
- skin t.
- SMA-12 profile t.
- sodium t.
- stat t.
- streptozyme t.
- sucrose hemolysis t.
- Sulkowitch's t.
- sweat t.
- Takata-Ara t.
- tanned red cell hemagglutination inhibition t.
- tetrazolium t.
- Thayer-Martin t.
- Thormählen's t.
- Thorn t.

Sia water test

test *(continued)*
- thromboplastin generation t.
- thymol turbidity t.
- thyroxine-binding index t.
- tine t.
- tolbutamide tolerance t.
- transaminase t. (SGOT-SGPT)
- *Treponema pallidum* immobilization t.
- TRH stimulation t.
- triiodothyronine resin uptake t.
- triiodothyronine suppression t.
- trypsin t.
- TSH stimulation t.
- T-3 uptake t.
- typhus antibody t.
- tyramine t.
- tyrosine t.
- Tzanck t.
- Uffelmann's t.
- urea clearance t.
- urea nitrogen t.
- urease t.
- uric acid t.
- urine acetone t.
- urobilinogen t.
- van den Bergh t.
- vanillylmandelic acid t.
- Van Slyke t.
- VDRL t.
- Voges-Proskauer t.
- Volhard's t.
- Wassermann t.
- Watson-Schwartz t.
- Weber's t.
- wire loop t.
- xylose concentration t.
- D-xylose absorption t.

test *(continued)*
- D-xylose tolerance t.
- zinc flocculation t.
- zinc turbidity t.

testicular
- t. agenesis
- t. artery
- t. dysgenesis
- t. feminization
- t. tumor
- t. vein

testis (testes)
- appendix of t.
- efferent ductule of t.
- gubernaculum of t.
- interstitial tissue of t.
- lobule of t.
- lymphatics of t.

testosterone
- t.-estradiol–binding globulin

Tet – tetanus
  tetralogy of Fallot

tetanic contraction

tetanolysin

tetanospasmin

tetanus
- t. bacillus
- t. toxin immunization reaction

tetany

TETD – tetraethylthiuram disulfide

tetrabromobenzoquinone

tetrabromo-*o*-cresol

tetracaine
- t. hydrochloride

tetrachlorobenzoquinone

tetrachlorodiphenyl sulfone

tetrachloroethane

tetrachloroethylene

tetrachlorophenol

tetrachloroquinone

n-tetracosanoic acid

tetracycline

tetrad

tetraethyl
- t. lead
- t. pyrophosphate

tetrahydrobiopterin

tetrahydrocannabinol

tetrahydro-compound S

tetrahydrocortisol

tetrahydro-11-deoxycortisol

tetrahydrofolate dehydrogenase

tetrahydrofolic acid

tetrahydrofuran

tetrahydronaphthalene

tetrahydropterolyglutamate methyltransferase

tetrahydrozoline hydrochloride

tetralogy
- t. of Eisenmenger
- t. of Fallot

tetramastigote

tetramer

tetramethyl lead

Tetramitidae

tetranitromethane

tetraplegia

tetraploid

tetraploidy

tetrasodium pyrophosphate

tetrasomic

tetrasomy

Tetratrichomonas
- *T. buccalis*
- *T. hominis*

tetravalent

tetrazolium salts

tetrodotoxin

tetrose

tetryl

TF — tactile fremitus
  tetralogy of Fallot
  thymol flocculation
  tissue-damaging factor
  transfer factor
  tuberculin filtrate
  tubular fluid
TFA — total fatty acids
TFE — polytetrafluoroethylene
  tetrafluoroethylene
Tfm — testicular feminization
  syndrome
TFS — testicular feminization
  syndrome
TG — thioguanine
  thyroglobulin
  toxic goiter
  triglyceride
TGA — transposition of the
  great arteries
TGAR — total graft area rejected
TGFA — triglyceride fatty acid
TGL — triglyceride
  triglyceride lipase
TGT — thromboplastin generation test
  thromboplastin generation time
TGV — thoracic gas volume
  transposition of the
  great vessels
TH — thyrohyoid
Th — thorium
th — thoracic
THA — total hydroxyapatite
thalamic fasciculus
thalamocortical
thalamogeniculate artery
thalamo-olivary tract
thalamosensory cortical fibers

thalamus (thalami)
  external medullary lamina of t.
  inferior peduncular interstitial nucleus of t.
  internal medullary lamina of t.
  interoanterodorsal nucleus of t.
  interoanteromedial nucleus of t.
  interoanteroventral nucleus of t.
  intralaminar nucleus of t.
  lateral ventral nucleus of t.
  medial nucleus of t.
  nucleus circularis of t.
  nucleus dorsointermedius externus of t.
  nucleus limitans of t.
  paracentral nucleus of t.
  parafascicular nucleus of t.
  posterolateral ventral nucleus of t.
  posteroventralis nucleus of t.
  reticular nucleus of t.
  rhomboid nucleus of t.
  superficial dorsal nucleus of t.
  ventral t.
thalassemia
  hemoglobin t.
  heterozygous t.
  homozygous t.
  t. intermedia
  t. major
  t. minor
  mixed t.
  sickle-cell t.
  t. trait

thalidomide
thallitoxicosis
thallium
thallospore
thallous chloride
thallus
THAM — tris(hydroxymethyl) aminomethane
thanite
thaumatropy
Thaumetopoea
Thaumetopoeidae
Thayer-Martin
    agar
    test
THC — tetrahydrocannabinol
THDOC — tetrahydrodeoxycorticosterone
THE — tetrahydrocortisone
thebaine
theca (thecae)
    t. cell–granulosa cell tumor
    t. cell tumor
    t. folliculi
    t. lutein cyst
    t. lutein tumor
thecal
thecoma
Theiler's virus
Thelazia
    T. callipaeda
thelaziasis
theliolymphocyte
thenar
thenyldiamine hydrochloride
thenylpyramine
theobromine
theolin
theophylline
theorem
    Bayes's t.

theoretical
theory
therapeutic
    t. abortion
thermal
    t. anesthesia
    t. conductivity detector
    t. death point
    t. death time
    t. hypesthesia
    t. neutron
thermistor
Thermoactinomyces
    T. vulgaris
thermocouple
thermodilution
thermoduric
thermodynamics
thermogram
thermograph
thermography
thermolabile
thermoluminescence
thermolysis
thermometer
    air t.
    alcohol t.
    axilla t.
    Beckmann t.
    bimetal t.
    Celsius t.
    centigrade t.
    clinical t.
    differential t.
    Fahrenheit t.
    gas t.
    Kelvin t.
    liquid-in-glass t.
    maximum t.
    mercurial t.
    metallic t.

thermometer *(continued)*
    metastatic t.
    minimum t.
    oral t.
    Rankine t.
    Réaumur t.
    recording t.
    rectal t.
    resistance t.
    thermocouple t.
thermometry
thermophile
thermoresistant
thermotaxis
thermotropism
thesaurismosis
thesaurocyte
theta antigen
THF — humoral thymic factor
       tetrahydrofolic acid
       tetrahydrofuran
THFA — tetrahydrofolic acid
thial
thiaminase
thiamine
    t. hydrochloride
    t. mononitrate
    t. nitrate
    phosphorylated t.
    t. pyrophosphokinase
thiamphenicol
thiamylal sodium
thiazide
thiazinamium chloride
thiazine dye
thiazole
thiazolsulfone
thickening
    hyaline t.
thiethylperazine
    t. maleate

thihexinol
    t. methylbromide
thimerosal
thin-layer chromatography
thioacid
thioaldehyde
thiobarbiturate
thiocarbarsone
thiocarbonyl group
thiochrome
thioctic acid
thiocyanate
    t. potassium
Thiodan
thiodiphenylamine
thioester
thioethanolamine
    t. acetyl-transferase
thioether
thioflavine T
thioglycolate
thioglycollic acid
thioketone
thiol
thiolaminopropionic acid
thiolestcrase
thiolester hydrolase
thioltransacetylase
thiolysis
thionamide
thioneb
thionin
thiopental sodium
thiophene
thiopropazate hydrochloride
thioproperazine mesylate
thioredoxin
thioridazine hydrochloride
thiosulfate
    t. citrate bile salts sucrose
    t. salt

thiosulfate *(continued)*
    t. sulfurtransferase
thiotepa
thiothixene
    t. hydrochloride
thiouracil
thiourea
thiram
third cranial nerve
third degree
    t. d. burn
    t. d. frostbite
    t. d. heart block
    t. d. radiation injury
third trimester pregnancy
thixotropic
thixotropy
THO — titrated water
Thomsen's disease
Thoms method
thonzylamine hydrochloride
thoracentesis
thoracic
    t. aorta
    t. artery
    t. branches, axillary artery
    t. cavity
    t. duct
    t. esophagus
    t. myotome
    t. nerve
    t. portion, sympathetic nervous system
    t. spinal cord
    t. sympathetic ganglion
    t. sympathetic nervous system
    t. sympathetic trunk
    t. vein
    t. vertebra
    t. viscera

thoracoacromial artery
thoracoepigastric vein
thoracolumbar
    t. fascia
    t. region
thoracopagus
    t. parasiticus
thoracoplasty
thoracostomy
thoracotomy
thorax (thoraces)
thorium
    t. isotope
Thormählen's test
Thorn test
THP — total hydroxyproline
Thr — threonine
thread
    mucous t's
threadworm
three-Hertz spike and slow waves
threonine
    t. aldolase
    t. dehydratase
threonyl-RNA synthetase
threose
threshold
    t. limit values
thrill
    aneurysmal t.
    aortic t.
    diastolic t.
    hydatid t.
    presystolic t.
    systolic t.
throat
    t. culture
thrombasthenia
    Glanzmann-Naegeli t.
    Glanzmann's t.

thrombin
    t. clotting time
thromboangiitis obliterans
thromboarteritis
    t. purulenta
thromboclasis
thrombocyte
thrombocythemia
    hemorrhagic t.
    primary t.
thrombocytic
    t. leukemia
    t. series
thrombocytin
thrombocytopathy
thrombocytopenia
thrombocytopenic purpura
    autoimmune t. p.
    idiopathic t. p.
    thrombotic t. p.
thrombocytopoiesis
thrombocytosis
thromboembolism
thromboendarterectomy
thromboendarteritis
thromboendocarditis
β-thromboglobulin
thrombolysis
thrombolytic
thrombometer
thrombonecrosis
    arteriolar t.
thrombopathy
    constitutional t.
thrombophlebitis
    migrating t.
thromboplastic
thromboplastin
    t. antecedent deficiency
    t. generation test
thromboplastinogen
thrombopoietin
thrombosed
    t. aneurysm
    t. arteriosclerotic aneurysm
    t. hemorrhoids
thrombosis
    agonal t.
    cardiac t.
    cerebral t.
    coronary t.
    dilatation t.
    marantic t.
    mesenteric t.
    placental t.
    propagating t.
    puerperal t.
    traumatic t.
    venous t.
thrombostasis
thrombosthenin
thrombotest
thrombotic
    t. nonbacterial endocarditis
    t. occlusion
    t. thrombocytopenic purpura
thromboxane
thrombus (thrombi)
    canalized t.
    marantic t.
    mural t.
    old t.
    organized t.
    platelet t.
    recent t.
    tumor t.
thrush
THS — tetrahydro-compound S
thulium
thumb
    metacarpophalangeal joint of t.
    phalanges of t.

Thy-1 antigen
thyme
thymic
    t. artery
    t. capsule
    t. carcinoma
    t. cortex
    t. leukemia
    t. lobule
    t. lymphocyte
    t. medulla
    t. reticulum cell
    t. vein
thymidine
    t. diphosphate
    t. monophosphate
    t. phosphate
    t. phosphorylase
    t. triphosphate
thymidylic acid
thymidylyl
thymin
thymine
    t. ribonucleoside
    t. ribonucleoside phosphate
thymocytotoxic autoantibody
thymol
    t. iodide
    t. phthalein
    t. turbidity
thymolphthalein
thymoma
    epithelial t.
    lymphocytic t.
thymopathy
thymopoietin
thymosin
thymus
    t.-dependent antigen
    t.-independent antigen
    t.-leukemia antigen
thyrocalcitonin
thyrocervical trunk
thyroglobulin
thyroglossal
    t. duct cyst
thyrohyoid muscle
thyroid
    t. artery
    t. capsule
    t. cartilage
    t. colloid
    t. crisis
    t. endocrine disorder
    t. extract
    t. follicle
    t. gland
    t. hormone
    t. isthmus
    lingual t.
    t. lobule
    t. microsomal antibodies
    t. nerve
    t. nodule
    t. radioiodine uptake
    t. scan
    t.-stimulating hormone
    t.-stimulating immunoglobulin
    t. storm
    t. suppression test
    t. tumor
    t. uptake of radioactive iodine
    t. vein
thyroidea
    t. accessoria
    t. ima
    t. ima artery
thyroiditis
    de Quervain's t.
    granulomatous t.
    Hashimoto's t.
    induced t.

thyroperoxidase antibody

thyroiditis *(continued)*
    ligneous t.
    Riedel's t.
    subacute t.
thyrosis
thyrotoxic
thyrotoxicosis
    t. factitia
thyrotrope
thyrotropic
thyrotropin
    t.-releasing hormone
thyroxin
thyroxine
    t.-binding albumin
    t.-binding globulin
    t.-binding prealbumin
THz — terahertz
TI — thoracic index
    time interval
    transverse inlet
    tricuspid incompetence
    tricuspid insufficiency
Ti — titanium
TIA — transient ischemic attack
TIBC — total iron-binding capacity
tibia
    saber t.
    t. valga
    t. vara
tibial
    t. anterior muscle bursa, subtendinous
    t. artery
    t. astragaloid joint
    t. nerve
    t. tuberosity of subcutaneous bursa
    t. vein

tibialis
    t. anterior muscle
    t. posterior muscle
tibiofibular
TIC — trypsin-inhibitory capacity
tic
    t. douloureux
ticarcillin
tick
    t.-borne fever, African
    t. fever, Colorado
    t. paralysis
tic-tac rhythm
TID — titrated initial dose
TIE — transient ischemic episode
Tietze's syndrome
tiglium
time
    Ivy's method of bleeding t.
    mean generation t.
    thermal death t.
timolol maleate
timothy bacillus
TIN — tubulointerstitial nephropathy
tin
    t. chloride
    t. oxide
tinctorial
tincture
tinea
    t. amiantacea
    t. barbae
    t. capitis
    t. ciliorum
    t. circinata
    t. corporis
    t. cruris
    t. favosa
    t. facialis

tinea *(continued)*
   t. glabrosa
   t. imbricata
   t. kerion
   t. manuum
   t. nigra
   t. pedis
   t. sycosis
   t. unguium
   t. versicolor
tinnitus
TIS — tumor in situ
tissue
   adipose t.
   areolar t.
   chondroid t.
   cicatricial t.
   connective t.
   endothelial t.
   extracellular t.
   fibrous t.
   hematopoietic t.
   homologous t.
   lymphoid t.
   mesenchymal t.
   myeloid t.
   nephrogenic t.
   osteogenic t.
   soft t.
   splenic t.
   subcutaneous t.
   t. thromboplastin
   tuberculosis granulation t.
TIT — triiodothyronine
titanium
   t. dioxide
titer
   agglutination t.
   antihyaluronidase t.
   CF antibody t.
titration

titrimetric
Tityus serrulatus
TIVC — thoracic inferior vena cava
TKA — transketolase activity
TKD — tokodynamometer
TKG — tokodynagraph
Tl — thallium
TLA — translumbar aortogram
TL antigen
TLC — thin-layer chromatography
      total L-chain concentration
      total lung capacity
      total lung compliance
TLD — thermoluminescent dosimeter
      tumor lethal dose
T/LD_{100} — minimum dose causing death or malformation of 100 per cent of fetuses
TLE — thin-layer electrophoresis
TLV — threshold limit values
TM — temporomandibular
     transmetatarsal
     tympanic membrane
Tm — thulium
T_m — maximal tubular excretory capacity of the kidneys
TMA — trimethoxyamphetamine
T_{max} — time of maximum concentration
T_{mg} or TmG — maximal tubular reabsorption of glucose
TMJ — temporomandibular joint
TML — tetramethyl lead

TMP — thymidine monophosphate
　　　thymine ribonucleoside phosphate
　　　trimethoprim
TMTD — tetramethylthiuram disulfide
TMV — tobacco mosaic virus
Tn — normal intraocular tension
TNF — tumor necrosis factor
TNI — total nodal irradiation
TNM — (primary) tumor, (regional lymph) nodes, (remote) metastases—cancer grading system
TNT — trinitrotoluene
TNTC — too numerous to count
TO — no evidence of primary tumor
　　　original tuberculin
　　　tincture of opium
TOA — tubo-ovarian abscess
toad toxins
Tobie, von Brand and Mehlman's diphasic medium
tobramycin
tocopherol
TOCP — triorthocresyl phosphate
Todd
　　bodies
　　units
Todd-Hewitt broth
toe
　　Morton's t
togavirus
tolazamide
tolazoline hydrochloride
tolbutamide

tolerance
　　immunologic t.
　　t. interval
tolerogen
o-tolidine
tolmetin sodium
tolnaftate
tolonium chloride
toluene
　　t. diisocyanate
toluic acid
toluidine
　　t. blue
p-toluidine
toluol
p-toluylenediamine
N-m-tolyl phthalamic acid
Tomes'
　　fibers
　　process
tomogram
tomography
　　axial transverse t.
　　computed t.
　　panoramic t.
　　plesiosectional t.
　　rotational t.
　　simultaneous multifilm t.
　　transversal t.
tomolaryngography
tongue
tonic-clonic attack
tonicity
tonofibril
tonofilament
tonography
tonotopic
tonsil
　　cerebellar t.
　　faucial t.
　　pharyngeal t.

tonsillar
- t. branch, glossopharyngeal nerve
- t. branch, ninth cranial nerve
- t. capsule
- t. crypts
- t. fossa
- t. pillar

tonsillectomy
tonsillitis
tooth
- deciduous t.
- developing t.
- permanent t.
- t. pulp
- t. root
- t. socket
- supporting structure t.

tophus (tophi)
topographic
topography
TOPV — trivalent oral poliovirus vaccine
TORCH — *to*xoplasmosis, *ru*bella, *c*ytomegalovirus, and *h*erpes simplex
torcular
- t. Herophili

Tornwaldt's disease
torocyte
TORP — total ossicular replacement prosthesis
torque
torr
torsion
- t. injury
- t. spasm

torticollis
Torula
- *T. capsulatus*
- *T. histolytica*

toruli tactiles
Torulopsis
- *T. glabrata*

torulopsosis
torulosis
torus (tori)
- mandibular t.
- t. palatinus

tosylate
total
- t. electromechanical systole
- t. iron-binding capacity
- t. lung capacity
- t. peripheral resistance
- t. ventilation

totipotential
Tourette's disease
tourniquet
Touton giant cells
Towne projection
toxalbumin
toxaphene
toxemia
- pregnancy t.

toxic
- t. adenoma
- t. cirrhosis
- t. dermatitis
- t. erythema
- t. goiter
- t. granulation
- t. nephrosis
- t. shock syndrome

toxicant
toxicity
toxicologic
toxicology
- analytical t.
- clinical t.
- environmental t.
- forensic t.
- industrial t.

toxicosis
toxigenic
toxigenicity
toxin
    Coley's t.
Toxocara
    T. canis
    T. cati
    T. mystax
toxocariasis
toxoid
toxoid-antitoxoid
Toxoplasma
    T. gondii
    T. pyrogenes
Toxoplasmea
toxoplasmin
toxoplasmosis
TP — temperature and pressure
    thrombocytopenic purpura
    total protein
    tryptophan
    tube precipitin
    tuberculin precipitation
TPA — *Treponema pallidum* agglutination
TPBF — total pulmonary blood flow
TPCF — *Treponema pallidum* complement-fixation
TPG — transplacental gradient
TPH — transplacental hemorrhage
TPI — treponemal immobilization test (cardiolipin)
    Treponema pallidum immobilization (test)
    triose phosphate isomerase
TPIA — *Treponema pallidum* immobilization (immune) adherence
TPM — triphenylmethane
TPN — triphosphopyridine nucleotide
TPNH — reduced triphosphopyridine nucleotide
TPP — thiamine pyrophosphate
TPR — temperature, pulse and respiration
    testosterone production rate
    total peripheral resistance
    total pulmonary resistance
TPS — tumor polysaccharide substance
TPT — typhoid-paratyphoid (vaccine)
TPTZ — tripyridyltriazine
TPVR — total pulmonary vascular resistance
TR — tetrazolium reduction
    total resistance
    total response
    tuberculin R (new tuberculin)
Tr — trace
TRA — transaldolase
trabecula (trabeculae)
    arachnoid trabeculae
    trabeculae carneae
    trabeculae cranii
    trabeculae lienis
    septomarginal t.
    splenic trabeculae
trabecular
    t. adenocarcinoma

trabecular *(continued)*
- t. adenoma
- t. bone
- t. carcinoma

trabeculation

tracé
- t. alternant
- t. discontinu

trace
- t. element

tracer

trachea

tracheal
- t. bifurcation
- t. cartilage
- t. gland
- t. lumen
- t. lymph node
- t. mucus
- t. muscle
- t. submucosa
- t. vein

tracheitis

tracheobronchial lymph node

tracheobronchitis

tracheobronchomegaly

tracheoesophageal

tracheostomy

tracheotomy

trachoma (trachomata)
- t. virus

Trachybdella bistriata

tract
- biliary t.
- Burdach's t.
- cerebellar t.
- cerebrospinal t.
- extrapyramidal t.
- Flechsig's t.
- gastrointestinal t.
- genitourinary t.

tract *(continued)*
- Goll's t.
- Gowers' t.
- Lissauer's t.
- motor t.
- olfactory t.
- pyramidal t.
- respiratory t.
- spinothalamic t.
- urinary t.

traction
- t. atrophy
- t. diverticulum

tractus solitarius nucleus

tragus (tragi)

trait
- secretor t.
- sickle cell t.

trance

transacylase

transaldolase

transamidinase

transaminase

transamination

transcarbamoylase

transcarboxylase

transcobalamin

transconfiguration

transcortical

transcortin

transcriptase

transcription

transducer
- electroacoustic t.
- neuroendocrine t.

transduction

transection

transfection

transfer
- t. factor
- group t.

transfer *(continued)*
- linear energy t.
- passive t.
- t. RNA

transferase

transferred antigen–cell-bound antibody reaction

transferred antigen–transferred antibody reaction

transferrin

transformation
- asbestos t.
- bacterial t.
- globular-fibrous t.
- lymphocytic t.
- t. mechanism

transformer

transformiminase

transformylase

transfusion
- autologous t.
- coagulation factor t.
- exchange t.
- intrauterine t.
- leukocyte t.
- massive t.
- platelet t.

transfusion reaction
- acute hemolytic t. r.
- allergic t. r.
- anaphylactic t. r.
- bacterial t. r.
- delayed hemolytic t. r.
- febrile nonhemolytic t. r.
- hemolytic t. r.

transglutaminase

transglycosylase

transhydrogenase

transhydroxymethylase

transient
- t. hypogammaglobulinemia
- t. ischemic attack

transillumination

transistor
- field effect t.
- insulated gate field effect t.
- junction field effect t.
- junction t.
- metal oxide semiconductor field effect t.
- t.-transistor logic
- unijunction t.

transition

transitional cell
- t. c. carcinoma
- t. c. papilloma

transketolase

translation
- t. control RNA
- inhibitors of t.

translocation
- balanced t.
- reciprocal t.
- robertsonian t.

translucent

transmandibular projection

transmethylase

transmethylation

transmissible

transmission
- t. electron microscope
- t. scan

transmittance
- peak t.

transmural

transmutation

transonic

transoral

transorbital

transoximinase

transphosphorylase

transplant

transplantation
- allogeneic t.

transplantation *(continued)*
    t. antigen
    heterotopic t.
    homotopic t.
    orthoptic t.
    t. rejection
    syngeneic t.
    syngenesioplastic t.
transport
    t. and secretion
    t. and storage
transposable
transposition
    t. of great vessels
transposon
transpulmonary pressure
transpyloric plane
transsexualism
transsynaptic degeneration
transtubercular plane
transudate
    acute inflammatory t.
transudation
transudative
transversalis fascia
transverse
    t. caudate vein
    t. colon
    t. fracture
    t. gyri
    t. mesocolon
    t. myelitis
    t. myelopathy
    t. peduncular tract nucleus
    t. presentation
    t. scapular artery
    t. sinus
transversion
transversospinalis muscle
transversus
    t. abdominis muscle
    t. perinei profundus muscle

transversus *(continued)*
    t. perinei superficialis muscle
tranylcypromine sulfate
trapezium bone
trapezius muscle
trapezoidal bone
trapezoid body
Traube-Hering waves
trauma (traumas, traumata)
traumatic
    t. abnormality
    t. agent
    t. asphyxial state
    t. atrophy
    t. neuroma
TRBF — total renal blood flow
TRC — tanned red cell
        total ridge count
Treacher Collins syndrome
trehalase
Treitz's fossa
Trematoda
trematode
tremor
    action t.
    intention t.
    static t.
trench
    t. fever
    t. foot
    t. mouth
Treponema
    T. buccale
    T. calligyrum
    T. carateum
    T. genitalis
    T. macrodentium
    T. microdentium
    T. mucosum
    T. orale
    T. pallidum

Treponema (continued)
   T. pertenue
   T. pintae
   T. refringens
   T. scoliodontum
   T. vincentii
Treponema pallidum immobiiization test
treponematosis
trepopnea
treppe
TRF — T-cell–replacing factor
   thyrotropin-releasing factor
TRH — thyrotropin-releasing hormone
TRH stimulation test
TRI — tetrazolium reduction inhibition
triacetin
triacetyloleandomycin
triacylglycerol
triad
   acute compression t.
   adrenomedullary t.
   Beck's t.
   Hutchinson's t.
   portal t's
   t. of retinal cone
   t. of skeletal muscle
triamcinolone
triamterene
triangle
   Codman's t.
   Einthoven's t.
triangular
   t. bone
   t. ligament
triarylmethane dye
Triatoma
triatomic
triatomid

Triatomidae
tribasic copper sulfate
tribe
tribromoethanol
TRIC — trachoma-inclusion conjunctivitis
tricarboxylic acid
triceps
   t. brachii muscle
   t. surae muscle
   t. tendon
Tricercomonas
Trichinella
   T. spiralis
trichinosis
trichloracetate
trichloracetic acid
trichlorethylene
trichlorfon
trichlormethiazide
trichloroacetic acid
trichlorobenzene
trichlorobenzoic acid
1,1,1-trichloroethane
trichloroethanol
trichloroethylene
bis-(trichlorohydroxy ethyl) urea
trichloronitromethane
trichlorophenol
trichlorophenoxyacetic acid
trichlorophenoxy ethyl sulfate
trichobezoar
Trichobilharzia
trichocephaliasis
Trichocephalus
   T. trichiura
Trichoderma
trichoepithelioma
Tricholoma
   T. pardinum
trichomonad

Trichomonas
   T. buccalis
   T. hominis
   T. intestinalis
   T. pulmonalis
   T. tenax
   T. vaginalis
trichomoniasis
trichomycosis
   t. axillaris
   t. chromatica
   t. favosa
   t. rubra
trichonodosis
Trichophyton
   T. concentricum
   T. crateriforme
   T. epilans
   T. ferrugineum
   T. gallinae
   T. glabrum
   T. gourvilii
   T. gypseum
   T. megninii
   T. mentagrophytes
   T. purpureum
   T. rosaceum
   T. rubrum
   T. sabouraudi
   T. schoenleini
   T. simii
   T. sulfureum
   T. tonsurans
   T. verrucosum
   T. violaceum
trichophytosis
Trichoptera
trichorrhexis
   t. nodosa
Trichosporon
   T. beigelii
   T. cutaneum

Trichosporon (continued)
   T. giganteum
   T. pedrosianum
trichosporosis
trichostrongyliasis
Trichostrongylidae
Trichostrongyloidea
Trichostrongylus
   T. axei
   T. brevis
   T. colubriformis
   T. instabilis
   T. orientalis
   T. probolurus
   T. vitrinus
Trichothecium
   T. roseum
trichotillomania
trichrome
trichuriasis
Trichuris
   T. trichiura
Trichuroidea
triclobisonium chloride
tricresol
tricresyl phosphate
tricuspid
   t. atresia
   t. orifice
   t. ring
   t. valve
tricuspid valve
   anterior leaflet of t. v.
   chordae tendineae of t. v.
   commissure of t. v.
   posterior leaflet of t. v.
   septal leaflet of t. v.
tricyclamol chloride
tricyclic
tridihexethyl
triethanolamine
triethylene glycol

Troponin

512 TRIETHYLENEMELAMINE – TRIT

triethylenemelamine
trifascicular
trifluoperazine hydrochloride
triflupromazine
    t. hydrochloride
trifluridine
trigeminal
    t. ganglion
    t. nerve
    t. neuralgia
triglyceride
trigone
    olfactory t.
    urinary bladder t.
trigonitis
trihexosylceramide galactosyl-
    hydrolase
trihexyphenidyl hydrochloride
3,4,5-trihydroxybenzoic acid
triiodothyronine
    t. resin uptake test
    t. suppression test
trilobate
trilostane
trimeprazine tartrate
trimer
trimetaphosphatase
trimethadione
trimethaphan camsylate
trimethidinium
trimethobenzamide
    t. hydrochloride
trimethoprim
trimethoxyamphetamine
bis-trimethylsilyltrifluoroaceta-
    mide
trinitroaniline
trinitrobenzene
trinitrophenol
trinitrophenylmethylnitramine
trinitrotoluene

Triodontophorus
    T. diminutus
triokinase
trioleandomycin
triolein I-131
triose
triosephosphate
    t. dehydrogenase
    t. isomerase
trioxymethylene
trioxypurine
tripelennamine
    t. citrate
    t. hydrochloride
triphenylmethane dye
triphenyl phosphate
Triphleps insidiosus
triphosphoric monoester hy-
    drolase
triple-blind
triplegia
triploid
triploidy
triprolidine hydrochloride
tris(hydroxymethyl)amino-
    methane
trismus
trisomic
trisomy
    t. C syndrome
    t. D syndrome
    t. E syndrome
    t. 8 syndrome
    t. 13 syndrome
    t. 13–15 syndrome
    t. 16–18 syndrome
    t. 18 syndrome
    t. 21 syndrome
    t. 22 syndrome
tristearin
trit – triturate

triterpene
tritiated
tritium
trivalent
TRK — transketolase
TRMC — tetramethylrhoda-mino-isothiocya-nate
tRNA — transfer RNA
tRNA suppressor
trochanter
trochanteric bursa
    t. b. of gluteus maximus muscle
    t. b. of gluteus medius muscle
    t. b. of gluteus minimus muscle
    subcutaneous t. b.
trochlea (trochleae)
trochlear
    t. nerve
    t. nucleus
Troglotrema
    T. salmincola
Troglotrematidae
Trolard's anastomosing vein
trolnitrate phosphate
Trombicula
    T. akamushi
    T. alfreddugèsi
    T. autumnalis
    T. deliensis
    T. irritans
    T. pallida
    T. scutellaris
    T. tsalsahuatl
    T. vandersandi
trombiculiasis
trombiculid
Trombiculidae
Trombidoidea
tromethamine
trophic
trophoblast
    syncytial t.
trophoblastic
    gestational t. disease
    t. neoplasia
    t. pseudomotor
trophonucleus
trophoplasm
trophotaxis
trophozoite
tropical sprue
tropicamide
tropinesterase
tropism
tropocollagen
tropoelastin
tropomyosin
troponin
Trousseau's sign
TRP — tubular reabsorption of phosphate
Trp — tryptophan
TRPT — theoretical renal phosphorus threshold
TRU — turbidity-reducing unit
T_3RU — triiodothyronine resin uptake (test)
Truant's stain
true
    t. bug
    t. knot
    t. oxygen
    t. yeast
truncate
truncation
truncus (trunci)
    t. arteriosus
    t. brachiocephalicus

truncus (trunci) *(continued)*
  t. corporis callosi
  t. costocervicalis
  trunci intestinales
  t. jugularis
  t. linguofacialis
  t. lumbosacralis
  t. pulmonalis
  t. subclavius
  t. sympathicus
  t. thyreocervicalis
  t. vagalis
trunk
  duplication t.
trypan blue
trypanocidal
Trypanosoma
  T. ariari
  T. brucei
  T. castellani
  T. cruzi
  T. gambiense
  T. hominis
  T. nigeriense
  T. rangeli
  T. rhodesiense
  T. triatomae
  T. ugandense
Trypanosomatidae
trypanosome
trypanosomiasis
  Gambian t.
  Rhodesian t.
trypanosomicidal
trypanosomicide
tryparsamide
trypsin
trypsinogen
tryptamine
Tryptar
tryptase

tryptophan
  t. 5-hydroxylase
  t. malabsorption syndrome
  t. peroxidase
tryptophanemia
tryptophanuria
tryptophanyl-RNA synthetase
tryptophyl
TS — test solution
  tropical sprue
TSA — trypticase soy agar
T_4SA — thyroxine-specific activity
TSB — trypticase soy broth
TSC — technetium sulfur colloid
  thiosemicarbizide
TSD — Tay-Sachs disease
TSE — trisodium edetate
tsetse fly
TSF — tissue-coding factor
TSH — thyroid-stimulating hormone
TSH-binding inhibitory immunoglobulin
TSH-displacing antibody
TSH-releasing hormone
TSH stimulation test
TSI — thyroid-stimulating immunoglobulin
  triple sugar iron (agar)
TSP — total serum protein
TSPAP — total serum prostatic acid phosphatase
TSR — thyroid-to-serum ratio
TSS — tropical splenomegaly syndrome
TST — tumor skin test
TSTA — tumor-specific transplantation antigen
T-strain mycoplasma

T-suppressor cells
tsutsugamushi disease
TSY — trypticase soy yeast
TT — tetrazol
    thrombin time
    thymol turbidity
    total thyroxine
    transthoracic
TTC — triphenyltetrazolium chloride
TTD — tissue tolerance dose
TTH — thyrotropic hormone
    tritiated thymidine
T-3 uptake test
TTI — time-tension index
TTP — thrombotic thrombocytopenic purpura
    thymidine triphosphate
TTS — temporary threshold shift
TTT — tolbutamide tolerance test
TU — thiouracil
    Todd units
    toxic unit
    tuberculin unit
tuaminoheptane
tubal
    t. epithelium
    t. insufflation
    t. muscularis
    t. ostium
    t. plica
    t. pregnancy
    t. serosa
    t. subserosa
    t. tonsil
tube
    auditory t.
    buccal t.
    corneal t.
    digestive t.

tube *(continued)*
    drainage t.
    Durham's t.
    endotracheal t.
    eustachian t.
    fallopian t.
    granulation t.
    intubation t.
    Miller-Abbott t.
    nasogastric t.
    nephrostomy t.
    NIXIE t.
    ovarian t's
    pharyngotympanic t.
    photomultiplier t.
    salivary t's
    Sengstaken-Blakemore t.
    thoracostomy t.
    x-ray t.
tuberal nucleus
tuberc — tuberculosis
tuber cinereum
tubercle
    caseous t.
    darwinian t.
    fibrous t.
    genital t.
    Ghon's t.
    hard t.
    otic t.
    soft t.
tubercle bacillus
    avian t. b.
    bovine t. b.
    human t. b.
tuberculid
    papulonecrotic t.
    rosacea-like t.
tuberculin
    t. reaction
    t.-type reaction
tuberculoid granuloma

tuberculoma
tuberculosis
    central nervous system t.
    t. cutis verrucosa
    endobronchial t.
    extrapulmonary t.
    gastrointestinal t.
    healed t.
    inactive t.
    laryngeal t.
    miliary t.
    pericardial t.
    pleural t.
    primary t.
    pulmonary t.
    secondary t.
tuberculostearic acid
tuberculous
    t. meningitis
tuberhypophyseal
tuberosity
    ischial t.
    pubic t.
    tibial t.
tuberous
    t. sclerosis
Tubifera
tubocurarine
    t. chloride
tubo-ovarian
tubular
    t. basement membrane
    t. interstitial nephritis
    Pick's t. adenoma
    t. vision
tubule
    caroticotympanic t's
    collecting t's
    connecting t's
    galactophorous t's
    lactiferous t's
    mesonephric t's

tubule *(continued)*
    renal t's
    seminiferous t's
    subtracheal t.
    tracheal t.
    transverse t.
    uriniferous t's
tubulin
tubulointerstitial
    t. nephropathy
tubulonecrosis
tubulorrhexis
tuftsin
TUG — total urinary gonadotropin
tularemia
    oculoglandular t.
    pneumonic t.
    typhoidal (enteric) t.
    ulceroglandular t.
tumor
    adenomatoid t.
    amyloid t.
    t. angiogenesis
    t.-associated rejection antigen
    benign t.
    Brenner t.
    Brooke's t.
    Burkitt's t.
    t. cells
    Codman's t.
    t. embolus
    endobronchial t.
    epithelial t., benign
    Ewing's t.
    giant cell t.
    Grawitz's t's
    Krukenberg's t.
    Leydig–Sertoli cell t.
    malignant t.
    metastatic t.

tumor *(continued)*
    monoclonal t.
    necrosis t.
    t. necrosis factor
    ovarian t.
    Pancoast's t.
    polyclonal t.
    Rathke's pouch t.
    t. registry
    Sertoli–Leydig cell t.
    t.-specific antigen
    t. staging
    thrombus t.
    turban t.
    Warthin's t.
    Wilms' t.
tumorigenic
tumorlets
Tunga
    T. penetrans
tungiasis
tungsten
tungstic acid
tunic
    fibrous t.
    mucous t.
    muscular t.
    pharyngeal t.
    serous t.
tunica (tunicae)
    t. adventitia
    t. albuginea
    t. fibrosa
    t. interna
    t. intima
    t. media
    t. vaginalis
    t. vasculosa
T-3 uptake test
turban tumor
Turbatrix
    T. aceti

turbidimetric
turbidimetry
turbidity
turbinate
    nasal t.
    sphenoid t.
Turcot's syndrome
Türk's cell
Turnbull blue
Turner's syndrome
TV — tidal volume
        tuberculin volutin
TVC — timed vital capacity
        total volume capacity
        transvaginal cone
T wave
twelfth cranial nerve
twin
    conjoined t's
    corporea lutea t.
    dichorionic placenta t's
    dizygotic t's
    fraternal t's
    heterokaryotic t's
    identical t's
    incomplete conjoined t's
    monoamniotic placenta t's
    monochorionic diamniotic placenta t.
    monochorionic placenta t's
    monozygotic t's
    parasitic t.
    placenta t.
    Siamese t's
TWL — transepidermal water loss
two-dimensional chromatography
Ty — typhoid
tympanic
    t. antrum
    t. cavity

tympanic *(continued)*
   t. membrane
   t. nerve
tympanic membrane
   fibrocartilaginous anulus of t. m.
   pars flaccida of t. m.
   pars tensa of t. m.
tympanites
tympanography
tympanosclerosis
tympanum
Tymphonotonus
type
   t. culture
   t. species
   t. strain
typhoid
   t. bacillus
   t. fever
   t. immunization reaction
typhous
typhus
   amarillic t.
   t. antibody test
   endemic t.
   epidemic t.
   louse-borne t.

typhus *(continued)*
   murine t.
   recrudescent t.
   scrub t.
typing
   ABO t.
   ABO-Rh t.
Tyr — tyrosine
tyramine test
Tyroglyphidae
Tyroglyphus
   T. siro
tyropanoate sodium
Tyrophagus
tyrosine
   t. aminotransferase
   t. decarboxylase
   t. hydroxylase
tyrosinemia
tyrosinosis
tyrosinuria
tyrosyl
   t.-RNA synthetase
tyrosyluria
tyrothricin
TZ — tuberculin zymoplastiche
Tzanck test

U

U — unit
   uranium
   urine
UA — umbilical artery
   unaggregated
   uric acid
   urinalysis
   uterine aspiration
UB — ultimobranchial body

UBBC — unsaturated vitamin B_{12}-binding capacity
UBF — uterine blood flow
UBG — urobilinogen
UBI — ultraviolet blood irradiation
ubiquinol
ubiquinone reductase
ubisemiquinone

UC — ulcerative colitis
  ultracentrifugal
  urea clearance
  urethral catheterization
  uterine contractions
U-cell lymphoma
UCG — urinary chorionic gonadotropin
UCP — urinary coproporphyrin
UD — urethral discharge
  uroporphyrinogen decarboxylase
UDP — uridine diphosphate
UDP-acetyl-galactosamine
UDP-acetyl-glucosamine
UDP-bilirubin glucuronosyltransferase
UDPG — uridine diphosphoglucose
UDPGA — uridine diphosphoglucuronic acid
UDP-galactose
UDP-glucose
UDP-glucose-hexose-1-phosphate uridylyltransferase
UDP-glucuronate
UDP-glucuronic acid
UDP-glucuronyl transferase
UDPGT — uridine diphosphoglycyronyl transferase
UDP-iduronate
UDP-iduronic acid
UDP-xylose
UFA — unesterified fatty acid
Uffelmann's test
"U" fibers
UG — urogenital
Uganda S virus
UGI — upper gastrointestinal
Uhl's anomaly
UI — uroporphyrin isomerase
UIBC — unsaturated iron-binding capacity
UICC — Union Internationale Contre Cancer
UIF — undegraded insulin factor
UIP — usual interstitial pneumonitis
UIQ — upper inner quadrant
UK — urokinase
UL — undifferentiated lymphoma
  upper lobe
ulatrophy
ulcer
  acute hemorrhagic u.
  acute u.
  amebic u.
  aphthous u.
  Barrett's u.
  chancroidal u.
  chronic u.
  corneal u.
  Curling's u.
  Cushing's u.
  decubitus u.
  diabetic u.
  duodenal u.
  focal u.
  gastric u.
  healed u.
  hemorrhagic u.
  Hunner's u.
  marginal u.
  penetrating u.
  peptic u.
  perforated u.
  serpiginous u.
  stasis u.
  stercoraceous u.
  stomal u.

ULCER – UNDULATION

ulcer *(continued)*
    trophic u.
    varicose u.
ulcerate
ulceration
ulcerative
    u. colitis
    u. cystitis
    u. inflammation
ulcerogenic
    u. tumor
ulceromembranous
ulcerous
ulegyria
ulerythema
    u. ophryogenes
Ullmann's line
Ullrich-Feichtiger syndrome
Ullrich's syndrome
Ullrich-Turner syndrome
ULN – upper limits of normal
ulna (ulnae)
ulnar
    u. artery
    u. nerve
    u. vein
ULQ – upper left quadrant
ultimobranchial bodies
ultrabrachycephalic
ultracentrifugation
ultradolichocephalic
ultrafiltration
ultrasonic
ultrasonication
ultrasonography
ultrasound
ultrastructure
ultraviolet
    u. burn
    u. light
    u. radiation
UM – uracil mustard

umb – umbilicus
umbilical
    u. artery
    u. cord
    u. ligament, middle
    u. mucous connective tissue
    u. polyp
    u. vein
umbilicus
umbrella cell
UMP – uridine monophosphate
UN – urea nitrogen
uncinariasis
uncinate
    u. epilepsy
    u. fasciculus
    u. process of pancreas
unconsciousness
uncrossed pyramidal tract
uncus
undecaprenol
    u. phosphate
undecoylium chloride–iodine
undecylenic acid
underflow
undernutrition
Underwood's disease
undescended testis
undifferentiated
    u. adenocarcinoma
    u. carcinoma
    u. epidermoid carcinoma
    u. lymphoma
    u. neuroepithelium
    u. sarcoma
    u. squamous cell carcinoma
undifferentiation
Undritz anomaly
undulant fever
undulation
    jugular u.
    respiratory u.

ung – unguentum (ointment)
unicellular
uniflagellate
unigravida
unilocular
    u. cyst
    u. echinococcosis
    u. hydatid
union
    faulty u.
    primary u.
    secondary u.
    vicious u.
Union Internationale Contre Cancer
unipara
unipolar
unit
    Behnken's u.
    Bessey-Lowry-Brock u.
    Bessey-Lowry u.
    Bethesda u.
    Bodansky u.
    Bowers-McComb u.
    British thermal u.
    u. cell
    Ehrlich's u.
    Gutman u.
    Holzknecht u.
    Hounsfield u.
    Karmen u's
    King-Armstrong u.
    Mache u.
    u. membrane
    mouse u.
    u. of neutron dosage
    rat u.
    Russell's u.
    Shinowara-Jones-Reinhard u.
    Sibley-Lehninger u.
    Somogyi u.

unit *(continued)*
    Svedberg flotation u.
    Todd u's
    Wohlgemuth u.
United States Public Health Service
unit of neutron dosage
univalent
univitelline
unknown
    u. etiology
    u. function
    u. morphology
    u. topographic site
unmedullated
unmyelinated
unresolved
    u. hepatitis
    u. lobar pneumonia
    u. pneumonia
unsaturated
    u. B_{12}-binding capacity
Unschuld's sign
ununited fracture
UOQ – upper outer quadrant
UP – ureteropelvic
        uroporphyrin
U/P – urine-plasma ratio
UPG – uroporphyrinogen
UPI – uteroplacental insufficiency
UPJ – ureteropelvic junction
uptake
    RAI scan u.
    resin u.
UR – upper respiratory
ur – urine
urachus
    patent u.
    persistent u.
uracil
    u. dehydrogenase

uracil *(continued)*
  u. mustard
  u. phosphoribosyltransferase
uracrasia
uragogue
uranium
  u. isotope
  u. nitrate
uranyl
urate
  u. crystals
  u. monosodium
  u. oxidase
uratemia
uratohistechia
Urbach-Oppenheim disease
Urbach-Wiethe disease
URD — upper respiratory disease
urea
  u. clearance
  u. cycle
  u. nitrogen
Ureaplasma urealyticum
ureapoiesis
urease
urecchysis
3-ureidopropionase
uremia
uremic
  u. colitis
  u. inflammation
  u. pericarditis
  u. pneumonia
ureotelic
ureter
  u. adventitia
  lamina propria of u.
  mucous membrane of u.
  u. muscularis
ureteral
  u. hyperperistalsis
  u. ileus
  u. lumen
  u. orifice
  u. peristalsis
ureteritis
  u. cystica
  u. glandularis
ureterocele
ureteroileostomy
ureterolith
ureterolysis
ureteropyelitis
ureterosigmoidostomy
ureterostenosis
ureterostomy
ureterovesical
urethan
urethane
urethra
  bulb of u.
  corpus cavernosum of u.
  mucous membrane of u.
urethral
  u. artery
  u. crista
  u. gland
  u. lacunae
  u. lumen
  u. meatus
  u. obstruction
  u. orifice
  u. tumor
urethrism
urethritis
  follicular u.
  granular u.
urethrocele
urethrostenosis
urginin

urhidrosis
URI — upper respiratory infection
uric acid
uricacidemia
uricosuria
uridine
    u. diphosphate galactose-4-epimerase
    u. diphosphate glucose epimerase
    u. diphosphoglucose
    u. diphosphoglucuronyltransferase
    u. monophosphate pyrophosphorylase
    u. phosphate
    u. phosphorylase
    u. triphosphate
uridylic acid
uridylyl
uridylyltransferase
urinalysis
urinary
    u. bladder
    u. cast
    u. pole, glomerular
    u. tract
    u. tract fluids
    u. tract infection
    u. tract spaces
urination
urine
    chylous u.
    diabetic u.
    gouty u.
    milky u.
    residual u.
urinophilous
urobenzoic acid
urobilin
urobilinogen
urobilinogenuria
urocanic acid
urocele
urochrome
urocortisol
uroerythrin
urogastrone
urogenital
    u. diaphragmatic fascia
    u. disorder
    u. ridge
    u. sinus
    u. system
urography
urokinase
urolith
urolithiasis
uromucoid
Uronema caudatum
uronephrosis
uronic acid
uronolactonase
uropepsin
uropepsinogen
uroporphyria
uroporphyrin
uroporphyrinogen I, III
uroporphyrinuria
uroreaction
urorosein
uroschesis
urothelial
URQ — upper right quadrant
URTI — upper respiratory tract infection
urticaria
    aquagenic u.
    cholinergic u.
    factitious u.
    giant u.

urticaria *(continued)*
    u. perstans
    u. pigmentosa
    solar u.
urticate
urticating caterpillar
Uruma virus
US — ultrasonic
USN — ultrasonic nebulizer
USO — unilateral salpingo-oophorectomy
USPHS — United States Public Health Service
USR — unheated serum reagin (test)
ustilaginism
Ustilago zeae
usual interstitial pneumonitis
uta
UTBG — unbound thyroxine-binding globulin
uteri herniae inguinale
uterine
    u. artery
    u. bleeding
    u. inertia
    u. ligament
    u. segment
    u. serosa
    u. subserosa
    u. tube
    u. vein
uteroabdominal
uterorectal
uterosacral

uterus (uteri)
    u. arcuatus
    u. bicornis unicollis
    u. didelphys
    duplex u. bicornis bicollis
    rudimentary u.
    septate u.
    u. unicornis
UTI — urinary tract infection
UTP — uridine triphosphate
utricle
    prostatic u.
utriculitis
utriculosaccular
UU — urine urobilinogen
UUN — urine urea nitrogen
UV — ultraviolet
    umbilical vein
    urinary volume
UVA — ultraviolet radiation
uvea
uveitis
uveomeningitis
uveoparotid
    u. fever
UVJ — ureterovesical junction
UVL — ultraviolet light
uvula
    bifid u.
    u. of bladder
    palatine u.
    u. vermis
    u. vesicae
uvular branch
U wave

V — vanadium
  vein
  volume
V_{co} — carbon monoxide (endogenous production)
V_d — apparent volume of distribution (V area)
V_T — tidal volume
V. — *Vibrio*
  vision
  visual acuity
v — volt
VA — vacuum aspiration
  ventriculoatrial
  vertebral artery
  visual acuity
  volt-ampere
Va — alveolar ventilation
vaccenic acid
vaccinate
vaccination
vaccine
  Cox v.
  RhoGAM v.
  Sabin v.
  Salk v.
vaccinia
  v. virus
vaccinoid
VACTERL — *v*ertebral, *a*nal, *c*ardiac, *t*racheal, *e*sophageal, *r*enal and *l*imb
vacuolar
vacuolation
vacuole
  autophagic v.
  condensing v's
  contractile v.

vacuole *(continued)*
  plasmocrine v.
  rhagiocrine v.
vacuolization
  cytoplasmic v.
  nuclear v.
vagabond's
  disease
  melanosis
vagina (vaginas, vaginae)
  cyclic v.
  fornix of v.
  menstrual v.
  pregnancy v.
  proliferative v.
  secretory v.
  septate v.
  vestibule of v.
vaginal
  v. apex
  v. artery
  v. canal
  v. discharge
  v. epithelium
  v. mucous membrane
  v. secretion
  v. vault
vaginismus
vaginitis
  emphysematous v.
vaginomycosis
vagotonia
vagus nerve
Vahlkampfia
Val — valine
valence
valeric acid
valethamate bromide

valgus
valine
    v. aminotransferase
    v. transaminase
valinemia
valinuria
vallate
vallecula
    v. cerebelli
    v. epiglottica
    v. ovata
    v. for petrosal ganglion
    v. sylvii
    v. unguis
valley fever
valproic acid
Valsalva's
    posterior sinus
    maneuver
value(s). *See* Appendix 1, Normal Laboratory Values.
valve
    anal v's
    aortic v.
    atrioventricular v.
    cardiac v's
    v. of coronary sinus
    v. of foramen ovale
    v. formation
    Heister's v.
    ileocecal v.
    v. of inferior vena cava
    Kerckring's v's
    mitral v.
    pulmonary v.
    pulmonic v. of commissure
    sinus v.
    spiral v.
    tricuspid v.
    v. of veins
    venous v.

valvular
    v. atresia
    v. incompetence
    v. malformation
    v. stenosis
    v. tissue embolus
valvulitis
    rheumatic v.
valylene
valyl-RNA synthetase
VAMP — *v*incristine, *a*methopterine, 6-*m*ercaptopurine and *p*rednisone
vanadium
van Bogaert's disease
van Buren's disease
vancomycin hydrochloride
van den Bergh test
van der Waals
    equation
    forces
van Gieson's stain
vanillic acid
vanillin
vanillylmandelic acid
Van Slyke test
vapor (vapores, vapors)
    burning v.
    v.-phase chromatography
vaporization
Vaquez-Osler disease
Vaquez's disease
var — variant
variant
variation
    meristic v.
    microbial v.
    R-S v.
    S-R v.
varicella
    v. virus

varicella *(continued)*
    v. zoster
    v.-zoster virus
varicelliform eruption
    Kaposi's v. e.
varices
    esophageal v.
varicocele
varicose
    v. ulcer
    v. vein
varicosity
variety
variola
    v. virus
varix (varices)
    esophageal v.
varus
vas (vasa)
    v. deferens
    vasa recta
    vasa vasorum
vasc — vascular
vascormone
vascular
    v. anomaly
    v. hemophilia
    v. leiomyoma
    v. pole
    v. ring
    v. sinusoid
vascularization
    corneal v.
vasculature
vasculitis
    necrotizing v.
    nodular v.
    segmented hyalinizing v.
vasculotoxic
vas deferens
    v. d. adventitia

vas deferens *(continued)*
    v. d. ampulla
    v. d. lumen
    v. d. mucosa
    v. d. muscularis
vasitis
vasoactive intestinal polypeptide
vasoactivity
vasoconstriction
vasodilatation
vasomotor
    v. dysfunction
    v. hypotonia
    v. rhinitis
vasopressin
vasopressor
vasospasm
vasotonin
vasovagal
vastus
    v. intermedius muscle
    v. lateralis muscle
    v. medialis muscle
VATER — *v*ertebral defects, imperforate *a*nus, *t*racheoesophageal fistula, and *r*adial and *r*enal dysplasia
Vater-Pacini corpuscles
Vater's ampulla
VB — vinblastine
VBL — vinblastine
VBP — vinblastine bleomycin and Platinol
VBS — veronal-buffered saline
VBS:FBS — veronal-buffered saline:fetal bovine serum
VC — vena cava
    ventilatory capacity
    vincristine
    vital capacity

VCA — viral capsid antigen
VCG — vectorcardiogram
VCR — vincristine
VCU — voiding cystourethrogram
VD — vapor density
venereal disease
VDA — visual discriminatory acuity
VDBR — volume of distribution of bilirubin
VDEL — Venereal Disease Experimental Laboratory
VDG — venereal disease – gonorrhea
VDH — valvular disease of the heart
VDM — vasodepressor material
VDP — vincristine, daunorubicin, prednisone
VDRL — Venereal Disease Research Laboratory
VDRL test
VDS — venereal disease – syphilis
VE — visual efficiency
volumic ejection
V & E — Vinethene and ether
vector
VEE virus — Venezuelan equine encephalomyelitis virus
vegan
vegetation
    bacterial v's
    verrucous v's
vegetative
    v. endocarditis
Veillonaceae
Veillonella
    V. alcalescens
    V. discoides
    V. orbiculus

Veillonella (continued)
    V. parvula
    V. reniformis
    V. vulvovaginitidis
vein
    Galen's great cerebral v.
    Galen's lesser v.
    Labbé's anastomosing v.
    Rosenthal's v.
    Trolard's anastomosing v.
    varicose v.
velamentous
velum (vela)
VEM — vasoexcitor material
vena (venae)
    v. cava
    v. caval syndrome
    venae cordis minimae
venereal
Venereal Disease Experimental Laboratory
Venereal Disease Research Laboratory
Venezuelan equine A encephalomyelitis virus
Venezuelan equine encephalitis
venipuncture
venography
    peripheral v.
    portal v.
    splenoportal v.
venom
    Russell's viper v.
venostasis
venous
    v. admixture
    v. anastomosis
    v. plexus
    v. pressure
    v. return
    v. sinus
    v. thrombosis

vent — ventricular
ventral
    v. cervical nerves
    v. column
    v. corticospinal tract
    v. displacement
    v. hernia
    v. horn
    v. lateral sulcus
    v. lumbar nerve
    v. medial fissure
    v. median fissure
    v. paraflocculus
    v. pontine syndrome
    v. proper fasciculus
    v. reticulospinal tract
    v. sacral nerve
    v. spinal nerve root
    v. spinocerebellar tract
    v. spinothalamic tract
    v. tegmental decussation
    v. thalamus
    v. thoracic nerve
ventricle
    aortic v.
    auxiliary v.
    cerebral v.
    double-outlet right v.
    fifth v.
    first v. of cerebrum
    fourth v.
    Galen's v.
    lateral v.
    left v.
    pineal v.
    right v.
    second v. of cerebrum
    sixth v.
    terminal v.
    third v. of cerebrum
    Verga's v.
ventricular
    v. contraction
    v. escape
    v. fibrillation
    v. fold
    v. premature beat
    v. premature contraction
    v. premature depolarization
    v. septal defect
    v. septum
    v. system
    v. tachycardia
    v. vein
ventriculoatrial
ventriculography
ventriculosubarachnoid
ventromedial nucleus
Venturi mask
venula (venulae)
venule
    postcapillary v.
VEP — visual evoked potential
VER — visual evoked response
verapamil
verbascose
Verga's ventricle
Verhoeff's stain
vermian
    v. lobule
    v. sublobule
vermicular
vermifuge
vermis
    cerebellar v.
    uvula v.
vernal
Verner-Morrison syndrome
Vernet's syndrome
vernix
    v. caseosa
Verocay bodies

verruca (verrucae)
    v. peruana
    v. plana
    v. plantaris
    v. seborrheica
    v. virus
    v. vulgaris
verrucal
    v. atypical endocarditis
    v. nonbacterial endocardiosis
verrucous
    v. carcinoma
    v. endocarditis
    v. papilloma
verruga
    v. peruana
vertebra (vertebrae)
    cervical v.
    dorsal v.
    lumbar v.
    sacral v.
    thoracic v.
vertebral
    v. artery
    v. basilar artery syndrome
    v. column
    v. joint
    v. nerve
    v. vein
vertex (vertices)
vertical occipital fasciculus
Verticillium
    V. graphii
vertigo
verumontanum
very-large-scale integration
very-low-density lipoprotein
ves — vesicular
vesical
    v. artery
    v. blood fluke

vesicle
vesicolithiasis
vesicoureteral
vesicourethral
vesicouterine
vesicovaginal
vesicular
    v. acute inflammation
    v. emphysema
    v. granulomatous inflammation
    v. inflammation
    v. nucleus
    v. pharyngitis
    v. stomatitis
vesiculin
vesiculitis
vessel
vestibular
    v. ganglion
    v. gland
    v. membrane
    v. nerve
    v. nucleus
    v. root
    v. window
vestibule
vestibulocochlear
    v. nerve
    v. organ
vestibulospinal
vestigial
VF — ventricular fibrillation
    ventricular fluid
    visual field
    vocal fremitus
V.f. — field of vision
VFP — ventricular fluid pressure
VG — ventricular gallop
VH — vaginal hysterectomy
    venous hematocrit

Vimentin (stain)

VH *(continued)*
    viral hepatitis
VHD — viral hematodepressive disease
VI — volume index
VIA — virus-inactivating agent
viability
viable
Vi agglutination
Vi antigen
vib — vibration
vibration
vibratory
    v. sense
    v. sense loss
Vibrio
    V. alginolyticus
    V. bubulus
    V. cholerae
    V. cholerae-asiaticae
    V. coli
    V. comma
    V. danubicus
    V. eltor
    V. fecalis
    V. fetus
    V. finkleri
    V. ghinda
    V. jejuni
    V. massauah
    V. metschnikovii
    V. niger
    V. parahaemolyticus
    V. phosphorescens
    V. proteus
    V. septicus
    V. sputorum
    V. tyrogenus
    V. vulnificus
vibrio
    Celebes v.
    cholera v.

vibrio *(continued)*
    El Tor v.
    nonagglutinating v's
    paracholera v's
vibrion
    v. septique
Vibrionaceae
vibriosis
vicarious menstruation
Vicia
    V. graminea
vicinal
Vidal's disease
vidarabine
VIG — vaccinia-immune globulin
Villaret's syndrome
villonodular
    v. pigmented synovitis
    v. pigmented tenosynovitis
villous
    v. adenoma
    v. papilloma
    v. tenosynovitis
villus (villi)
    arachnoid v.
    intestinal v.
    synovial v.
vinbarbital
vinblastine sulfate
Vincent's
    angina
    organism
    stomatitis
vincristine sulfate
vindesine
vinegar acid
Vinson-Plummer syndrome
vinyl
    v. chloride
    v. ether
    v. polymers

532 VINYL – VIRUS (VIRUSES)

vinyl *(continued)*
    v. trichloride
violet
    amethyst v.
    Bensley's safranin acid v.
    Bernthsen's methylene v.
    chrome v.
    cresyl v.
    gentian v.
    hexamethyl v.
    methylene v.
    pentamethyl v.
viomycin sulfate
viosterol
VIP — vasoactive intestinal polypeptide
    voluntary interruption of pregnancy
viral
    v. capsid antigen
    v. hepatitis
    v. pneumonia
Virchow-Robin space
Virchow's
    hydatid
    node
viremia
virginal
viridans streptococcus
virilism
    adrenal v.
virility
virilization
    adrenal v.
virilizing syndrome
virion
virogene
virology
virulence
virulent
viruria

virus (viruses)
    animal v's
    v. animatum
    APC v.
    apeu v.
    arbor v's, groups A, B, C, unclassified
    Argentinian hemorrhagic fever v.
    attenuated v.
    Australian X disease v.
    Australian X encephalitis v.
    bacterial v.
    biundulant milk fever v.
    Brunhilde v.
    Bunyamwera v.
    Bwamba fever v.
    C v.
    CA v.
    Cache Valley v.
    California encephalitis v.
    Central European encephalitis v.
    chickenpox v.
    chikungunya fever v.
    Coe v.
    Colorado tick fever v.
    Columbia SK v.
    common cold v.
    coryza v.
    cowpox v.
    Coxsackie v., A, type 1; B, type 1
    Crimean hemorrhagic fever v.
    croup-associated v.
    cytomegalic inclusion disease v.
    dengue v., types 1, 2, 3, 4
    diphasic meningoencephalitis v.

virus (viruses) *(continued)*
- diphasic milk fever v.
- distemper v.
- eastern equine encephalomyelitis v.
- Ebola v.
- EBV v.
- ECBO v.
- ECDO v.
- ECHO v., type 1, type 12, type 28
- ECMO v.
- ECSO v.
- ecthyma infectiosum v.
- EEE v.
- EMC v.
- encephalomyocarditis v.
- enteric cytopathogenic human orphan v.
- entomopox v.
- epidemic keratoconjunctivitis v.
- epidemic parotitis v.
- Epstein-Barr v.
- equine encephalomyelitis v.
- erythema infectiosum v.
- exanthem subitum v.
- fifth disease v.
- filterable v.
- fixed v.
- foot-and-mouth disease v., types A, B, C
- German measles v.
- Guama v.
- Guaroa v.
- hemadsorption v., types 1, 2
- hepatitis v.
- herpangina v.
- herpes simplex v., I, II
- herpes zoster v.

virus (viruses) *(continued)*
- human T cell leukemia-lymphoma v.
- Ilheus v.
- inclusion conjunctivitis v.
- infectious hepatitis v.
- influenza v., types A, B, C
- Itaqui v.
- Japanese B encephalitis v.
- JH v.
- Junin v.
- Kumba v.
- Kyasanur Forest disease v.
- Lansing v.
- Lassa v.
- latent v.
- LCM v.
- Leon v.
- lepori pox v.
- louping ill v.
- Lunyo v.
- lymphocytic choriomeningitis v.
- lymphogranuloma venereum v.
- Marituba v.
- masked v.
- Mayaro v.
- measles v.
- Mengo v.
- MM v.
- molluscum contagiosum v.
- molluscum sebaceum v.
- monkey B v.
- mumps v.
- Murray Valley encephalitis v.
- Newcastle disease v.
- nonbacterial gastroenteritis v.
- Norwalk v.

534 VIRUS (VIRUSES) – VISCID

virus (viruses) *(continued)*
    Ntaya v.
    Omsk hemorrhagic fever v.
    O'nyong-nyong fever v.
    orf v.
    Oriboca v.
    ornithosis v.
    Oropouche v.
    orphan v's
    pappataci fever v.
    parainfluenza v., types 1, 2, 3, 4
    parapox v.
    parrot v.
    pharyngoconjunctival fever v.
    phlebotomus fever v.
    pneumonitis v.
    poliomyelitis v.
    polyoma v.
    Powassan v.
    pox v.
    psittacosis v.
    rabies v.
    respiratory exanthematous v.
    respiratory infection v.
    respiratory syncytial v.
    Rift Valley fever v.
    roseola infantum v.
    Rous sarcoma v.
    RS v.
    rubella v.
    rubeola v.
    Russian spring-summer encephalitis v.
    St. Louis encephalitis v.
    Salisbury common cold v.
    salivary gland v.
    sand-fly fever v.
    Semliki Forest v.
    Sendai v.

virus (viruses) *(continued)*
    serum hepatitis v.
    Simbu v.
    simian sarcoma v.
    Sindbis v.
    smallpox v.
    street v.
    Teschen v.
    Theiler's v.
    tickborne v's
    trachoma v.
    Uganda S v.
    unorganized v.
    Uruma v.
    vaccinia v.
    varicella v.
    varicella-zoster v.
    variola v.
    VEE v.
    Venezuelan equine A encephalomyelitis v.
    verruca v.
    vesicular stomatitis v.
    WEE v.
    Wesselsbron v.
    western equine encephalomyelitis v.
    West Nile v.
    Willowbrook v.
    yellow fever v.
    Zika v.
    2060 v.
VIS – vaginal irrigation smear
viscera
    abdominal v.
    thoracic v.
visceral
    v. membrane
    v. pericardium
    v. peritoneum
visceromegaly
viscid

viscidosis
viscosimeter
    Ostwald v.
    Stormer v.
viscosity
viscous
viscus (viscera)
visual
    v. cortex
    v. disorder
    v. evoked potential
    v. field defect
vit — vitamin
vital
    v. capacity
    v. red
    v. signs
    v. staining
vitamin
    v. A
    v. A_1 (retinol)
    v. A_2 (dehydroretinol)
    v. B
    v. B complex
    v. B_1 (thiamine)
    v. B_2 (riboflavin)
    v. B_6
    v. B_{12} (cyanocobalamin)
    v. B_{12b} (hydroxocobalamine)
    v. B_c (folic acid)
    v. B_c conjugate (folic acid)
    v. C (ascorbic acid)
    v. D (calciferol)
    v. D_2 (ergocalciferol)
    v. D_3 (cholecalciferol)
    v. E (alpha-tocopherol)
    v. G (riboflavin)
    v. H (biotin)
    v. K
    v. K_1 (phytonadione)
    v. K_2 (menaquinone)

vitamin *(continued)*
    v. K_3 (menadione)
    v. L
    v. L_1
    v. L_2
    v. M (folic acid)
vit cap — vital capacity
vitellin
vitelline
    v. duct
vitellointestinal
    v. duct
vitiligo
vitreous
    v. body
    v. humor
vitriol oil
vivax malaria
VLDL or VLDLP — very low density lipoprotein
VLSI — very large scale integration
VM — viomycin
        voltmeter
VMA — vanillylmandelic acid
VMR — vasomotor rhinitis
VN — virus-neutralizing
vocal
    v. cord
    v. fold
Voges-Proskauer
    broth
    test
Vogt-Koyanagi disease
volar
    v. artery
    v. digital vein
    v. metacarpal artery
    v. metacarpal vein
volatile
volatilization
vole bacillus

Volhard's test
Volkmann's
   canal
   contracture
   paralysis
volt
voltage
volt-ohm-milliammeter
volume
   atomic v.
   blood v.
   end-diastolic v.
   end-systolic v.
   expiratory reserve v.
   inspiratory reserve v.
   mean corpuscular v.
   packed-cell v.
   residual v.
   stroke v.
   tidal v.
volumetric
voluntary
   v. activity
   v. muscle
Volutella
   V. cinerescens
volutin
volvulus
VOM — volt-ohm-milliammeter
vomer
vomeronasal
   v. cartilage
   v. organ
vomiting
vomitus
von Bechterew's (Bekhterev's) disease
von Economo's disease
von Gierke's disease
von Hippel–Lindau disease
von Hippel's disease
von Kossa's method
von Kupffer cell
von Meyenburg's complex
von Recklinghausen's disease
von Willebrand's
   antigen
   disease
   factor
vortex (vortices)
voxel — volume element
voyeurism
VP — vasopressin
   venipuncture
   venous pressure
   Voges-Proskauer (reaction)
   volume-pressure
VPB — ventricular premature beat
VPC — vapor-phase chromatography
   ventricular premature contraction
   volume per cent
VPD — ventricular premature depolarization
VPRC — volume of packed red cells
V/Q — ventilation-perfusion
VR — valve replacement
   vascular resistance
   venous return
   ventilation ratio
   vocal resonance
VRBC — red blood cell volume
VRI   viral respiratory infection
VS — venisection
   vital signs
   volumetric solution
v.s. — vibration seconds
VSD — ventricular septal defect
VSS — vital signs stable

VSV — vesicular stomatitis
    virus
VSW — ventricular stroke work
VT — tidal volume
    vacuum tuberculin
    ventricular tachycardia
V & T — volume and tension
V_T — tidal volume
vulva
vulvar
    v. connective tissue
    v. mucous membrane

vulvitis
    chronic hypertrophic v.
vulvovaginitis
VV — viper venom
vv — veins
v/v — volume for volume
VW — vessel wall
    von Willebrand's disease
VZ — varicella-zoster
VZV — varicella-zoster virus

W

W — tungsten
    water
    Weber (test)
    wehnelt (unit of roentgen
      ray penetrating ability)
W+ — weakly positive
w — watt
Waardenburg's syndrome
Wade-Fite-Faraco stain
Waldenström's macroglobulinemia
Waldeyer's tonsillar ring
Wallenberg's syndrome
wallerian degeneration
Walsh's average
Walthard's cell rests
wandering pacemaker
warfarin
    w. potassium
    w. sodium
wart
    plantar w.
Warthin-Finkeldey giant cells
Warthin's tumor
warty dyskeratosis

wash
    Gravlee jet w.
washing
    bronchial w.
WASP — World Association of Societies of Pathology
wasserhelle
    w. cell
    w. hyperplasia
Wassermann
    antigen
    reaction
    test
water
    w. brash
    w.-clear-cell hyperplasia
    w. gas
Waterhouse-Friderichsen syndrome
watershed
    abdominal w's
    w. infarct
Watsonius watsoni
Watson-Schwartz test
watt

wave
- alpha w's
- beta w's
- brain w's
- C w.
- contraction w.
- delta w's
- dicrotic w.
- diphasic w.
- Erb's w's
- E w.
- F w's
- H w.
- monophasic w.
- M w.
- P w.
- polyphasic w.
- positive rolandic sharp w.
- Q w.
- R w.
- S w.
- sawtooth w.
- sine w.
- T w.
- theta w's
- three-hertz spike and slow w's
- Traube-Hering w's
- tricrotic w.
- triphasic w.
- U w.
- v w.
- ventricular w.
- x w.
- y w.

wax
- bone w.
- w. gland

waxy degeneration
Wayson stain
WB — weight bearing
    whole blood

WB *(continued)*
    whole body
    Willowbrook (virus)
Wb — Weber
WBC — white blood cell
    white blood count
WBC/hpf — white blood cells per high power field
WBF — whole-blood folate
WBH — whole-blood hematocrit
WBR — whole-body radiation
WC — white cell
    white cell casts
    whooping cough
WC' — whole complement
WCC — white cell count
WD — wallerian degeneration
WDLL — well-differentiated lymphocytic lymphoma
WE — western encephalitis
    western encephalomyelitis

web
- cell w.
- esophageal w.
- laryngeal w.
- terminal w.

webbed
- w. fingers
- w. neck
- w. toes

Weber-Christian disease
Weber's test
WEE — western equine encephalomyelitis
WEE virus — western equine encephalomyelitis virus
Wegener's granulomatosis
Weibel-Palade body
Weichselbaum's diplococcus

Western blot

Weigert's
  iron hematoxylin stain
  stain
weights and measures. *See* Appendix 5, Table of Weights and Measures.
Weil-Felix reaction
Weil's disease
Weinman's medium
Welch's bacillus
well-differentiated lymphocytic lymphoma
wen
Wenckebach block
Werdnig-Hoffmann
  disease
  paralysis
Wermer's syndrome
Werner's syndrome
Wernicke-Korsakoff syndrome
Wernicke's
  disease
  encephalopathy
Wesenberg-Hamazaki body
Wesselsbron virus
Westergren's sedimentation rate
western
  w. equine encephalitis
  w. equine encephalomyelitis virus
West Nile fever
West Nile virus
Westphal-Strümpell pseudosclerosis
WF — Weil-Felix (reaction)
WFR — Weil-Felix reaction
WGA — wheat germ agglutinin
Wharton's duct
wheal
wheat germ agglutinin
wheeze
whey
  litmus w.
whiplash
Whipple's disease
whipworm
white
  w. blood cell
  w. blood cell count
  w. lead
  w. line
  w. matter
  w. muscle
  w. pulp
  w. ramus
whitehead
white substance
  Schwann's w. s.
whitlow
Whitmore's bacillus
Whitten effect
WHO — World Health Organization
  WHO histologic classification of ovarian tumors
whole blood
whooping cough
Wickham's striae
Widal reaction
Wilkins-Chilgren agar
Willis's circle
Willowbrook virus
Wilms' tumor
Wilson-Mikity syndrome
Wilson's disease
window
  cochlear w.
  vestibular w.
Winslow's epiploic foramen
Wintrobe's
  macromethod
  sedimentation rate

wire-loop lesion
Wirsung's duct
Wiskott-Aldrich syndrome
WK — Wernicke-Korsakoff (syndrome)
wk — week(s)
WMA — World Medical Association
WMR — work metabolic rate
WNL — within normal limits
W/O — water in oil
Wohlfahrtia
   W. magnifica
   W. opaca
   W. vigil
Wohlgemuth unit
Wolff-Chaikoff effect
wolffian
   w. duct
   w. duct carcinoma
   w. rest
Wolff-Parkinson-White syndrome
Wolman's disease
woolsorter's disease
World Association of Societies of Pathology
World Health Organization
   WHO histologic classification of ovarian tumors
World Medical Association
wound
   abraded w.
   avulsed w.
   contused w.

wound *(continued)*
   gunshot w.
   incised w.
   lacerated w.
   missile w.
   mutilating w.
   penetrating w.
   perforating w.
   stab w.
   superficial w.
   surgical w.
WP — weakly positive
WPW — Wolff-Parkinson-White (syndrome)
WR — Wassermann reaction
   weakly reactive
W rays
WRC — washed red cells
WRE — whole ragweed extract
Wright respirometer
Wright's stain
wrinkled nucleus
Wrisberg's nerve
wrist
   tennis w.
wryneck
ws — watts-second
wt — weight
Wuchereria
   W. bancrofti
   W. malayi
   W. pacifica
wuchereriasis
w/v — weight per volume
Wyeomyia

X Y Z

X — homeopathic symbol for the decimal scale of potencies
  Kienböck's unit of x-ray dosage
  magnification
  respirations (anesthesia chart)
X
  X chromatin b's
  X chromatin
  X chromosome
xanthate
xanthelasma
xanthene
xanthine
  x. dimethyl
  x. oxidase
  x. trimethyl
xanthinuria
xanthochromatic
xanthochromia
xanthochromic
xanthocyte
xanthogranuloma
  juvenile x.
xanthogranulomatous
xanthoma
  x. cell
  x. diabeticorum
  x. disseminatum
  juvenile x.
  x. striatum palmare
  x. tendinosum
  x. tuberosum simplex
xanthomatosis
xanthomatous
Xanthomonas
xanthopsia
xanthopterin
xanthosine
  x. monophosphate
  x. phosphate
xanthurenic
  x. acid
  x. aciduria
xanthuria
xanthylic acid
XC — excretory cystogram
X chromatin bodies
X chromosome
XDP — xeroderma pigmentosum
Xe — xenon
xenobiotic
xenodiagnosis
xenogenetic
xenon
xenoparasite
Xenopsylla
  X. astia
  X. brasiliensis
  X. cheopis
Xenopus
  X. laevis
xerocytosis
xeroderma
  x. pigmentosum
xerophthalmia
xeroradiography
xerosis
xerostomia
xiphisternum
xiphoid process
XLD — xylose-lysine-deoxycholate (agar)

X-linked
- X-l. character
- X-l. dominant inheritance
- X-l. familial hypophosphatemia
- X-l. gene
- X-l. heredity
- X-l. hypogammaglobulinemia
- X-l. recessive inheritance

XM — crossmatch
XMP — xanthosine monophosphate
XP — xeroderma pigmentosum
XR — x-ray
x-ray
XS — excess
    xiphisternum
XT — exotropia
XU — excretory urogram
Xu — x-unit
XX karyotype
XXX karyotype
XY karyotype
xylanase
xylene
xylenol
xylitol
- x. dehydrogenase (NADP-linked)
- x. oxidoreductase

xylometazoline hydrochloride
xylose
- D-x. absorption test
- x. concentration test
- D-x. tolerance test

xylosuria
xylulokinase
xylulose
- x. dehydrogenase
- x. 5-phosphate
- x. reductase

xylulosuria
xylyl
XYY karyotype
XYZ syndrome

Y — yttrium
Y
- Y body
- Y chromatin
- Y chromosome

y — year(s)
yaws
- crab y.
- forest y.

Yb — ytterbium
yeast — *Torulopsis glabrata*
yellow
- alizarin y.
- fast y.
- y. fat
- y. fever
- y. fever virus
- metaniline y.
- y. phosphorus

yerbine
Yersinia
- *Y. enterocolitica*
- *Y. pestis*
- *Y. pseudotuberculosis*

Yersinieae
YF — yellow fever
Y-linked character
yohimbine
Yokogawa's fluke
yolk
- accessory y.
- formative y.
- y. sac
- y. stalk

yperite
ypsiliform
YS — yellow spot

YS *(continued)*
  yolk sac
ytterbium
yttrium

Z — atomic number
  zero
  Zuckung (contraction)
Zahn's
  infarct
  lines
Z/D — zero defects
ZE — Zollinger-Ellison (syndrome)
Zebrina
Zeeman's effect
Zener's
  breakdown
  diode
Zenker's
  degeneration
  diverticulum
  dysplasia
  fixative
zeolite
zeta
  z. potential
  z. sedimentation rate
Ziehl-Neelsen stain
ZIG — zoster immune globulin
Zika virus
Zimmermann's
  pericyte
  reaction
zinc
  z. arsenate
  z. arsenite
  z. bacitracin
  z. caprylate
  z. chloride
  z. cyanide
  z. dimethyldithiocarbamate

zinc *(continued)*
  z. gelatin
  z. isotope
  z. oxide
  z. pelargonate
  z. peroxide
  z. phenolsulfonate
  z. phosphide
  z. propionate
  z. stearate
  z. sulfate
  z. trichlorophenate
  z. undecylenate
zincalism
Zinn's
  artery
  zonule
zinterol hydrochloride
ziram
zirconium
  z. dioxide
  z. oxide
Zn — zinc
Zollinger-Ellison syndrome
zona (zonae)
  z. fasciculata
  z. glomerulosa
  z. incerta
  z. pellucida
  z. reticularis
zonal
zone
  epileptogenic z.
  hemorrhoidal z.
  hyperesthetic z.
  interpalpebral z.
  motor z.
  nephrogenic z.
  placental z.
  visual z.
zonula (zonulae)
  z. adherens

zonula (zonulae) *(continued)*
    z. ciliaris
    z. occludens
zonular
zonule
    ciliary z.
    lens z.
    Zinn's z.
Zoogloea
Zoomastigophora
zoonosis
zooprophylaxis
zoster
    z. immune globulin
ZR — zirconium
ZSR — zeta sedimentation rate
Zuberella
Zuckerkandl's organs
Zwischenferment
zwitterion
zygoma
zygomatic
    z. bone

zygomatic *(continued)*
    z. branch of facial nerve
    z. nerve
zygomaticomaxillary
Zygomycetes
zygomycosis
zygonema
zygote
zygotene
Zymobacterium
zymogen
zymogenic cell
zymohexase
zymolysis
Zymomonas
zymophore
zymosis
zymosthenic
zytase
Zz. — *zingiber*, ginger
Z.Z. 'Z" — increasing degrees of contraction

PART II
APPENDICES

REFERENCE VALUES IN HEMATOLOGY

	CONVENTIONAL UNITS	FACTOR	S.I. UNITS	NOTES
Acid hemolysis test (Ham)	No hemolysis	—	No hemolysis	
Alkaline phosphatase, leukocyte	Total score 14–100	—	Total score 14–100	
Carboxyhemoglobin	Up to 5% of total	0.01	0.05 of total	a
Cell counts				
Erythrocytes				
Males	4.6–6.2 million/cu. mm.	10^6	4.6–$6.2 \times 10^{12}/l$	
Females	4.2–5.4 million/cu. mm.		4.2–$5.4 \times 10^{12}/l$	
Children (varies with age)	4.5–5.1 million/cu. mm.		4.5–$5.1 \times 10^{12}/l$	
Leukocytes				
Total	4500–11,000/cu. mm.	10^6	4.5–$11.0 \times 10^9/l$	
Differential	Percentage Absolute	10^6		b
Myelocytes	0 0/cu. mm.		0/l	
Band neutrophils	3–5 150–400/cu. mm.		150–$400 \times 10^6/l$	
Segmented neutrophils	54–62 3000–5800/cu. mm.		3000–$5800 \times 10^6/l$	
Lymphocytes	25–33 1500–3000/cu. mm.		1500–$3000 \times 10^6/l$	
Monocytes	3–7 300–500/cu. mm.		300–$500 \times 10^6/l$	
Eosinophils	1–3 50–250/cu. mm.		50–$250 \times 10^6/l$	
Basophils	0–0.75 15–50/cu. mm.		15–$50 \times 10^6/l$	
Platelets	150,000–350,000/cu. mm.	10^6	150–$350 \times 10^9/l$	
Reticulocytes	25,000–75,000/cu. mm.	10^6	25–$75 \times 10^9/l$	b
	0.5–1.5% of erythrocytes			
Coagulation tests				
Bleeding time (Duke)	1–5 min.	—	1–5 min	
Bleeding time (Ivy)	Less than 5 min.	—	Less than 5 min	
Clot retraction, qualitative	Begins in 30–60 min	—	Begins in 30–60 min	
	Complete in 24 hrs.	—	Complete in 24 h	
Coagulation time (Lee-White)	5–15 min. (glass tubes)	—	5–15 min (glass tubes)	
	19–60 min. (siliconized tubes)	—	19–60 min (siliconized tubes)	
Euglobulin lysis time	2–6 hr. at 37°	—	2–6 h at 37 C	
Factor VIII and other coagulation factors	50–150% of normal	—	0.50–1.5 of normal	a

Fibrin split products (Thrombo-Wellco test)	Negative at 1:4 dilution	—	Negative at 1:4 dilution	
Fibrinogen	200–400 mg/100 ml.	0.0293	5.9–11.7 µmol/l	
Fibrinolysins	0	—	0	
Partial thromboplastin time, activated (APTT)	35–45 sec.	—	35–45 s	c
Prothrombin consumption	Over 80% consumed in 1 hr.	0.01	Over 0.80 consumed in 1 h	a
Prothrombin content	100% (calculated from prothrombin time)	0.01	1.0 (calculated from prothrombin time)	a
Prothrombin time (one stage)	12.0–14.0 sec.	—	12.0–14.0 s	
Thromboplastin generation test	Compared to normal control	—	Compared to normal control	
Tourniquet test	Ten or fewer petechiae in a 2.5 cm. circle after 5 min.	—	Ten or fewer petechiae in a 2.5 cm circle after 5 min	
Cold hemolysin test (Donath-Landsteiner)	No hemolysis	—	No hemolysis	
Coombs test				
Direct	Negative	—	Negative	
Indirect	Negative	—	Negative	
Corpuscular values of erythrocytes (values are for adults; in children, values vary with age)				
M.C.H. (mean corpuscular hemoglobin)	27–31 picogm.	0.0155	0.42–0.48 fmol	d
M.C.V. (mean corpuscular volume)	80–105 cu. micra	1.0	80–105 fl	
M.C.H.C. (mean corpuscular hemoglobin concentration)	32–36%	0.01	0.32–0.36	a
Haptoglobin (as hemoglobin binding capacity)	100–200 mg/100 ml.	0.155	16–31 µmol/l	d
Hematocrit				
Males	40–54 ml/100 ml.	0.01	0.40–0.54	a
Females	37–47 ml/100 ml.		0.37–0.47	
Newborn	49–54 ml/100 ml.		0.49–0.54	
Children (varies with age)	35–49 ml/100 ml.		0.35–0.49	
Hemoglobin				
Males	14.0–18.0 grams/100 ml.	0.155	2.17–2.79 mmol/l	d
Females	12.0–16.0 grams/100 ml.		1.86–2.48 mmol/l	
Newborn	16.5–19.5 grams/100 ml.		2.56–3.02 mmol/l	
Children (varies with age)	11.2–16.5 grams/100 ml.		1.74–2.56 mmol/l	

REFERENCE VALUES IN HEMATOLOGY (Continued)

	CONVENTIONAL UNITS	FACTOR	S.I. UNITS	NOTES
Hemoglobin, fetal	Less than 1% of total	0.01	Less than 0.01 of total	a
Hemoglobin A_{1c}	3–5% of total	0.01	0.03–0.05 of total	a
Hemoglobin A_2	1.5–3.0% of total	0.01	0.015–0.03 of total	a
Hemoglobin, plasma	0–5.0 mg./100 ml.	0.155	0–0.8 μmol/l	d
Methemoglobin	0–130 mg/100 ml	0.155	4.7–20 μmol/l	e
Osmotic fragility of erythrocytes	Begins in 0.45–0.39% NaCl	171	Begins in 77–67 mmol/l NaCl	
	Complete in 0.33–0.30% NaCl		Complete in 56–51 mmol/l NaCl	
Sedimentation rate				
Wintrobe: Males	0–5 mm. in 1 hr.	—	0–5 mm/h	
Females	0–15 mm. in 1 hr.	—	0–15 mm/h	
Westergren: Males	0–15 mm. in 1 hr.	—	0–15 mm/h	
Females	0–20 mm. in 1 hr.	—	0–20 mm/h	
(May be slightly higher in children and during pregnancy)				
Bone marrow, differential cell count				
	Range *Average*		*Range* *Average*	
Myeloblasts	0.3–5.0% 2.0%	0.01	0.003–0.05 0.02	a
Promyelocytes	1.0–8.0% 5.0%		0.01–0.08 0.05	
Myelocytes: Neutrophilic	5.0–19.0% 12.0%		0.05–0.19 0.12	
Eosinophilic	0.5–3.0% 1.5%		0.005–0.03 0.015	
Basophilic	0.0–0.5% 0.3%		0.00–0.005 0.003	
Metamyelocytes	13.0–32.0% 22.0%		0.13–0.32 0.22	
Polymorphonuclear neutrophils	7.0–30.0% 20.0%		0.07–0.30 0.20	
Polymorphonuclear eosinophils	0.5–4.0% 2.0%		0.005–0.04 0.02	
Polymorphonuclear basophils	0.0–0.7% 0.2%		0.00–0.007 0.002	
Lymphocytes	3.0–17.0% 10.0%		0.03–0.17 0.10	
Plasma cells	0.0–2.0% 0.4%		0.00–0.02 0.004	
Monocytes	0.5–5.0% 2.0%		0.005–0.05 0.02	
Reticulum cells	0.1–2.0% 0.2%		0.001–0.02 0.002	
Megakaryocytes	0.3–3.0% 0.4%		0.003–0.03 0.004	
Pronormoblasts	1.0–8.0% 4.0%		0.01–0.08 0.04	
Normoblasts	7.0–32.0% 18.0%		0.07–0.32 0.18	

REFERENCE VALUES FOR BLOOD, PLASMA AND SERUM

(For some procedures the reference values may vary depending upon the method used)

	CONVENTIONAL UNITS	FACTOR	S.I. UNITS	NOTES
Acetoacetate plus acetone, serum				
Qualitative	Negative	—	Negative	
Quantitative	0.3–2.0 mg./100 ml.	10	3–20 mg/l	
Adrenocorticotropin (ACTH), plasma	10–80 picogm./ml.	1.0	10–80 ng/l	
Aldolase, serum	0–11 milliunits/ml. (I.U.) (30°)	1.0	0–11 units/l (30 C)	f
Alpha amino nitrogen, serum	3.0–5.5 mg./100 ml.	0.714	2.1–3.9 mmol/l	
Ammonia, plasma	20–120 mcg./100 ml.	0.554	11–67 µmol/l	
Amylase, serum	Less than 160 Caraway units/100 ml.	—	Less than 160 Caraway units/dl	f
Anion gap	8–16 mEq./l.	1.0	8–16 mmol/l	
Ascorbic acid, blood	0.4–1.5 mg./100 ml.	56.8	23–85 µmol/l	
Base excess, blood	0 ± 2 mEq./liter	1.0	0 ± 2 mmol/l	
Bicarbonate, serum	23–29 mEq./liter	1.0	23–29 mmol/l	
Bile acids, serum	0.3–3.0 mg./dl.	10	3.0–30.0 mg/l	
Bilirubin, serum				
Direct	0.1–0.4 mg./100 ml.	17.1	1.7–6.8 µmol/l	
Indirect	0.2–0.7 mg./100 ml. (Total minus direct)	17.1	3.4–12 µmol/l (Total minus direct)	
Total	0.3–1.1 mg./100 ml.	17.1	5.1–19 µmol/l	
Bromsulphalein (BSP) (Inject 5 mg./kg. body weight, draw sample at 45 min.)	Less than 5%	0.01	Less than 0.05	a
Calcium, serum	4.5–5.5 mEq./liter	0.50	2.25–2.75 mmol/l	
	9.0–11.0 mg./100 ml.	0.25	2.25–2.75 mmol/l	
	(Slightly higher in children)		(Slightly higher in children)	
	(Varies with protein concentration)		(Varies with protein concentration)	
Calcium, ionized, serum	2.1–2.6 mEq./liter	0.50	1.05–1.30 mmol/l	
	4.25–5.25 mg./100 ml.	0.25	1.05–1.30 mmol/l	
Carbon dioxide content, serum				
Adults	24–30 mEq./liter	1.0	24–30 mmol/l	
Infants	20–28 mEq./liter	1.0	20–28 mmol/l	

APPENDIX 1 549

REFERENCE VALUES FOR BLOOD, PLASMA AND SERUM (Continued)

(For some procedures the reference values may vary depending upon the method used)

	CONVENTIONAL UNITS	FACTOR	S.I. UNITS	NOTES
Carbon dioxide tension (PCO_2), blood	35–45 mm. Hg		35–45 mm Hg	
Carotene, serum	50–300 mcg./100 ml.	0.0186	0.93–5.58 μmol/l	g
Ceruloplasmin, serum	23–44 mg./100 ml.	0.0662	1.5–2.9 mmol/l	h
Chloride, serum	96–106 mEq./liter	1.0	96–106 mmol/l	
Cholesterol, serum				
Total	150–250 mg./100 ml.	0.0259	3.9–6.5 mmol/l	
Esters	68–76% of total cholesterol	0.01	0.68–0.76 of total cholesterol	a
Cholinesterase				
Serum	0.5–1.3 pH units	—	0.5–1.3 pH units	f
Erythrocytes	0.5–1.0 pH unit	—	0.5–1.0 pH unit	f
Copper, serum				
Males	70–140 mcg/100 ml.	0.157	11–22 μmol/l	
Females	85–155 mcg./100 ml.	0.157	13–24 μmol/l	
Cortisol, plasma (8 A.M.)	6–23 mcg./100 ml.	27.6	170–635 nmol/l	
Creatine, serum	0.2–0.8 mg./100 ml.	76.3	15–61 μmol/l	
Creatine phosphokinase, serum				
Males	0–50 milliunits/ml. (I.U.) (30°)	1.0	0–50 units/l (30 C)	f
Females	0–30 milliunits/ml. (I.U.) (30°) (Oliver-Rosalki)	1.0	0–30 units/l (30 C) (Oliver-Rosalki)	f
Creatine phosphokinase isoenzymes, serum				
CPK-MM	Present	—	Present	
CPK-MB	Absent	—	Absent	
CPK-BB	Absent	—	Absent	
Creatinine, serum	0.7–1.5 mg./100 ml.	88.4	62–133 μmol/l	
Cryoglobulins, serum	0	—	0	
Fatty acids, total, serum	190–420 mg./100 ml.	0.0352	7–15 mmol/l	
Ferritin, serum	20–200 nanogm./ml.	1.0	20–200 μg/l	i
Fibrinogen, plasma	200–400 mg./100 ml.	0.0293	5.9–11.7 μmol/l	
Folate, serum	5–21 nanogm./ml.	2.27	11–48 nmol/l	c

Follicle stimulating hormone (FSH), plasma			
Males	4–25 milliunits/ml. (I.U.)	1.0	4–25 IU/l
Females	4–30 milliunits/ml. (I.U.)		4–30 IU/l
Postmenopausal	40–250 milliunits/ml. (I.U.)		40–250 IU/l
Gamma glutamyltransferase				
Males	6–32 milliunits/ml. (I.U.) (30°)	1.0	6–32 units/l (30 C)	f
Females	4–18 milliunits/ml. (I.U.) (30°)	1.0	4–18 units/l (30 C)	f
Gastrin, serum	0–200 picogm/ml.	1.0	0–200 ng/l	
Glucose (fasting)				
Blood	60–100 mg./100 ml.	0.0555	3.33–5.55 mmol/l	
Plasma or serum	70–115 mg./100 ml.	0.0555	3.89–6.38 mmol/l	
Growth hormone, serum	0–10 nanogm/ml.	1.0	0–10 µg/l	
Haptoglobin, serum	100–200 mg/100 ml.	0.155	16–31 µmol/l	d
	(As hemoglobin binding capacity)		(As hemoglobin binding capacity)	
	0–180 milliunits/ml. (I.U.) (Rosalki-Wilkinson)		0–180 units/l (30 C) (Rosalki-Wilkinson)	f
Hydroxybutyric dehydrogenase, serum	114–290 units/ml. (Wroblewski)	1.0	114–290 units/ml (Wroblewski)	f
	8–18 mcg./100 ml.	0.0276	0.22–0.50 µmol/l	j
17-Hydroxycorticosteroids, plasma				
Immunoglobulins, serum				
IgG	550–1900 mg./100 ml.	0.01	5.5–19.0 g/l	
IgA	60–333 mg./100 ml.	0.01	0.60–3.3 g/l	
IgM	45–145 mg./100 ml.	0.01	0.45–1.5 g/l	
	(Varies with age in children)		(Varies with age in children)	
Insulin, plasma (fasting)	5–25 microunits/ml.	1.0	5–25 milliunits/l	
Iodine, protein bound, serum	3.5–8.0 mcg./100 ml.	0.0788	0.28–0.63 µmol/l	
Iron, serum	75–175 mcg./100 ml.	0.179	13–31 µmol/l	
Iron binding capacity, serum				
Total	250–410 mcg./100 ml.	0.179	45–73 µmol/l	k
Saturation	20–55%	0.01	0.20–0.55	
17-Ketosteroids, plasma	25–125 mcg./100 ml.	0.0347	0.87–4.34 µmol/l	a
Lactate, blood, venous	0.6–1.8 mEq/liter	1.0	0.6–1.8 mmol/l	—
Lactate dehydrogenase, serum	0–300 milliunits/ml. (I.U.) (30°) (Wroblewski modified)	1.0	0–300 units/l (30 C) (Wroblewski modified)	f
	150–450 units/ml. (Wroblewski)	—	150–450 units/ml (Wroblewski)	
	80–120 units/ml. (Wacker)	—	80–120 units/ml (Wacker)	

REFERENCE VALUES FOR BLOOD, PLASMA AND SERUM (Continued)

(For some procedures the reference values may vary depending upon the method used)

	CONVENTIONAL UNITS	FACTOR	S.I. UNITS	NOTES
Lactate dehydrogenase isoenzymes, serum				
LDH_1	22–37% of total	0.01	0.22–0.37 of total	a
LDH_2	30–46% of total		0.30–0.46 of total	
LDH_3	14–29% of total		0.14–0.29 of total	
LDH_4	5–11% of total		0.05–0.11 of total	
LDH_5	2–11% of total		0.02–0.11 of total	
Leucine aminopeptidase, serum	14–40 milliunits/ml. (I.U.) (30°)	1.0	14–40 units/l (30 C)	f
Lipase, serum	0–1.5 units (Cherry-Crandall)	—	0–1.5 units (Cherry-Crandall)	f
Lipids, total, serum	450–850 mg/100 ml.	0.01	4.5–8.5 g/l	m
Luteinizing hormone (LH), serum				
Males	6–18 milliunits/ml. (I.U.)	1.0	6–18 IU/l	
Females, premenopausal	5–22 milliunits/ml. (I.U.)	1.0	5–22 IU/l	
midcycle	3 times baseline	—	3 times baseline	
postmenopausal	Greater than 30 milliunits/ml. (I.U.)	—	Greater than 30 IU/l	
Magnesium, serum	1.5–2.5 mEq/liter	0.50	0.75–1.25 mmol/l	
	1.8–3.0 mg/100 ml.	0.411		
5'-Nucleotidase, serum	Less than 1.6 milliunits/ml. (I.U.) (30°)	1.0	Less than 1.6 units/l (30 C)	f
Nitrogen, nonprotein, serum	15–35 mg/100 ml.	0.714	10.7–25.0 mmol/l	
Osmolality, serum	285–295 mOsm/kg. serum water		285–295 mmol/kg serum water	n
Oxygen, blood				
Capacity	16–24 vol.% (varies with hemoglobin)	0.446	7.14–10.7 mmol/l (varies with hemoglobin)	o
Content Arterial	15–23 vol.%	0.446	6.69–10.3 mmol/l	o
Venous	10–16 vol.%	0.446	4.46–7.14 mmol/l	o
Saturation Arterial	94–100% of capacity	0.01	0.94–1.00 of capacity	a
Venous	60–85% of capacity	0.01	0.60–0.85 of capacity	a
Tension, pO_2 Arterial	75–100 mm. Hg	—	75–100 mm Hg	g
P_{50} blood	26–27 mm. Hg	—	26–27 mm Hg	g
pH, arterial, blood	7.35–7.45	—	7.35–7.45	p
Phenylalanine, serum	Less than 3 mg/100 ml.	0.0605	Less than 0.18 mmol/l	
Phosphatase, acid, serum	0–7.0 milliunits/ml. (I.U.) (30°)	1.0	0–7.0 units/l (30 C)	f
	1.0–5.0 units (King-Armstrong)	—	1.0–5.0 units (King-Armstrong)	f
Phosphatase, alkaline, serum	10–32 milliunits/ml. (I.U.) (30°)	1.0	1.0–32 units/l (30 C)	
	5.0–13.0 units (King-Armstrong) (Values are higher in children)	—	5.0–13.0 units (King-Armstrong) (Values are higher in children)	

APPENDIX 1   553

Phosphate, inorganic, serum				
Adults	3.0–4.5 mg/100 ml.	0.323	1.0–1.5 mmol/l	
Children	4.0–7.0 mg/100 ml.	0.323	1.3–2.3 mmol/l	
Phospholipids, serum	6–12 mg/100 ml.		1.9–3.9 mmol/l	
	(As lipid phosphorus)		(As lipid phosphorus)	
	3.5–5.0 mEq./liter	1.0	3.5–5.0 mmol/l	
Potassium, serum				
Protein, serum				
Total	6.0–8.0 grams/100 ml.	10	60–80 g/l	
Albumin	3.5–5.5 grams/100 ml.	10	35–55 g/l	
		0.154	0.54–0.85 mmol/l	
Phosphate, inorganic, serum				m
Adults	3.0–4.5 mg/100 ml.	0.323	1.0–1.5 mmol/l	q
Children	4.0–7.0 mg/100 ml.	0.323	1.3–2.3 mmol/l	
Phospholipids, serum	6–12 mg/100 ml.		1.9–3.9 mmol/l	
	(As lipid phosphorus)		(As lipid phosphorus)	
	3.5–5.0 mEq./liter	1.0	3.5–5.0 mmol/l	
Potassium, serum				
Protein, serum				
Total	6.0–8.0 grams/100 ml.	10	60–80 g/l	m
Albumin	3.5–5.5 grams/100 ml.	10	35–55 g/l	q
		0.154	0.54–0.85 mmol/l	
Globulin	2.5–3.5 grams/100 ml.	10	25–35 g/l	
Electrophoresis				
Albumin	3.5–5.5 grams/100 ml.	10	35–55 g/l	q
	52–68% of toal	0.01	0.52–0.68 of toal	a
Globulin				
Alpha₁	0.2–0.4 gram/100 ml.	10	2–4 g/l	m
	2–5% of total	0.01	0.02–0.05 of total	a
Alpha₂	0.5–0.9 gram/100 ml.	10	5–9 g/l	m
	7–14% of total	0.01	0.07–0.14 of total	a
Beta	0.6–1.1 grams/100 ml.	10	6–11 g/l	m
	9–15% of total	0.01	0.09–0.15 of total	a
Gamma	0.7–1.7 grams/100 ml.	10	7–17 g/l	m
	11–21% of total	0.01	0.11–0.21 of total	a
Protoporphyrin, erythrocyte	27–61 mcg./100 ml. packed RBC	0.0178	0.48–1.09 µmol/l packed RBC	
Pyruvate, blood	0.01–0.11 mEq./liter	1.0	0.01–0.11 mmol/l	
Sodium, serum	136–145 mEq./liter	1.0	136–145 mmol/l	
Sulfates, inorganic, serum	0.8–1.2 mg/100 ml.	104	83–125 µmol/l	
Testosterone, plasma				
Males	275–875 nanogm./100 ml.	0.0347	9.5–30 nmol/l	
Females	23–75 nanogm./100 ml.	0.0347	0.8–2.6 nmol/l	
Pregnant	38–190 nanogm./100 ml.	0.0347	1.3–6.6 nmol/l	

REFERENCE VALUES FOR BLOOD, PLASMA AND SERUM (Continued)

(For some procedures the reference values may vary depending upon the method used)

	CONVENTIONAL UNITS	FACTOR	S.I. UNITS	NOTES
Thyroid stimulating hormone (TSH), serum	0–7 microunits/ml.	1.0	0–7 milliunits/l	
Thyroxine, free, serum	1.0–2.1 nanogm./100 ml.	12.9	13–27 pmol/l	
Thyroxine (T_4), serum	4.4–9.9 mcg./100 ml.	12.9	57–128 nmol/l	
Thyroxine binding globulin (TBG), serum (as thyroxine)	10–26 mcg./100 ml.	12.9	129–335 nmol/l	
Thyroxine iodine, serum	2.9–6.4 mcg./100 ml.	78.8	229–504 nmol/l	k
Tri-iodothyronine (T_3), serum	150–250 nanogm./100 ml.	0.0154	2.3–3.9 nmol/l	a
Tri-iodothyronine (T_3) uptake, resin (T_3RU)	25–38%	0.01	0.25–0.38 uptake	
Transaminase, serum				
SGOT (aspartate aminotransferase)	0–19 milliunits/ml. (I.U.) (30°) (Karmen modified)	1.0	0–19 units/l (30 C) (Karmen modified)	f
	15–40 units/ml. (Karmen)		15–40 units/ml (Karmen)	
	18–40 units/ml. (Reitman-Frankel)		18–40 units/ml (Reitman-Frankel)	
SGPT (alanine aminotransferase)	0–17 milliunits/ml. (I.U.) (30°) (Karmen modified)	1.0	0–17 units/l (30 C) (Karmen modified)	f
	6–35 units/ml. (Karmen)		6–35 units/ml (Karmen)	
	5–35 units/ml. (Reitman-Frankel)		5–35 units/ml (Reitman-Frankel)	
Triglycerides, serum	40–150 mg./100 ml.	0.01	0.4–1.5 g/l	
		0.0114	0.45–1.71 mmol/l	r
Urate (serum)				
Males	2.5–8.0 mg./100 ml.	0.0595	0.15–0.48 mmol/l	
Females	1.5–7.0 mg./100 ml.	0.0595	0.09–0.42 mmol/l	
Urea				
Blood	21–43 mg./100 ml.	0.167	3.5–7.2 mmol/l	
Plasma or serum	24–49 mg./100 ml.	0.167	4.0–8.2 mmol/l	
Urea nitrogen				
Blood	10–20 mg./100 ml.	0.714	7.1–14.3 mmol/l	
Plasma or serum	11–23 mg./100 ml.	0.714	7.9–16.4 mmol/l	
Vitamin A, serum	20–80 mcg./100 ml.	0.0349	0.70–2.8 μmol/l	
Vitamin B_{12}, serum	180–900 picogm./ml.	0.738	133–664 pmol/l	k

REFERENCE VALUES FOR URINE

(For some procedures the reference values may vary depending upon the method used)

	CONVENTIONAL UNITS	FACTOR	S.I. UNITS	NOTES
Acetone and acetoacetate, qualitative	Negative	—	Negative	
Addis count				
Erythrocytes	0–130,000/24 hrs.	—	0–130 000/24 h	
Leukocytes	0–650,000/24 hrs.	—	0–650 000/24 h	
Casts (hyaline)	0–2000/24 hrs.	—	0–2000/24 h	
Albumin				
Qualitative	Negative	—	Negative	
Quantitative	10–100 mg./24 hrs.	—	10–100 mg/24 h	q
Aldosterone	3–20 mcg./24 hrs.	2.77	8.3–55 nmol/24 h	
Alpha amino nitrogen	50–200 mg./24 hrs.	0.0714	3.6–14.3 mmol/24 h	
Ammonia nitrogen	20–70 mEq./24 hrs.	1.0	20–70 mmol/24 h	
Amylase	35–260 Caraway units/hr.	—	35–260 Caraway units/h	
Bilirubin, qualitative	Negative	—	Negative	f
Calcium				
Low Ca diet	Less than 150 mg./24 hrs.	0.025	Less than 3.8 mmol/24 h	
Usual diet	Less than 250 mg./24 hrs.	0.025	Less than 6.3 mmol/24 h	
Catecholamines				
Epinephrine	Less than 10 mcg./24 hrs.	5.46	Less than 55 nmol/24 h	
Norepinephrine	Less than 100 mcg./24 hrs.	5.91	Less than 590 nmol/24 h	
Total free catecholamines	4–126 mcg./24 hrs.	5.91	24–745 nmol/24 h	
Total metanephrines	0.1–1.6 mg./24 hrs.	5.07	0.5–8.1 µmol/24 h	
Chloride	110–250 mEq./24 hrs. (Varies with intake)	1.0	110–250 mmol/24 h (Varies with intake)	
Chorionic gonadotropin	0	—	0	
Copper	0–50 mcg./24 hrs.	0.0157	0–0.80 µmol/24 h	
Creatine				
Males	0–40 mg./24 hrs.	0.00762	0–0.30 mmol/24 h	s
Females	0–100 mg./24 hrs. (Higher in children and during pregnancy)	0.00762	0–0.76 mmol/24 h (Higher in children and during pregnancy)	t
Creatinine	15–25 mg./kg. body weight/24 hrs.	0.00884	0.13–0.22 mmol · kg^{-1} body weight/24 h	

APPENDIX 1   555

REFERENCE VALUES FOR URINE (Continued)

(For some procedures the reference values may vary depending upon the method used)

	CONVENTIONAL UNITS	FACTOR	S.I. UNITS	NOTES
Creatinine clearance				
Males	110–150 ml/min.	—	110–150 ml/min	
Females	105–132 ml/min. (1.73 sq. meter surface area)	—	105–132 ml/min (1.73 m² surface area)	
Cystine or cysteine, qualitative	Negative		Negative	
Dehydroepiandrosterone	Less than 15% of total 17-ketosteroids	0.01	Less than 0.15 of total 17-ketosteroids	a
Delta aminolevulinic acid	1.3–7.0 mg/24 hrs.	7.63	10–53 µmol/24 h	
Estrogens				
Males				
Estrone	3–8 µg/24 hrs.	3.70	11–30 nmol/24 h	
Estradiol	0–6 µg/24 hrs.	3.67	0–22 nmol/24 h	
Estriol	1–11 µg/24 hrs.	3.47	3–38 nmol/24 h	
Total	4–25 µg/24 hrs.	3.60	14–90 nmol/24 h	
Females				
Estrone	4–31 µg/24 hrs.	3.70	15–115 nmol/24 h	
Estradiol	0–14 µg/24 hrs.	3.67	0–51 nmol/24 h	
Estriol	0–72 µg/24 hrs.	3.47	0–250 nmol/24 h	
Total	5–100 µg/24 hrs.	3.60	18–360 nmol/24 h	u
	(Markedly increased during pregnancy)		(Markedly increased during pregnancy)	
Glucose (as reducing substance)	Less than 250 mg./24 hrs.	—	Less than 250 mg/24 h	
Gonadotropins, pituitary	10–50 mouse units/24 hrs.	—	10–50 mouse units/24 h	
Hemoglobin and myoglobin, qualitative	Negative	—	Negative	
Hemogentisic acid, qualitative	Negative	—	Negative	
17-Hydroxycorticosteroids				
Males	3–9 mg/24 hrs.	2.76	8.3–25 µmol/24 h	
Females	2–8 mg/24 hrs.		5.5–22 µmol/24 h	
5-Hydroxyindoleacetic acid				
Qualitative	Negative		Negative	j
Quantitative	Less than 9 mg/24 hrs.	5.23	Less than 47 µmol/24 h	
17-Ketosteroids				
Males	6–18 mg/24 hrs.	3.47	21–62 µmol/24 h	l
Females	4–13 mg/24 hrs.		14–45 µmol/24 h	
	(Varies with age)		(Varies with age)	

Magnesium	6.0–8.5 mEq./24 hrs.	0.5	3.0–4.3 mmol/24 h
Metanephrines (see Catecholamines)			
Osmolality	38–1400 mOsm./kg. water	—	38–1400 mmol/kg water	n
pH	4.6–8.0, average 6.0	—	4.6–8.0, average 6.0	p
	(Depends on diet)		(Depends on diet)
Phenolsulfonphthalein excretion (PSP)	25% or more in 15 min.	0.01	0.25 or more in 15 min	a
	40% or more in 30 min.		0.40 or more in 30 min
	55% or more in 2 hrs.		0.55 or more in 2 h
	(After injection of 1 ml PSP intravenously)		(After injection of 1 ml PSP intravenously)
Phenylpyruvic acid, qualitative	Negative	—	Negative
Phosphorus	0.9–1.3 gm./24 hrs.	32.3	29–42 mmol/24 h
Porphobilinogen			
Qualitative	Negative	—	Negative
Quantitative	0–0.2 mg/100 ml.	4.42	0–0.9 µmol/l
	Less than 2.0 mg/24 hrs.		Less than 9 µmol/24 h
Porphyrins			
Coproporphyrin	50–250 mcg/24 hrs.	1.53	77–380 nmol/24 h
Uroporphyrin	10–30 mcg./24 hrs.	1.20	12–36 nmol/24 h
Potassium	25–100 mEq./24 hrs.	1.0	25–100 mmol/24 h
	(Varies with intake)		(Varies with intake)
Pregnanediol			
Males	0.4–1.4 mg./24 hrs.	3.12	1.2–4.4 µmol/24 h
Females			
Proliferative phase	0.5–1.5 mg./24 hrs.		1.6–4.7 µmol/24 h
Luteal phase	2.0–7.0 mg./24 hrs.		6.2–22 µmol/24 h
Postmenopausal phase	0.2–1.0 mg./24 hrs.		0.6–3.1 µmol/24 h
Pregnanetriol	Less than 2.5 mg/24 hrs. in adults	2.97	Less than 7.4 µmol/24 h in adults
Protein			
Qualitative	Negative	—	Negative
Quantitative	10–150 mg./24 hrs.	1.0	10–150 mg/24 h
Sodium	130–260 mEq./24 hrs.		130–260 mmol/24 h	m
	(Varies with intake)		(Varies with intake)
Specific gravity	1.003–1.030	1.0	1.003–1.030
Titratable acidity	20–40 mEq./24 hrs.		20–40 mmol/24 h
Urate	200–500 mg./24 hrs.	0.00595	1.2–3.0 mmol/24 h
	(With normal diet)		(With normal diet)
Urobilinogen	Up to 1.0 Ehrlich unit/2 hrs.	—	Up to 1.0 Ehrlich unit/2 h
	(1–3 P.M.)		(1–3 P.M.)
Vanillylmandelic acid (VMA)	0–4.0 mg/24 hrs.		0–4.0 mg/24 h
(4-hydroxy-3-methoxymandelic acid)	1–8 mg./24 hrs.	5.05	5–40 µmol/24 h

APPENDIX 1   557

REFERENCE VALUES FOR THERAPEUTIC DRUG MONITORING

DRUG	THERAPEUTIC RANGE	TOXIC LEVELS	PROPRIETARY NAMES
Antibiotics			
Amikacin, serum	15–25 mcg./ml.	Peak: >35 mcg./ml. Trough: >5 mcg./ml.	Amikin
Chloramphenicol, serum	10–20 mcg./ml.	>25 mcg./ml.	Chloromycetin
Gentamicin, serum	5–10 mcg./ml.	Peak: >12 mcg./ml. Trough: >2 mcg./ml.	Garamycin
Tobramycin, serum	5–10 mcg./ml.	Peak: >12 mcg./ml. Trough: >2 mcg./ml.	Nebcin
Anticonvulsants			
Carbamazepine, serum	5–12 mcg./ml.	>15 mcg./ml.	Tegretol
Ethosuximide, serum	40–80 mcg./ml.	>150 mcg./ml.	Zarontin
Phenobarbital, serum	10–25 mcg./ml.	Vary widely because of developed tolerance	
Phenytoin, serum (diphenylhydantoin)	10–20 mcg./ml.	>20 mcg./ml.	Dilantin
Primidone, serum	4–12 mcg./ml.	>15 mcg./ml.	Mysoline
Valproic acid, serum	50–100 mcg./ml.	>200 mcg./ml.	Depakene
Anti-inflammatory agents			
Acetaminophen, serum	10–20 mcg./ml.	>250 mcg./ml.	Tylenol Datril
Salicylate, serum	100–250 mcg./ml.	>300 mcg./ml.	
Bronchodilator			
Theophylline (aminophylline)	10–20 mcg./ml.	>20 mcg./ml.	

Cardiovascular drugs

Digitoxin, serum	15–25 nanogm./ml. > 25 nanogm./ml. (Specimen obtained 12–24 hrs. after last dose)	Crystodigin
Digoxin, serum	0.8–2 nanogm./ml. > 2.4 nanogm./ml. (Specimen obtained 12–24 hrs. after last dose)	Lanoxin
Disopyramide, serum	2–4 mcg./ml. > 7 mcg./ml.	Norpace
Lidocaine, serum	1.5–5 mcg./ml. > 7 nanogm./ml.	Anestacon, Xylocaine, Pronestyl
Procainamide, serum	4–10 mcg./ml. > 16 mcg./ml. *8–16 mcg./ml. *> 20 mcg./ml. (*Procainamide + N-Acetyl Procainamide)	
Propranolol, serum	50–100 nanogm./ml. Variable	Inderal
Quinidine, serum	2–5 mcg./ml. > 10 mcg./ml.	Cardioquin, Quinaglute, Quinidex, Quinora

Psychopharmacologic drugs

Amitriptyline, serum	*120–150 nanogm./ml. *> 500 nanogm./ml. (*Amitriptyline + Nortriptyline)	Amitril, Elavil, Endep, Etrafon, Limbitrol, Triavil
Chlordiazepoxide, serum	1–3 mcg./ml. > 5 mcg./ml.	Librium
Desipramine, serum	*150–250 nanogm./ml. *> 500 nanogm./ml. (*Desipramine + Imipramine)	Norpramin, Pertofrane
Diazepam, serum	0.5–2.5 mcg./ml. > 5 mcg./ml.	Valium
Imipramine, serum	*150–250 nanogm./ml. *> 500 nanogm./ml. (*Imipramine + Desipramine)	Antipress, Imavate, Janimine, Presamine, Tofranil
Lithium, serum	0.8–1.5 mEq./liter > 2.0 mEq./liter (Specimen obtained 12 hrs. after last dose)	
Nortriptyline, serum	50–150 nanogm./ml. > 500 nanogm./ml.	Aventyl, Pamelor

REFERENCE VALUES IN TOXICOLOGY

	CONVENTIONAL UNITS	FACTOR	S.I. UNITS	NOTES
Arsenic, blood	3.5–7.2 mcg./100 ml.	0.133	0.47–0.96 μmol/l	
Arsenic, urine	Less than 100 mcg./24 hrs.	0.0133	Less than 1.3 μmol/24 h	
Bromides, serum	0	1.0	0	
	Toxic levels:		Toxic levels:	
	Above 17 mEq./liter		Above 17 mmol/l	
Carbon monoxide, blood	Up to 5% saturation	—	Up to 0.05 saturation	a
	Symptoms occur with 20% saturation		Symptoms occur with 0.20 saturation	
Ethanol, blood	Less than 0.005%	217	Less than 1 mmol/l	
Marked intoxication	0.3–0.4%		65–87 mmol/l	
Alcoholic stupor	0.4–0.5%		87–109 mmol/l	
Coma	Above 0.5%		Above 109 mmol/l	
Lead, blood	0–40 mcg/100 ml.	0.0483	0–2 μmol/l	
Lead, urine	Less than 100 mcg./24 hrs.	0.00483	Less than 0.48 μmol/24 h	
Mercury, urine	Less than 10 mcg./24 hrs.	4.98	Less than 50 nmol/24 h	

REFERENCE VALUES FOR CEREBROSPINAL FLUID

	CONVENTIONAL UNITS	FACTOR	S.I. UNITS	NOTES
Cells	Fewer than 5/cu. mm.; all mononuclear	—	Fewer than 5/μl; all mononuclear	
Chloride	120–130 mEq./liter	1.0	120–130 mmol/l	
	(20 mEq./liter higher than serum)		(20 mmol/l higher than serum)	
Electrophoresis	Predominantly albumin	—	Predominantly albumin	
Glucose	50–75 mg./100 ml.	0.0555	2.8–4.2 mmol/l	
	(20 mg./100 ml. less than serum)		(1.1 mmol/l less than serum)	
IgG				
Children under 14	Less than 8% of total protein	—	Less than 0.08 of total protein	a,m
Adults	Less than 14% of total protein		Less than 0.14 of total protein	
Pressure	70–180 mm. water		70–180 mm water	g
Protein, total	15–45 mg./100 ml.	0.01	0.150–0.450 g/l	m
	(Higher, up to 70 mg./100 ml. in elderly adults and children)		(Higher, up to 0.70 g/l, in elderly adults and children)	

REFERENCE VALUES FOR GASTRIC ANALYSIS

	CONVENTIONAL UNITS	FACTOR	S.I. UNITS	NOTES
Basal gastric secretion (1 hour)				
Concentration	(Mean ± 1 S.D.)	1.0	(Mean ± 1 S.D.)	
Males	25.8 ± 1.8 mEq/liter		25.8 ± 1.8 mmol/l	
Females	20.3 ± 3.0 mEq/liter		20.3 ± 3.0 mmol/l	
Output	(Mean ± 1 S.D.)	1.0	(Mean ± 1 S.D.)	
Males	2.57 ± 0.16 mEq/hr.		2.57 ± 0.16 mmol/h	
Females	1.61 ± 0.18 mEq/hr.		1.61 ± 0.18 mmol/h	
After histamine stimulation		1.0		
Normal	Mean output 11.8 mEq/hr.		Mean output 11.8 mmol/h	
Duodenal ulcer	Mean output 15.2 mEq/hr.		Mean output 15.2 mmol/h	
After maximal histamine stimulation		1.0		
Normal	Mean output 22.6 mEq/hr.		Mean output 22.6 mmol/h	
Duodenal ulcer	Mean output 44.6 mEq/hr.		Mean output 44.6 mmol/h	
Diagnex blue (Squibb): Anacidity	0–0.3 mg. in 2 hrs.	1.0	0–0.3 mg in 2 h	
Doubtful	0.3–0.6 mg. in 2 hrs.		0.3–0.6 mg in 2 h	
Normal	Greater than 0.6 mg. in 2 hrs.		Greater than 0.6 mg in 2 h	
Volume, fasting stomach content	50–100 ml.	—	0.05–0.1 l	
Emptying time	3–6 hrs.	—	3–6 h	
Color	Opalescent or colorless	—	Opalescent or colorless	
Specific gravity	1.006–1.009	—	1.006–1.009	
pH (adults)	0.9–1.5	—	0.9–1.5	p

GASTROINTESTINAL ABSORPTION TESTS

	CONVENTIONAL UNITS	FACTOR	S.I. UNITS	NOTES
d-Xylose absorption test	After an 8 hour fast, 10 ml/kg body weight of a 0.05 solution of d-xylose is given by mouth. Nothing further by mouth is given until the test has been completed. All urine voided during the following 5 hours is pooled, and blood samples are taken at 0, 60, and 120 minutes. Normally 0.26 (range 0.16–0.33) of ingested xylose is excreted within 5 hours, and the serum xylose reaches a level between 25 and 40 mg./100 ml. after 1 hour and is maintained at this level for another 60 minutes.		No change	
Vitamin A absorption	A fasting blood specimen is obtained and 200,000 units of vitamin A in oil is given by mouth. Serum vitamin A level should rise to twice fasting level in 3 to 5 hours.		No change	

REFERENCE VALUES FOR FECES

	CONVENTIONAL UNITS	FACTOR	S.I. UNITS	NOTES
Bulk	100–200 grams/24 hrs.	—	100–200 g/24 h	
Dry matter	23–32 grams/24 hrs.	—	23–32 g/24 h	
Fat, total	Less than 6.0 grams/24 hrs.	—	Less than 6.0 g/24 h	
Nitrogen, total	Less than 2.0 grams/24 hrs.	—	Less than 2.0 g/24 h	
Urobilinogen	40–280 mg./24 hrs.	0.01	40–280 mg/24 h	
Water	Approximately 65%		Approximately 0.65	a

REFERENCE VALUES FOR SEMEN ANALYSIS

	CONVENTIONAL UNITS	FACTOR	S.I. UNITS	NOTES
Volume	2–5 ml; usually 3–4 ml	—	2–5 ml; usually 3–4 ml	
Liquefaction	Complete in 15 min.	—	Complete in 15 min	
pH	7.2–8.0; average 7.8	—	7.2–8.0; average 7.8	
Leukocytes	Occasional or absent	—	Occasional or absent	
Count	60–150 million/ml.	—	60–150 million/ml	p
	Below 60 million/ml. is abnormal	—	Below 60 million/ml is abnormal	
Motility	80% or more motile	—	0.80 or more motile	a
Morphology	80–90% normal forms	—	0.80–0.90 normal forms	a

PANCREATIC (ISLET) FUNCTION TESTS

Glucose tolerance tests	
Oral	Patient should be on a diet containing 300 grams of carbohydrate per day for 3 days prior to test. After ingestion of 100 grams of glucose or 1.75 grams glucose/kg. body weight, blood glucose is not more than 160 mg./100 ml. after 60 minutes, 140 mg./100 ml. after 90 minutes, and 120 mg./100 ml. after 120 minutes. Values are for blood; serum measurements are approximately 15% higher.
Intravenous	Blood glucose does not exceed 200 mg./100 ml. after infusion of 0.5 gram of glucose/kg. body weight over 30 minutes. Glucose concentration falls below initial level at 2 hours and returns to preinfusion levels in 3 or 4 hours. Values are for blood; serum measurements are approximately 15% higher.
Cortisone-glucose tolerance test	The patient should be on a diet containing 300 grams of carbohydrate per day for 3 days prior to test. At 8½ and again 2 hours prior to glucose load patient is given cortisone acetate by mouth (50 mg. if patient's ideal weight is less than 160 lb., 62.5 mg. if ideal weight is greater than 160 lb.). An oral dose of glucose, 1.75 grams/kg. body weight, is given and blood samples are taken at 0, 30, 60, 90, and 120 minutes. Test is considered positive if true blood glucose exceeds 160 mg./100 ml. at 60 minutes, 140 mg./100 ml. at 90 minutes, and 120 mg./100 ml. at 120 minutes. Values are for blood; serum measurements are approximately 15% higher.

REFERENCE VALUES FOR IMMUNOLOGIC PROCEDURES

	CONVENTIONAL UNITS	FACTOR	S.I. UNITS	NOTES
Syphilis serology (RPR and VDRL)	Negative		No change	
Mono screen	Negative		No change	
R.A. test (latex)	1:40 Negative 1:80–1:160 Doubtful 1:320 Positive		No change	
Rose test	1:10 Negative 1:20–1:40 Doubtful 1:80 Positive		No change	
Anti-streptolysin O titer	Normal up to 1:128. Single test usually has little significance. Rise in titer or persistently elevated titer is significant.		No change	
Anti-hyaluronidase titer	Less than 1:200. Significant if rising titer can be demonstrated at weekly intervals.		No change	
C-reactive protein	Negative		No change	
Anti-nuclear antibody	One specimen is sufficient, unless the result is inconsistent with the clinical impression. Most patients with active lupus have high ANA titers (160 or greater); some have lower titers (20–40). Patients with inactive lupus may have a negative test. Antinuclear antibodies are occasionally present in patients with no evidence of systemic lupus, usually in lower titers (20–40).		No change	
Febrile agglutinins	Titers of 1:80 or greater may be significant, particularly if subsequent samples show rise in titer.		No change	
Tularemia agglutinins	1:80 Negative 1:160 Doubtful 1:320 Positive		No change	
Proteus OX-19 agglutinins	Titers of 1:80 or greater may be significant, particularly if subsequent samples show rise in titer.		No change	
Complement fixation tests	Titers of 1:8 or less are usually not significant. Paired sera showing rise in titer of more than two tubes are usually considered significant.		No change	
C3 Test	80–140 mg/100 ml.	0.01	0.80–1.40 g/l	
C4 Test	11–75 mg/100 ml.	0.01	0.11–0.75 g/l	q

NOTES

a. Percentage is expressed as a decimal fraction.
b. Percentage may be expressed as a decimal fraction; however, when the result expressed is itself a variable fraction of another variable, the absolute value is more meaningful. There is no reason, other than custom, for expressing reticulocyte counts and differential leukocyte counts in percentages or decimal fractions rather than in absolute numbers.
c. Molecular weight of fibrinogen = 341,000 daltons.
d. Molecular weight of hemoglobin = 64,500 daltons. Because of disagreement as to whether the monomer or tetramer of hemoglobin should be used in the conversion, it has been recommended that the conventional grams per deciliter be retained. The tetramer is used in the table; values given should be multiplied by 4 to obtain concentration of the monomer.
e. Molecular weight of methemoglobin = 64,500 daltons. See note d above.
f. Enzyme units have not been changed in these tables because the proposed enzyme unit, the katal, has not been universally adopted (1 International Unit = 16.7 nkat).
g. It has been proposed that pressure be expressed in the Pascal (1 mm Hg = 0.133 kPa); however, this convention has not been universally accepted.
h. Molecular weight of ceruloplasmin = 151,000.
i. "Fatty acids" includes a mixture of different aliphatic acids of varying molecular weight. A mean molecular weight of 284 has been assumed in calculating the conversion factor.

j. Based upon molecular weight of cortisol 362.47.
k. The practice of expressing concentration of an organic molecule in terms of one of its constituent elements originated when measurements included a heterogeneous class of compounds (nonprotein nitrogenous compounds, iodine-containing compounds bound to serum proteins). It was carried over to expressing measurements of specific substances (urea, thyroxine), but the practice should be discarded. For iodine and nitrogen 1 mole is taken as the monoatomic form, although they occur as diatomic molecules.
l. Based upon molecular weight of dehydroepiandrosterone 288.41.
m. Weight per volume is retained as the unit because of the heterogeneous nature of the material measured.
n. The proposal that osmolality be reported as freezing point depression using the millikelvin as the unit has not been received with universal enthusiasm. The milliosmole is not an S.I. unit, and the unit used here is the millimole.
o. Volumes per cent might be converted to a decimal fraction; however, this would not permit direct correlation with hemoglobin content, which is possible when oxygen content and capacity are expressed in molar quantities. One millimole of hemoglobin combines with 4 millimoles of oxygen.
p. Hydrogen ion concentration in S.I. units would be expressed in nanomoles per liter; however, this change has not received general approval. Conversion can be calculated as antilog ($-$pH).
q. Albumin is expressed in grams per liter to be consistent with units used for other proteins.

Concentration of albumin may be expressed in mmol/l also, an expression that permits assessment of binding capacity of albumin for substances such as bilirubin. Molecular weight of albumin is 65,000.

r. Most techniques for quantitating triglycerides measure the glycerol moiety, and the total mass is calculated using an average molecular weight. The factor given assumes a mean molecular weight of 875 for triglycerides.

s. Calculated as norepinephrine, molecular weight 169.18.

t. Calculated as metanephrine, molecular weight 197.23.

u. Conversion factor calculated from molecular weights of estrone, estradiol, and estriol in proportions of 2:1:2.

REFERENCES

1. AMA Drug Evaluations. 4th ed. Chicago, American Medical Association, 1980.
2. Baron, D. N., Broughton, P. M. G., Cohen, M., Lansley, T. S., Lewis, S. M., and Shinton, N. K.: J. Clin. Path. 27:590, 1974.
3. Dybkaer, R.: Am. J. Clin. Path. 52:637, 1969.
4. Goodman, L. S., and Gilman, A.: Pharmacologic Basis of Therapeutics. 5th ed. New York, Macmillan, 1975.
5. Henry, J. B.: Clinical Diagnosis and Management by Laboratory Methods, 16th ed. Philadelphia, W. B. Saunders Company, 1979.
6. Henry, R. J., Cannon, D. C., and Winkleman, J. W.: Clinical Chemistry—Principles and Techniques, 2nd ed. New York, Harper & Row, 1974.
7. International Committee for Standardization in Hematology, International Federation of Clinical Chemistry and World Association of Pathology Societies: Clin. Chem. 19:135, 1973.
8. Lehmann, H. P.: Amer. J. Clin. Path. 65:2, 1976.

9. Miale, J. B.: Laboratory Medicine—Hematology, 5th ed. St. Louis, C. V. Mosby, 1977.
10. Page, C. H., and Vigoureux, P.: The International System of Units (S.I.). U.S. Department of Commerce, National Bureau of Standards, Special Publication 330, 1974.
11. Physicians' Desk Reference. 34th ed. Oradell, N.J., Medical Economics Company, 1980.
12. Scully, R. E., McNeely, B. U., and Galdabini, J. J.: N. Engl. J. Med. *302*:37, 1980.
13. Tietz, N. W.: Fundamentals of Clinical Chemistry, 2nd ed. Philadelphia, W. B. Saunders Company, 1976.
14. Wintrobe, M. D., Lee, G. R., Boggs, D. R., Bithell, T. C., Athens, J. W., and Foerster, J.: Clinical Hematology. 7th ed. Philadelphia, Lea & Febiger, 1974.
15. Young, D. S.: N. Engl. J. Med., *292*:795, 1975.

EPONYMIC DISEASES AND SYNDROMES

Aarskog-Scott s.
Aarskog's s.
Abercrombie's s.
Achard s.
Achard-Thiers s.
Acosta's d.
Adair-Dighton s.
Adams' d.
Adams-Stokes d.
Addison's d.
Addison-Biermer d.
addisonian s.
Adie's s.
Ahumada–del Castillo s.
Aicardi's s.
Akureyri d.
Albarrán's d.
Albers-Schönberg d.
Albert's d.
Albright-McCune-Sternberg s.
Albright's s.
Aldrich's s.
Alexander's d.
Alezzandrini's s.
Alibert's d.
Allen-Masters s.
Almeida's d.
Alper's d.
Alport's s.
Alström's s.
Alzheimer's d.
amniotic infection s. of Blane
Anders' d.
Andersen's d., s.
Andes d.
Andrews' d.
Angelucci's s.
Anton's s.
Apert-Crouzon d.
Apert's d., s.
Aran-Duchenne d.

Argonz–del Castillo s.
Armstrong's d.
Arndt-Gottron s.
Arnold-Chiari s.
Arnold's nerve reflex cough s.
Ascher's s.
Asherman's s.
Aufrecht's d.
Aujeszky's d.
Avellis' s.
Axenfeld's s.
Ayerza's d., s.
Baastrup's d.
Babinski-Fröhlich s.
s. of Babinski-Nageotte
Babinski's s.
Babinski-Vaquez s.
Baelz's d.
Bäfverstedt's s.
Balfour's d.
Balint's s.
Ballet's d.
Ballingall's d.
Baló's d.
Bamberger-Marie d.
Bamberger's d.
Bamle d.
Bang's d.
Bannister's d.
Banti's d., s.
Barclay-Baron d.
Barcoo d.
Bardet-Biedl s.
Barlow's d., s.
Barraquer's d.
Barré-Guillain s.
Barrett's s.
Barthélemy's d.
Bartter's s.
Basedow's d.
Basel d.

Bassen-Kornzweig s.
Bateman's d.
Batten-Mayou d.
Batten's d.
Bayle's d.
Bazin's d.
Beard's d.
Beau's d., s.
Beauvais' d.
Bechterew's (Bekhterev's) d.
Becker's d.
Beck's d.
Beckwith's s.
Beckwith-Wiedemann s.
Begbie's d.
Béguez César d.
Behçet's s.
Behr's d.
Beigel's d.
Bekhterev's d.
Bell's d.
s. of Benedikt
Benson's d.
Bergeron's d.
Berger's d.
Berlin's d.
Bernard-Horner s.
Bernard-Sergent s.
Bernard-Soulier s.
Bernard's s.
Bernhardt-Roth s.
Bernhardt's d.
Bernheim's s.
Bertolotti's s.
Besnier-Boeck d.
Besnier-Boeck-Schaumann d., s.
Best's d.
Bianchi's s.
Biedl's d.
Bielschowsky-Jansky d.
Bielschowsky's d.
Biemond's s.
Biermer's d.
Biett's d.
Bilderbeck's d.
Billroth's d.

Binswanger's d.
Bird's d.
Björnstad's s.
Blatin's s.
Bloch-Sulzberger s.
Blocq's d.
Bloodgood's d.
Bloom's s.
Blount-Barber d.
Blount's d.
Blum's s.
body of Luys s.
Boeck's d.
Boerhaave's s.
Bogaert's d.
Bonnet-Dechaume-Blanc s.
Bonnevie-Ullrich s.
Bonnier's s.
Böök's s.
Börjeson-Forssman-Lehmann s.
Börjeson's s.
Bornholm d.
Bostock's d.
Bouchard's d.
Bouchet-Gsell d.
Bouillaud's d., s.
Bourneville-Pringle d.
Bourneville's d.
Bouveret's d., s.
Bowen's d.
Brachmann–de Lange s.
Bradley's d.
Brailsford-Morquio d.
Breda's d.
Breisky's d.
Brennemann's s.
Bretonneau's d.
Bright's d.
Brill's d.
Brill-Symmers d.
Brill-Zinsser d.
Brinton's d.
Brion-Kayser d.
Briquet's s.
Brissaud-Marie s.
Brissaud's d.

APPENDIX 2 571

Brissaud-Sicard s.
Bristowe's s.
Brock s.
Brocq's d.
Brodie's d.
Brooke's d.
Brown-Séquard d., s.
Brown's vertical retraction s.
Brown-Symmers d.
Bruck's d.
Brugsch's s.
Bruns' s.
Brunsting's s.
Brushfield-Wyatt d., s.
Bruton's d.
Budd-Chiari s.
Budd's d.
Buerger-Grütz d.
Buerger's d.
Buhl's d.
Bürger-Grütz s.
Burnett's s.
Bury's d.
Buschke-Ollendorff s.
Buschke's d.
Busquet's d.
Buss d.
Busse-Buschke d.
Byler's d.
Bywaters' s.
Cacchi-Ricci d.
Caffey's d., s.
Caffey-Silverman s.
Calvé-Perthes d.
Camurati-Engelmann d.
Canada-Cronkhite s.
Canavan's d.
Capdepont's d.
Capgras' s.
Caplan's s.
Caroli's d.
Carpenter's s.
Carrión's d.
Castellani's d.
Cavare's d.
Cazenave's d.

s. of Cestan-Chenais
Cestan-Raymond s.
Cestan's s.
Chabert's d.
Chagas-Cruz d.
Chagas' d.
Championniére's d.
Charcot-Marie-Tooth d.
Charcot's d., s.
Charcot-Weiss-Barker s.
Charlin's s.
Charlouis' d.
Charrin's d.
Chauffard's s.
Chauffard-Still s.
Cheadle's d.
Chédiak-Higashi s.
Chédiak-Steinbrinck-Higashi s.
Cheney s.
Cherchevski's d.
Chester's d.
Chiari-Arnold s.
Chiari-Budd s.
Chiari-Frommel s.
Chiari II s.
Chiari's s.
Chilaiditi's s.
Chotzen's s.
Christensen-Krabbe d.
Christian's d., s.
Christian-Weber d.
Christmas d.
Christ-Siemens s.
Christ-Siemens-Touraine s.
Churg-Strauss s.
Ciarrocchi's d.
Citelli's s.
Civatte's d.
Clarke-Hadfield s.
Claude Bernard–Horner s.
Claude's s.
Clérambault-Kandinsky s.
Clough and Richter's s.
Clouston's s.
Coats' d.
Cockayne's s.

Coffin-Lowry s.
Coffin-Siris s.
Cogan's s.
Collet-Sicard s.
Collet's s.
Concato's d.
Conn's s.
Conor and Bruch's d.
Conradi's d., s.
Cooley's d.
Cooper's d.
Corbus' d.
Cori's d.
Cornelia de Lange's s.
Corrigan's d.
Corvisart's d.
Costen's s.
Cotard's d.
Cottunius' d.
Cotugno's d.
Courvoisier-Terrier s.
Cowden's d.
Crandall's s.
Creutzfeldt-Jakob d., s.
Crigler-Najjar s.
Crocq's d.
Crohn's d.
Cronkhite-Canada s.
Cronkhite's s.
Crouzon's d.
Cruveilhier-Baumgarten s.
Cruveilhier's d.
Cruz-Chagas d.
Csillag's d.
Curschmann's d.
Curtius' s.
Cushing's d., s.
Cyriax's s.
Czerny's d.
Daae-Finsen d.
Daae's d.
DaCosta's d., s.
Dalrymple's d.
Danbolt-Closs s.
Dandy-Walker s.
Danielssen-Boeck d.

Danielssen's d.
Danlos' s.
Darier's d.
Darling's d.
David's d.
Debré-Sémélaigne s.
de Clerambault s.
Degos' d., s.
Déjérine-Klumpke s.
s. of Déjérine-Roussy
Déjérine's d., s.
Déjérine-Sottas d., s.
de Lange's s.
del Castillo s.
Dennie-Marfan s.
de Quervain's d.
Dercum's d.
De Sanctis-Cacchione s.
de Toni–Fanconi s.
Deutschländer's d.
Devergie's d.
Devic's d.
DiGeorge's s.
Dighton-Adair s.
Di Guglielmo d., s.
Dimitri's d.
Döhle d.
Donohue's s.
Down's s.
Dresbach's s.
Dressler's s.
Duane's s.
Dubini's d.
Dubin-Johnson s.
Dubin-Sprinz d., s.
Dubois' d.
Dubreuil-Chambardel s.
Duchenne-Aran d.
Duchenne-Erb s.
Duchenne-Griesinger d.
Duchenne's d., s.
Duhring's d.
Dukes' d.
Duplay's s.
Dupré's s.
Dupuytren's d.

APPENDIX 2   573

Durand-Nicolas-Favre d.
Durand's d.
Durante's d.
Duroziez's d.
Dutton's d.
Dyggve-Melchior-Clausen s.
Dyke-Davidoff s.
Eagle s.
Eales's d.
Eaton-Lambert s.
Ebstein's d.
Economo's d.
Eddowes' s.
Edsall's d.
Edwards-Patau s.
Edwards' s.
Ehlers-Danlos s.
Eichstedt's d.
Eisenlohr's s.
Eisenmenger's s.
Ekbom s.
Ellis–van Creveld s.
Engelmann's d.
Engel-Recklinghausen d.
English d.
Engman's d.
Epstein's d., s.
Erb-Charcot d.
Erb-Goldflam d.
Erb-Landouzy d.
Erb's d., s.
Erdheim d.
Eulenburg's d.
Faber's s.
Fabry's d.
Fahr's d.
Fahr-Volhard d.
Fallot's s.
Fanconi's s.
Farber's d., s.
Farber-Uzman s.
Fauchard's d.
Favre-Durand-Nicholas d.
Favre-Racouchot s.
Fede's d.
Feer's d.

Felty's s.
Fenwick's d.
Fiedler's d.
Fiessinger-Leroy-Reiter s.
Fiessinger's s.
Figueira's s.
Filatov-Dukes d.
Filatov's d.
Fisher's d.
Fitz-Hugh-Curtis s.
Fitz's s.
Flajani's d.
Flatau-Schilder d.
Fleischner's d.
Flynn-Aird s.
Foix's s.
Fölling's d.
Forbes-Albright s.
Forbes' d.
Fordyce's d.
Forney's s.
Forssman's carotid s.
Förster's d.
Foster Kennedy s.
Fothergill's d.
Fournier's d.
Foville's s.
Fox-Fordyce d.
Fraley s.
Franceschetti-Jadassohn s.
Franceschetti s.
Francis' d.
François' s.
Frankl-Hochwart's d.
Franklin's d.
Fraser's s.
Freeman-Sheldon s.
Frei's d.
Freiberg's d.
Frenkel's anterior ocular traumatic s.
Frey's s.
Friderichsen-Waterhouse s.
Friedländer's d.
Friedmann's d.
Friedmann's vasomotor s.

APPENDIX 2

Friedreich's d.
Friend d.
Fröhlich's s.
Froin's s.
Frommel-Chiari s.
Frommel's d.
Fuchs's s.
Fürstner's d.
Gailliard's s.
Gairdner's d.
Gaisböck's d.
Gamna's d.
Gamstorp's d.
Gandy-Nanta d.
Ganser's s.
Gardner-Diamond s.
Gardner's s.
Garré's d.
Gasser's s.
Gaucher's d.
Gee-Herter d.
Gee-Herter-Heubner d.
Gee's d.
Gee-Thaysen d.
Gélineau's s.
Gensoul's d.
Gerhardt's d., s.
Gerlier's d.
Gerstmann's s.
Gianotti-Crosti s.
Gibert's d.
Gibney's d.
Gierke's d.
Gilbert's d., s.
Gilchrist's d.
Gilles de la Tourette's s.
Glanzmann-Riniker s.
Glanzmann's d.
Glasser's d.
Glénard's d.
Glisson's d.
Goldberg-Maxwell s.
Goldenhar's s.
Goldflam-Erb d.
Goldflam's d.
Goldscheider's d.

Goldstein's d.
Goltz-Gorlin s.
Goltz's s.
Goodpasture's s.
Good's s.
Gopalan's s.
Gorham's d.
Gorlin-Chaudhry-Moss s.
Gorlin-Goltz s.
Gorlin-Psaume s.
Gorlin's s.
Gougerot and Blum d.
Gougerot-Carteaud s.
Gougerot-Nulock-Houwer s.
Gougerot-Sjögren d.
Gowers' s.
Gradenigo's s.
Graefe's d.
Graham Little s.
Graves' d.
Greenfield's d.
Greenhow's d.
Greig's s.
Griesinger's d.
Grönblad-Strandberg s.
Gross's d.
Grover's d.
Gruber's s.
Gubler's s.
di Guglielmo's d.
Guillain-Barré s.
Guinon's d.
Gull's d.
Gull-Sutton d.
Gunn's s.
Günther's d.
Habermann's d.
Haber's s.
Hadfield-Clarke s.
Haff d.
Haglund's d.
Hagner's s.
Hailey-Hailey d.
Hakim's s.
Hallermann-Streiff s.
Hallermann-Streiff-Francois s.

APPENDIX 2 575

Hallervorden s.
Hallervorden-Spatz d., s.
Hallgren's s.
Hallopeau's d.
Hallopeau-Siemens s.
Hall's d.
Hamman-Rich s.
Hamman's d.
Hammond's d.
Hand-Schüller-Christian d.
Hand's d.
Hanhart's s.
Hanot-Chauffard s.
Hanot's d.
Hansen's d.
d. of the Hapsburgs
Harada's s.
Hare's s.
Harris' s.
Hartnup d., s.
Hashimoto's d.
Hassin's s.
Hayem-Widal s.
Heberden's d.
Hebra's d.
Heerfordt's d., s.
Hegglin's s.
Heidenhaim's s.
Heine-Medin d.
Heller-Döhle d.
Helweg-Larssen s.
Hench-Rosenberg s.
Henderson-Jones d.
Henoch-Schönlein s.
Herrmann's s.
Hers' d.
Herter-Heubner d.
Herter's d.
Heubner's d.
Hildenbrand's d.
Hines-Bannick s.
Hippel-Lindau d.
Hippel's d.
Hirschfeld's d.
Hirschsprung's d.
His's d.

His-Werner d.
Hjärre's d.
Hodara's d.
Hodgkin's d.
Hodgson's d.
Hoffa's d.
Hoffmann-Werdnig s.
Holmes-Adie s.
Holt-Oram s.
Homén's s.
Hoppe-Goldflam d.
Horner-Bernard s.
Horner's s.
Horton's d., s.
Houssay s.
Huchard's d.
Hünermann's d.
Hunter-Hurler s.
Hunter's s.
Huntington's d.
Hunt's d., s.
Hurler-Pfaundler s.
Hurler's d., s.
Hutchinson-Boeck d.
Hutchinson-Gilford d.
Hutchinson's d.
Hutchison s.
Hutinel's d.
Hyde's d.
Irvine's s.
Isambert's d.
Ivemark's s.
Jaccoud's s.
Jackson's s.
Jacod's s.
Jadassohn-Lewandowsky s.
Jaffe-Lichtenstein d., s.
Jahnke's s.
Jakob-Creutzfeldt d.
Jakob's d.
Jaksch's d.
Janet's d.
Jansen's d.
Jansky-Bielschowsky d.
Jensen's d.
Jervell and Lange-Nielsen s.

APPENDIX 2

Jeune's s.
Job's s.
Johne's d.
Johnson-Stevens d.
Jourdain's d.
Jüngling's d.
juvenile Paget's d.
Kahlbaum's d.
Kahler's d.
Kaiserstuhl d.
Kalischer's d.
Kallmann's s.
Kanner's s.
Kartagener's s.
Kasabach-Merritt s.
Kashin-Beck d.
Kast's s.
Kawasaki d.
Kayser's d.
Kearns' s.
Kedani d.
Kennedy's s.
Kienböck's d.
Kiloh-Nevin s.
Kimmelstiel-Wilson s.
Kimura's d.
Kinnier Wilson d.
Kinsbourne s.
Kirkland's d.
Klauder's s.
Klebs' d.
Kleine-Levin s.
Klemperer's d.
Klinefelter's s.
Klippel-Feil s.
Klippel's d.
Klippel-Trenaunay s.
Klippel-Trenaunay-Weber s.
Klumpke-Déjérine s.
Klüver-Bucy s.
Kneist s.
Kocher-Debré-Sémélaigne s.
Kocher's s.
Koenig's s.
Koenig-Wichman d.
Koerber-Salus-Elschnig s.

Köhler-Pellegrini-Stieda d.
Köhler's bone d.
Köhlmeier-Degos d.
Kokka d.
König's s.
Korsakoff's d., s.
Koshevnikoff's d.
Krabbe's d., s.
Krause's s.
Krishaber's d.
Kufs' d.
Kugelberg-Welander d.
Kuhnt-Junius d.
Kümmell's d.
Kümmell-Verneuil d.
Kunkel's s.
Kuskokwim s.
Kussmaul-Maier d.
Kussmaul's d.
Kyrle's d.
Laband's s.
Labbé's neurocirculatory s.
Ladd's s.
Laennec's d.
Lafora's d.
Lambert-Eaton s.
Lancereaux-Mathieu d.
Landouzy's d.
Landry's d., s.
Lane's d.
Langdon-Down's d.
Larrey-Weil d.
Larsen-Johansson d.
Larsen's d., s.
Lasègue's d.
Lauber's d.
Laubry-Soulle s.
Launois' s.
Launois-Cléret s.
Laurence-Biedl s.
Laurence-Moon s.
Laurence-Moon-Bardet-Biedl s.
Laurence-Moon-Biedl s.
Läwen-Roth s.
Lawford's s.
Lawrence-Seip s.

APPENDIX 2 577

Leber's d.
Legal's d.
Legg-Calvé d.
Legg-Calvé-Perthes d.
Legg-Calvé-Waldenström d.
Legg's d.
Leigh's d.
Leiner's d.
Leloir's d.
Lenegre's d.
Lennox s.
Lenz's s.
Leredde's s.
Leriche's d., s.
Leri-Weill d., s.
Lermoyez's s.
Leroy's d.
Lesch-Nyhan s.
Letterer-Siwe d.
Lévi's s.
Lev's d.
Lévy-Roussy s.
Lewandowsky-Lutz d.
Leyden-Moebius s.
Leyden's d.
Lhermitte and McAlpine s.
Libman-Sacks d., s.
Lichtheim's d., s.
Lightwood's s.
Lignac-Fanconi d., s.
Liganc's d., s.
Lindau's d.
Lindau–von Hippel d.
Lipschütz's d.
Little's d.
Lobo's d.
Lobstein's d., s.
Löffler's s.
Looser-Milkman s.
Lorain-Lévi s.
Lorain's d.
Louis-Bar s.
Lowe's d., s.
Lowe-Terrey-MacLachlan s.
Lown-Ganong-Levine s.
Lucas-Championniére d.

Lucey-Driscoll s.
Luft's d.
Lutembacher's s.
Lutz-Splendore-Almeida d.
Lyell's d., s.
Mackenzie's d., s.
MacLean-Maxwell d.
Macleod's s.
Madelung's d.
Maffucci's s.
Magitot's d.
Maher's d.
Majocchi's d.
Malassez's d.
Malherbe's d.
Malibu d.
Malin's s.
Mallory-Weiss s.
Manson's d.
Marañón's s.
Marburg virus d.
Marchesani's s.
Marchiafava-Bignami d.
Marchiafava-Micheli d.
March's d.
Marcus Gunn's s.
Marek's d.
Marfan's s.
Margolis s.
Marinesco-Garland s.
Marie-Bamberger d., s.
Marie-Robinson s.
Marie's d., s.
Marie-Strümpell d.
Marie-Tooth d.
Marinesco-Sjögren's s.
Marion's d.
Maroteaux-Lamy s.
Marshall's s.
Marsh's d.
Martin's d.
Martorell's s.
Mathieu's d.
Maunier-Kuhn d.
Mauriac s.
Maxcy's d.

578 APPENDIX 2

Mayer-Rokitansky-Küster s.
McArdle-Schmid-Pearson d.
McArdle's d.
McCune-Albright s.
Meckel-Gruber s.
Meckel's s.
Medin's d.
Meige's d.
Meigs' s.
Meleda d.
Melkersson-Rosenthal s.
Melkersson's s.
Melnick-Needles s.
Menetrier's d., s.
Mengert's shock s.
Meniere's d., s.
Menkes' s.
Merzbacher-Pelizaeus d.
Meyenburg-Altherr-Uehlinger s.
Meyenburg's d.
Meyer-Betz d.
Meyer-Schwickerath and Weyers s.
Meyer's d.
Mibelli's d.
Miescher's d.
Mikulicz's d., s.
Milkman's s.
Millard-Gubler s.
Miller's d.
Mills' d.
Milroy's d.
Milton's d.
Minamata d.
Minkowski-Chauffard s.
Minor's d.
Minot–von Willebrand s.
Mitchell's d.
Möbius' d., s.
Moeller-Barlow d.
Molten's d
Monakow's s.
Mondor's d.
Monge's d.
Moore's s.
Morel-Kraepelin d.
Morel's s.

Morgagni-Adams-Stokes s.
Morgagni's d., s.
Morgagni-Stewart-Morel s.
Morquio-Brailsford d.
Morquio's s.
Morquio-Ullrich s.
Morris s.
Morton's d., s.
Morvan's d., s.
Moschcowitz's d.
Mosse's s.
Mounier-Kuhn s.
Mozer's d.
Mucha-Habermann d., s.
Mucha's d.
Muckle-Wells s.
Munchausen's s.
Munchmeyer's d.
Murchison-Sanderson s.
Myá's d.
Nadia d.
Naegeli's s.
Naffziger's s.
Neftel's d.
Nelson's s.
Netherton's s.
Neumann's d.
Nezelof's s.
Nicolas-Favre d.
Nidoko d.
Nieden's s.
Niemann-Pick d.
Niemann's d.
Noack's s.
Nonne-Milroy-Meige s.
Nonne's s.
Noonan's s.
Nordau's d.
Norrie's d.
Norum's d.
Nothnagel's s.
Novy's rat d.
Ogilvie's s.
Oguchi's d.
Ohara's d.
Ollier's d.

APPENDIX 2 579

Olmer's d.
Opitz's d.
Oppenheim's d., s.
Ormond's d.
Osgood-Schlatter d.
Osler's d.
Osler-Vaquez d.
Osler-Weber-Rendu d.
Ostrum-Furst s.
Otto's d.
Owren's d.
Paas's d.
Paget's d.
Paget's d., extramammary
Pancoast's s.
Panner's d.
Papillon-Léage and Psaume s.
Papillon-Lefévre s.
Parinaud's oculoglandular s.
Parinaud's s.
parkinsonian s.
Parkinson's d.
Parrot's d.
Parry-Romberg s.
Parry's d.
Parsons' d.
Patau's s.
Patella's d.
Paterson-Brown-Kelly s.
Paterson-Kelly s.
Paterson's s.
Pauzat's d.
Pavy's d.
Payr's d.
Pel-Ebstein d.
Pelizaeus-Merzbacher d.
Pellegrini's d.
Pellegrini-Stieda d.
Pellizzi's s.
Pendred's s.
Pepper s.
Perrin-Ferraton d.
Perthes' d.
Pette-Döring d.
Peutz-Jeghers s.
Peutz s.

Peyronie's d.
Pfaundler-Hurler s.
Pfeiffer's d., s.
Phocas' d.
Picchini's s.
Pick's d.
pickwickian s.
Pictou d.
Pierre Robin s.
Pinkus' d.
Plummer's d.
Plummer-Vinson s.
Poland's s.
Polhemus-Schafer-Ivemark s.
Pompe's d.
Poncet's d.
Posada's d.
Posada-Wernicke d.
Potter's s.
Pott's d.
Poulet's d.
Prader-Willi s.
Preiser's d.
Pringle's d.
Profichet's s.
pseudo-Turner's s.
Purtscher's d.
Putnam-Dana s.
Pyle's d.
Quervain's d.
Quincke's d.
Quinquaud's d.
Raeder's paratrigeminal s.
Ramsay Hunt s.
Ranikhet d.
Rayer's d.
Raymond-Cestan s.
Raynaud's d.
Recklinghausen-Applebaum d.
Recklinghausen's d.
Recklinghausen's d. of bone
Reclus' d.
Reed-Hodgkin d.
Refetoff s.
Refsum's d.
Reichmann's d., s.

Reifenstein's s.
Reiter's d., s.
Rendu-Osler d.
Rendu-Osler-Weber d.
Renpenning's s.
Reye's s.
Ribas-Torres d.
Richards-Rundle s.
Richter's s.
Riedel's d.
Rieger's s.
Riga-Fede d.
Riga's d.
Riggs' d.
Riley-Day s.
Riley-Smith s.
Ritter's d.
Roaf's s.
Robert's s.
Robinow's s.
Robinson's d.
Robin's s.
Robles' d.
Roger's d., s.
Rokitansky-Küster-Hauser s.
Rokitansky's d.
Romano-Ward s.
Romberg's d., s.
Rose d.
Rosenbach's s.
Rosenthal-Kloepfer s.
Rosenthal's s.
Rosewater's s.
Rossbach's d.
Rot-Bernhardt d., s.
Roth-Bernhardt d., s.
Rothmann-Makai s.
Rothmund-Thomson s.
Roth's d., s.
Rotor's s.
Rot's d., s.
Rotter's s.
Rougnon-Heberden d.
Roussy-Déjérine s.
Roussy-Lévy's d., s.
Rovsing s.

Rubarth's d.
Rubinstein's s.
Rubinstein-Taybi s.
Rud's s.
Rummo's d.
Russell's s.
Rust's d., s.
Ruysch's d.
Sabin-Feldman s.
Sachs' d.
Saethre-Chotzen s.
St. Agatha's d.
St. Aignon's d.
St. Anthony's d.
St. Appolonia's d.
St. Avertin's d.
St. Avidus' d.
St. Blasius' d.
St. Dymphna's d.
St. Erasmus' d.
St. Fiacre's d.
St. Gervasius' d.
St. Gotthard's tunnel d.
St. Hubert's d.
St. Job's d.
St. Mathurin's d.
St. Modestus' d.
St. Roch's d.
St. Sement's d.
St. Valentine's d.
St. Zachary's d.
Sanchez Salorio s.
Sander's d.
Sanders' d.
Sandhoff's d.
Sanfilippo's s.
Saunders' d.
Savill's d.
Schafer's s.
Schamberg's d.
Schanz's d., s.
Schaumann's d., s.
Scheie's s.
Schenck's d.
Scheuermann's d.
Schilder's d.

APPENDIX 2 581

Schimmelbusch's d.
Schirmer's s.
Schlatter-Osgood d.
Schlatter's d.
Schmid-Fraccaro s.
Schmidt's s.
Schmorl's d.
Scholz's d.
Schönlein-Henoch d., s.
Schönlein's d.
Schottmüller's d.
Schridde's d.
Schroeder's d., s.
Schüller-Christian d., s.
Schüller's d., s.
Schultz s.
Schultz's d.
Schwartz s.
Schwediauer's d.
Schweninger-Buzzi d.
Seckel's s.
Seitelberger's d.
Selter's d.
Selye s.
Senear-Usher s.
Sertoli-cell-only s.
Sever's d.
Sézary reticulosis s.
Sézary s.
Shaver's d.
Sheehan's s.
Shichito d.
Shwachman s.
Shwachman-Diamond s.
Shy-Drager s.
Sicard's s.
Silverskiöld's s.
Silver's s.
Silvestrini-Corda s.
Simmonds' d.
Simons' d.
Sipple's s.
Sjögren-Larsson s.
Sjögren's d., s.
Skevas-Zerfus d.
Sluder's s.

Sly d.
Smith-Lemli-Opitz s.
Smith's d.
Smith-Strang d.
Sneddon-Wilkinson d.
Sohval-Soffer s.
Sorsby's s.
Sotos' s.
Sotos' s. of cerebral gigantism
Spencer's d.
Spens's s.
Speransky-Richen-Siegmund s.
Spielmeyer-Stock d.
Spielmeyer-Vogt d.
Sprinz-Dubin s.
Sprinz-Nelson s.
Spurway s.
Stanton's d.
Stargardt's d.
Steele-Richardson-Olszewski s.
Steinbrocker's s.
Steiner's s.
Steinert's d.
Stein-Leventhal s.
Sterbe d.
Sternberg's d.
Stevens-Johnson s.
Stewart-Morel s.
Stewart-Treves s.
Sticker's d.
Stickler s.
Stieda's d.
Still-Chauffard s.
Stilling s.
Stilling-Turk-Duane s.
Still's d.
Stokes-Adams d.
Stokes' d.
Stokvis' d.
Stokvis-Talma s.
Strümpell-Leichtenstern d.
Strümpell-Lorrain d.
Strümpell-Marie d.
Strümpell's d.
Strümpell-Westphal d.
Stryker-Halbeisen s.

Stühmer's d.
Sturge-Kalischer-Weber s.
Sturge's s.
Sturge-Weber s.
Sudeck-Leriche s.
Sudeck's d.
Sulzberger-Garbe s.
Sutton and Gull's d.
Sutton's d.
Swediaur's d.
Sweet's d., s.
Swift-Feer d.
Swift's d.
Sydenham's d.
Sylvest's d.
Symmers' d.
Takahara's d.
Takayasu's d., s.
Talfan d.
Talma's d.
Tangier d.
Tapia's s.
Taussig-Bing s.
Tay-Sachs d.
Tay's d.
Terry's s.
Teschen d.
Thaysen's d.
Theiler's d.
Thibierge-Weissenbach s.
Thiele s.
Thiemann's d.
Thomsen's d.
Thomson's d.
Thorn's s.
Thornwaldt's d., s.
Thygeson's d.
Tietze's s.
Tillaux's d.
Timme's s.
Tolosa-Hunt s.
Tommaselli's d.
Tooth d.
Tornwaldt's d.
Torre's s.
Torsten-Sjögren's s.
Touraine-Solente-Golé s.
Tourette's d.
Treacher Collins s.
Trevor's d.
Troisier's s.
Trousseau's s.
Turcot s.
Turner's s.
Tyzzer's d.
Uehlinger's s.
Ullrich-Feichtiger s.
Ullrich-Turner s.
Ulysses s.
Underwood's d.
Unna's d.
Unverricht's d.
Urbach-Oppenheim d.
Urbach-Wiethe d.
Usher's s.
van Bogaert's d.
van Buchem's s.
van Buren's d.
van der Hoeve's s.
Van der Woude's s.
Vaquez-Osler d.
Vaquez's d.
Verner-Morrison s.
Vernet's s.
Verneuil's d.
Verse's d.
Vidal's d.
Villaret's s.
Vincent's d.
Vinson-Plummer s.
Vinson's s.
Virchow's d.
Vogt-Koyanagi s.
Vogt-Spielmeyer d.
Vogt's s.
Volkmann's d., s.
Voltolini's d.
von Bechterew's (Bekhterev's) d.
von Economo's d.
von Gierke's d.
von Hippel–Lindau d.
von Hippel's d.

von Jaksch's d.
von Meyenburg's d.
von Recklinghausen's d.
von Willebrand's d., s.
Voorhoeve's d.
Vrolik's d.
Waardenburg's s.
Wagner's d.
Waldenström's d.
Wallenberg's s.
Wardrop's d.
Wartenberg's d.
Wassilieff's d.
Waterhouse-Friderichsen s.
s. of Weber
Weber-Christian d.
Weber-Cockayne s.
Weber-Dimitri d.
Weber-Dubler s.
Weber's d.
Wegener's s.
Wegner's d.
Weill-Marchesani s.
Weil's d., s.
Weir Mitchell's d.
Wenckebach's d.
Werdnig-Hoffmann d., s.
Werlhof's d.
Wermer's s.
Werner-His d.
Werner-Schultz d.
Werner's s.
Wernicke-Korsakoff s.
Wernicke's d., s.
Wesselsbron d.
Westphal's d.
Westphal-Strümpell d.
West's s.

Weyers' oligodactyly s.
Weyers-Thier s.
Whipple's d.
White's d.
Whitmore's d.
Whytt's d.
Widal s.
Wildervanck s.
Wilkie's d.
Willebrand's s.
Williams-Campbell s.
Williams s.
Willis' d.
Wilson-Mikity s.
Wilson's d., s.
Winckel's d.
Windscheid's d.
Winiwarter-Buerger d.
Winkler's d.
Winter's s.
Winton d.
Wiskott-Aldrich s.
Witkop's d.
Witkop–Von Sallmann d.
Wohlfart-Kugelberg-Welander d.
Wolff-Parkinson-White s.
Wolf-Hirschhorn s.
Wolfram s.
Wolman's d.
Woringer-Kolopp d.
Wright's s.
Young's s.
Zahorsky's d.
Zellweger s.
Ziehen-Oppenheim d.
Zieve s.
Zollinger-Ellison s.

CULTURE MEDIA*

(a. = agar; b. = broth; c. = culture medium; m. = medium)

acetate differential a.
agar c.
albumin b. (Dubos)
Anderson's m.
antibiotic c.
Aronson's c.
asparagin c.
Avery's c.
azide violet blood a.
bacteriostasis a.
Balamuth's c.
Barile-Yaguchi-Eveland (BYE) a.
basal c.
beef infusion c.
beer wort c.
bile c., bile salt c.
bismuth sulfite a.
blood c. (Kracke)
Boeck and Drbohlav's c.
Bordet-Gengou a.
boric acid b.
brain-heart infusion m.
Braun's c.
brilliant green a.
brilliant green–bile a.
bromcresol purple desoxycholate (BCP-D) a.
Brucella a.
buffered desoxycholate glucose (BDG) b.
carbohydrate b.
Cary-Blair transport m.

Casman b.
cell c.
Chapman-Stone a.
charcoal a.
chlamydospore a.
chocolate c.
Clark and Lubs c.
Clauberg's a.
clearing m.
clostrisel a.
coagulase-mannitol a.
corn meal a.
Corper's c.
Craig's c.
cystine-heart a.
Czapek-Dox a.
decarboxylase c.
deoxycholate-citrate m.
deoxycholate citrate lactose saccharose (DCLS) a.
dextrose a.
dextrose starch a.
Dieudonné's c.
differential c.
Dorset's egg c.
Dubos' c.
Durham's c.
Eagle's basal m.
egg c.
egg albumin c.
egg-meat c.
Eijkman lactose b.

---

*Adapted from Dorland's Illustrated Medical Dictionary, 26th ed. Philadelphia, W. B. Saunders Company, 1981.

APPENDIX 3   585

Eisenberg's milk-rice c.
EMB a.
Emerson a.
Endo a.
enriched c.
eosin-methylene blue (EMB) a.
eosin-methylthionine chloride c.
esculin c.
ethyl violet azide b.
extract a.
FDA m.
Fildes c.
fish b.
Fletcher m.
Forget-Fredette a.
formate ricinoleate m.
Fränkel and Voges' asparagin c.
fuchsin a., fuchsin sulfite a.
gelatin a., c.
glucose-formate b.
glycerin b.
glycerinated potato c.
glycerin-potato b.
hanging block m.
haricot b.
Hershell's c.
hormone c.
Hoyle's m.
indicator c.
infusion m.
inosite-free b.
iron b.
Jordan tartrate c.
Kendall's c.
KF streptococcal m.
Kitasato's b.
Kligler iron a.
Koser citrate b.
Krumwiede triple sugar a.
Kulp c.
lactose-litmus b.
lauryl sulfate b.
lead b.
Les c.
Levine's EMB a., Levine's eosin-methylene blue a.

Li-Rivers c.
litmus-milk c.
litmus-whey c.
Littman a.
Loeffler m.
Löwenstein-Jensen c.
Löwenstein's c.
L.S.U. m.
MacConkey a., b.
malachite green b.
malt a.
malt extract a., b.
mannitol salt a.
Martin's b.
meat extract m.
meat infusion m.
membrane filter m.
milk c.
milk-rice c.
mineral salts a.
Monsur's a.
motility test m.
MR-VP b.
Mueller-Hinton a.
Mycoplasma a.
Naegeli's c.
Neill's m.
neomycin assay a.
neutral red c.
NIH agar m.
nitrate b.
N.N.N. c.
Noguchi's c.
nutrient c.
nystatin assay a.
oleic a. (Dubos)
Omeliansky's nutritive c.
Pai's c.
Parietti's b.
Park and Williams' chocolate c.
Pasteur's c.
peptone water c.
Petragnani c.
Petroff's synthetic c.
Petruschky's c.
phenol red m.

phenylalanine a.
Pike streptococcal b.
polymyxin test a.'s
potato blood a.
potato dextrose a.
proof a.
Proskauer-Beck m.
protein-free c.
rice extract a.
Robertson's c.
Rogosa SL m.
Rosenow's veal-brain b.
rosolic acid-peptone c.
Russell's double sugar a.
Sabouraud a.
saccharose-mannitol a.
Salmonella-Shigella (SS) a.
seed a.
selective c.
selenite b.
selenite-cystine b.
semisolid c.
serum b.
silicate jelly c.
Simmons' citrate a.
Snyder a.
Soyka's milk-rice c.
spirit blue a.
Spirolate b.
standard methods a.
sterility test b., c.
streptomycin assay a. with yeast extract

Stuart b.
sugar b.
sulfite a.
sulfite polymyxin sulfadiazine (SPS) a.
tartrate c.
TB charcoal a.
TCBS a.
tellurite a.
tellurite glycine a.
tetrathionate b.
tetrathionate enrichment b.
Thayer-Martin m.
thiosulfate citrate bile salts sucrose (TCBS) a.
Tindale's m.
Todd-Hewitt b.
tomato juice a.
triple sugar iron a.
Trudeau m.
urea a.
urease test b.
Uschinsky's c.
veal infusion c.
Venkatraman-Ramikrishnan m.
wheat b.
Wilson-Blair c.
Winogradsky's c.
wort a., b.
yeast autolysate c.
zein a.

TABLE OF ELEMENTS

NAME	SYMBOL	AT. NO.	AT. WT.*
Actinium	Ac	89	(227)
Aluminum	Al	13	26.982
Americium	Am	95	(243)
Antimony	Sb	51	121.75
Argon	Ar	18	39.948
Arsenic	As	33	74.922
Astatine	At	85	(210)
Barium	Ba	56	137.34
Berkelium	Bk	97	(247)
Beryllium	Be	4	9.012
Bismuth	Bi	83	208.980
Boron	B	5	10.811
Bromine	Br	35	79.909
Cadmium	Cd	48	112.40
Calcium	Ca	20	40.08
Californium	Cf	98	(249)
Carbon	C	6	12.011
Cerium	Ce	58	140.12
Cesium	Cs	55	132.905
Chlorine	Cl	17	35.453
Chromium	Cr	24	51.996
Cobalt	Co	27	58.933
Copper	Cu	29	63.54
Curium	Cm	96	(247)
Dysprosium	Dy	66	162.50
Einsteinium	Es	99	(254)
Erbium	Er	68	167.26
Europium	Eu	63	151.96
Fermium	Fm	100	(253)
Fluorine	F	9	18.998
Francium	Fr	87	(223)
Gadolinium	Gd	64	157.25
Gallium	Ga	31	69.72
Germanium	Ge	32	72.59
Gold	Au	79	196.967
Hafnium	Hf	72	178.49
Hahnium	Ha	105	(260)
Helium	He	2	4.003
Holmium	Ho	67	164.930
Hydrogen	H	1	1.008
Indium	In	49	114.82
Iodine	I	53	126.904
Iridium	Ir	77	192.2
Iron	Fe	26	55.847
Krypton	Kr	36	83.80
Lanthanum	La	57	138.91
Lawrencium	Lw	103	(257)
Lead	Pb	82	207.19
Lithium	Li	3	6.939
Lutetium	Lu	71	174.97
Magnesium	Mg	12	24.312

*Atomic weights are corrected to conform with the 1961 values of the Commission on Atomic Weights, expressed to the fourth decimal point, rounded off to the nearest thousandth. The numbers in parentheses are the mass numbers of the most stable or most common isotopes.

NAME	SYMBOL	AT. NO.	AT. WT.*
Manganese	Mn	25	54.938
Mendelevium	Md	101	(256)
Mercury	Hg	80	200.59
Molybdenum	Mo	42	95.94
Neodymium	Nd	60	144.24
Neon	Ne	10	20.183
Neptunium	Np	93	(237)
Nickel	Ni	28	58.71
Niobium	Nb	41	92.906
Nitrogen	N	7	14.007
Nobelium	No	102	(253)
Osmium	Os	76	190.2
Oxygen	O	8	15.999
Palladium	Pd	46	106.4
Phosphorus	P	15	30.974
Platinum	Pt	78	195.09
Plutonium	Pu	94	(242)
Polonium	Po	84	(210)
Potassium	K	19	39.102
Praseodymium	Pr	59	140.907
Promethium	Pm	61	(147)
Protactinium	Pa	91	(231)
Radium	Ra	88	(226)
Radon	Rn	86	(222)
Rhenium	Re	75	186.2
Rhodium	Rh	45	102.905
Rubidium	Rb	37	85.47
Ruthenium	Ru	44	101.07
Rutherfordium	Rf	104	(261)
Samarium	Sm	62	150.35
Scandium	Sc	21	44.956
Selenium	Se	34	78.96
Silicon	Si	14	28.086
Silver	Ag	47	107.870
Sodium	Na	11	22.990
Strontium	Sr	38	87.62
Sulfur	S	16	32.064
Tantalum	Ta	73	180.948
Technetium	Tc	43	(99)
Tellurium	Te	52	127.60
Terbium	Tb	65	158.924
Thallium	Tl	81	204.37
Thorium	Th	90	232.038
Thulium	Tm	69	168.934
Tin	Sn	50	118.69
Titanium	Ti	22	47.90
Tungsten	W	74	183.85
Uranium	U	92	238.03
Vanadium	V	23	50.942
Xenon	Xe	54	131.30
Ytterbium	Yb	70	173.04
Yttrium	Y	39	88.905
Zinc	Zn	30	65.37
Zirconium	Zr	40	91.22

*Atomic weights are corrected to conform with the 1961 values of the Commission on Atomic Weights, expressed to the fourth decimal point, rounded off to the nearest thousandth. The numbers in parentheses are the mass numbers of the most stable or most common isotopes.

(Courtesy of Dorland's Illustrated Medical Dictionary, 26th ed. P. 429. Philadelphia, W.B. Saunders Company, 1981.)

TABLES OF WEIGHTS AND MEASURES*

Measures of Mass

AVOIRDUPOIS WEIGHT

GRAINS	DRAMS	OUNCES	POUNDS	METRIC EQUIVALENTS, GRAMS
1	0.0366	0.0023	0.00014	0.0647989
27.34	1	0.0625	0.0039	1.772
437.5	16	1	0.0625	28.350
7000	256	16	1	453.5924277

APOTHECARIES' WEIGHT

GRAINS	SCRUPLES (Ͽ)	DRAMS (ʒ)	OUNCES (℥)	POUNDS (lb.)	METRIC EQUIVALENTS, GRAMS
1	0.05	0.0167	0.0021	0.00017	0.0647989
20	1	0.333	0.042	0.0035	1.296
60	3	1	0.125	0.0104	3.888
480	24	8	1	0.0833	31.103
5760	288	96	12	1	373.24177

*Courtesy of Miller, B. F., and Keane, C. B.: Encyclopedia and Dictionary of Medicine, Nursing, and Allied Health, 2nd ed. Philadelphia, W. B. Saunders Company, 1978.

Troy Weight

GRAINS	PENNYWEIGHTS	OUNCES	POUNDS	METRIC EQUIVALENTS, GRAMS
1	0.042	0.002	0.00017	0.0647989
24	1	0.05	0.0042	1.555
480	20	1	0.083	31.103
5760	240	12	1	373.24177

Metric Weight

MICROGRAM	MILLIGRAM	CENTIGRAM	DECIGRAM	GRAM	DECAGRAM	HECTOGRAM	KILOGRAM	EQUIVALENTS AVOIRDUPOIS	APOTHECARIES'
1	...	...	...	...	...	...	...	0.000015 grains	
10^3	1	...	...	...	...	...	...	0.015432 grains	
10^4	10	1	...	...	...	...	...	0.154323 grains	
10^5	10^2	10	1	...	...	...	...	1.543235 grains	
10^6	10^3	10^2	10	1	...	...	...	15.432356 grains	
10^7	10^4	10^3	10^2	10	1	...	...	5.6438 dr.	7.7162 scr.
10^8	10^5	10^4	10^3	10^2	10	1	...	3.527 oz.	3.215 oz.
10^9	10^6	10^5	10^4	10^3	10^2	10	1	2.2046 lb.	2.6792 lb.
10^{12}	10^9	10^8	10^7	10^6	10^5	10^4	10^3	2204.6223 lb.	2679.2285 lb.

TABLES OF WEIGHTS AND MEASURES—*Continued*

Measures of Capacity

APOTHECARIES' (WINE) MEASURE

MINIMS	FLUID DRAMS	FLUID OUNCES	GILLS	PINTS	QUARTS	GALLONS	CUBIC INCHES	EQUIVALENTS MILLI-LITERS	CUBIC CENTIMETERS
1	0.0166	0.002	0.0005	0.00013	...	...	0.00376	0.06161	0.06161
60	1	0.125	0.0312	0.0078	0.0039	...	0.22558	3.6967	3.6967
480	8	1	0.25	0.0625	0.0312	0.0078	1.80468	29.5737	29.5737
1920	32	4	1	0.25	0.125	0.0312	7.21875	118.2948	118.2948
7680	128	16	4	1	0.5	0.125	28.875	473.179	473.179
15360	256	32	8	2	1	0.25	57.75	946.358	946.358
61440	1024	128	32	8	4	1	231	3785.434	3785.434

METRIC MEASURE

MICROLITER	MILLILITER	CENTILITER	DECILITER	LITER	DEKALITER	HECTOLITER	KILOLITER	MYRIALITER	EQUIVALENTS (APOTHECARIES' FLUID)
1	...	...	...	...	...	...	...	...	0.01623108 min.
10^3	1	...	...	...	...	...	...	...	16.23 min.
10^4	10	1	...	...	...	...	...	...	2.7 fl. dr.
10^5	10^2	10	1	...	...	...	...	...	3.38 fl. oz.
10^6	10^3	10^2	10	1	...	...	...	...	2.11 pts.
10^7	10^4	10^3	10^2	10	1	...	...	...	2.64 gal.
10^8	10^5	10^4	10^3	10^2	10	1	...	...	26.418 gal.
10^9	10^6	10^5	10^4	10^3	10^2	10	1	...	264.18 gal.
10^{10}	10^7	10^6	10^5	10^4	10^3	10^2	10	1	2611.8 gal.

1 liter = 2.113363738 pints (Apothecaries).

TABLES OF WEIGHTS AND MEASURES — *Continued*

Measures of Length

Metric Measure

MICRON	MILLI-METER	CENTI-METER	DECI-METER	METER	DEKA-METER	HECTO-METER	KILO-METER	MYRIA-METER	MEGA-METER	EQUIVALENTS
1	0.001	10^{-4}	...	...	...	...	...	...	...	0.000039 inch
10^3	1	10^{-1}	...	...	...	...	...	...	...	0.03937 inch
10^4	10	1	...	...	...	...	...	...	...	0.3937 inch
10^5	10^2	10	1	...	...	...	...	...	...	3.937 inch
10^6	10^3	10^2	10	1	...	...	...	...	...	39.37 inch
10^7	10^4	10^3	10^2	10	1	...	...	...	...	10.9361 yards
10^8	10^5	10^4	10^3	10^2	10	1	...	...	...	109.3612 yards
10^9	10^6	10^5	10^4	10^3	10^2	10	1	...	...	1093.6121 yards
10^{10}	10^7	10^6	10^5	10^4	10^3	10^2	10	1	...	6.2137 miles
10^{11}	10^8	10^7	10^6	10^5	10^4	10^3	10^2	10	1	62.1370 miles

Conversion Tables

AVOIRDUPOIS – METRIC WEIGHT

Ounces	Grams
1/16	1.772
1/8	3.544
1/4	7.088
1/2	14.175
1	28.350
2	56.699
3	85.049
4	113.398
5	141.748
6	170.097
7	198.447
8	226.796
9	255.146
10	283.495
11	311.845
12	340.194
13	368.544
14	396.893
15	425.243
16 (1 lb.)	453.59

Pounds	
1 (16 oz.)	453.59
2	907.18
3	1360.78 (1.36 kg.)
4	1814.37 (1.81 ")
5	2267.96 (2.27 ")
6	2721.55 (2.72 ")
7	3175.15 (3.18 ")
8	3628.74 (3.63 ")
9	4082.33 (4.08 ")
10	4535.92 (4.54 ")

APOTHECARIES' – METRIC LIQUID MEASURE

Minims	Milliliters
1	0.06
2	0.12
3	0.19
4	0.25
5	0.31
10	0.62
15	0.92
20	1.23
25	1.54
30	1.85
35	2.16
40	2.46
45	2.77
50	3.08
55	3.39
60 (1 fl.dr.)	3.70

Fluid drams	
1	3.70
2	7.39
3	11.09
4	14.79
5	18.48
6	22.18
7	25.88
8 (1 fl.oz.)	29.57

Fluid ounces	
1	29.57
2	59.15
3	88.72
4	118.29
5	147.87
6	177.44
7	207.01
8	236.58
9	266.16
10	295.73
11	325.30
12	354.88
13	384.45
14	414.02
15	443.59
16 (1 pt.)	473.18
32 (1 qt.)	946.36
128 (1 gal.)	3785.43

METRIC – AVOIRDUPOIS WEIGHT

GRAMS	OUNCES
0.001 (1 mg.)	0.000035274
1	0.035274
1000 (1 kg.)	35.274 (2.2046 lb.)

METRIC – APOTHECARIES' LIQUID MEASURE

MILLILITERS	MINIMS	MILLILITERS	FLUID DRAMS	MILLILITERS	FLUID OUNCES
1	16.231	5	1.35	30	1.01
2	32.5	10	2.71	40	1.35
3	48.7	15	4.06	50	1.69
4	64.9	20	5.4	500	16.91
5	81.1	25	6.76	1000 (1 L.)	33.815
		30	7.1		

APPENDIX 5

TABLES OF WEIGHTS AND MEASURES – Continued

CONVERSION TABLES

APOTHECARIES' – METRIC WEIGHT		METRIC – APOTHECARIES' WEIGHT	
Grains	Grams	Milligrams	Grains
1/150	0.0004	1	0.015432
1/120	0.0005	2	0.030864
1/100	0.0006	3	0.046296
1/80	0.0008	4	0.061728
1/64	0.001	5	0.077160
1/50	0.0013	6	0.092592
1/48	0.0014	7	0.108024
1/30	0.0022	8	0.123456
1/25	0.0026	9	0.138888
1/16	0.004	10	0.154320
1/12	0.005	15	0.231480
1/10	0.006	20	0.308640
1/9	0.007	25	0.385800
1/8	0.008	30	0.462960
1/7	0.009	35	0.540120
1/6	0.01	40	0.617280
1/5	0.013	45	0.694440
1/4	0.016	50	0.771600
1/3	0.02	100	1.543240
1/2	0.032		
1	0.065	Grams	
1 1/2	0.097 (0.1)	0.1	1.5432
2	0.12	0.2	3.0864
3	0.20	0.3	4.6296
4	0.24	0.4	6.1728
5	0.30	0.5	7.7160
6	0.40	0.6	9.2592
7	0.45	0.7	10.8024
8	0.50	0.8	12.3456
9	0.60	0.9	13.8888
10	0.65	1.0	15.4320
15	1.00	1.5	23.1480
20 (1ʒ)	1.30	2.0	30.8640
30	2.00	2.5	38.5800
Scruples		3.0	46.2960
1	1.296 (1.3)	3.5	54.0120
2	2.592 (2.6)	4.0	61.728
3 (1ʒ)	3.888 (3.9)	4.5	69.444
Drams		5.0	77.162
1	3.888	10.0	154.324
2	7.776		
3	11.664		Equivalents
4	15.552	10	2.572 drams
5	19.440	15	3.858 "
6	23.328	20	5.144 "
7	27.216	25	6.430 "
8 (1ʒ)	31.103	30	7.716 "
Ounces		40	1.286 oz.
1	31.103	45	1.447 "
2	62.207	50	1.607 "
3	93.310	100	3.215 "
4	124.414	200	6.430 "
5	155.517	300	9.644 "
6	186.621	400	12.859 "
7	217.724	500	1.34 lb.
8	248.828	600	1.61 "
9	279.931	700	1.88 "
10	311.035	800	2.14 "
11	342.138	900	2.41 "
12 (1 lb.)	373.242	1000	2.68 "

Tables of Weights and Measures—Concluded

Metric Doses With Approximate Apothecary Equivalents*

These *approximate* dose equivalents represent the quantities usually prescribed, under identical conditions, by physicians trained, respectively, in the metric or in the apothecary system of weights and measures. In labeling dosage forms in both the metric and the apothecary systems, if one is the approximate equivalent of the other, the approximate figure shall be enclosed in parentheses.

When prepared dosage forms such as tablets, capsules, pills, etc., are prescribed in the metric system, the pharmacist may dispense the corresponding *approximate* equivalent in the apothecary system, and vice versa, as indicated in the following table.

Caution—For the conversion of specific quantities in a prescription which requires compounding, or in converting a pharmaceutical formula from one system of weights or measures to the other, *exact* equivalents must be used.

LIQUID MEASURE METRIC	APPROX. APOTHECARY EQUIVALENTS	LIQUID MEASURE METRIC	APPROX. APOTHECARY EQUIVALENTS
1000 ml.	1 quart	3 ml.	45 minims
750 ml.	1 1/2 pints	2 ml.	30 minims
500 ml.	1 pint	1 ml.	15 minims
250 ml.	8 fluid ounces	0.75 ml.	12 minims
200 ml.	7 fluid ounces	0.6 ml.	10 minims
100 ml.	3 1/2 fluid ounces	0.5 ml.	8 minims
50 ml.	1 3/4 fluid ounces	0.3 ml.	5 minims
30 ml.	1 fluid ounce	0.25 ml.	4 minims
15 ml.	4 fluid drams	0.2 ml.	3 minims
10 ml.	2 1/2 fluid drams	0.1 ml.	1 1/2 minims
8 ml.	2 fluid drams	0.06 ml.	1 minim
5 ml.	1 1/4 fluid drams	0.05 ml.	3/4 minim
4 ml.	1 fluid dram	0.03 ml.	1/2 minim

WEIGHT METRIC	APPROX. APOTHECARY EQUIVALENTS	WEIGHT METRIC	APPROX. APOTHECARY EQUIVALENTS
30 Gm.	1 ounce	30 mg.	1/2 grain
15 Gm.	4 drams	25 mg.	3/8 grain
10 Gm.	2 1/2 drams	20 mg.	1/3 grain
7.5 Gm.	2 drams	15 mg.	1/4 grain
6 Gm.	90 grains	12 mg.	1/5 grain
5 Gm.	75 grains	10 mg.	1/6 grain
4 Gm.	60 grains (1 dram)	8 mg.	1/8 grain
3 Gm.	45 grains	6 mg.	1/10 grain
2 Gm.	30 grains (1/2 dram)	5 mg.	1/12 grain
1.5 Gm.	22 grains	4 mg.	1/15 grain
1 Gm.	15 grains	3 mg.	1/20 grain
0.75 Gm.	12 grains	2 mg.	1/30 grain
0.6 Gm.	10 grains	1.5 mg.	1/40 grain
0.5 Gm.	7 1/2 grains	1.2 mg.	1/50 grain
0.4 Gm.	6 grains	1 mg.	1/60 grain
0.3 Gm.	5 grains	0.8 mg.	1/80 grain
0.25 Gm.	4 grains	0.6 mg.	1/100 grain
0.2 Gm.	3 grains	0.5 mg.	1/120 grain
0.15 Gm.	2 1/2 grains	0.4 mg.	1/150 grain
0.12 Gm.	2 grains	0.3 mg.	1/200 grain
0.1 Gm.	1 1/2 grains	0.25 mg.	1/250 grain
75 mg.	1 1/4 grains	0.2 mg.	1/300 grain
60 mg.	1 grain	0.15 mg.	1/400 grain
50 mg.	3/4 grain	0.12 mg.	1/500 grain
40 mg.	2/3 grain	0.1 mg.	1/600 grain

Note—A milliliter (ml.) is the approximate equivalent of a cubic centimeter (cc.).

*Adopted by the latest Pharmacopeia, National Formulary, and New and Nonofficial Remedies, and approved by the Federal Food and Drug Administration.

COMBINING FORMS IN MEDICAL TERMINOLOGY*

The following is a list of combining forms encountered frequently in the vocabulary of medicine. A dash or dashes are appended to indicate whether the form usually precedes (as ante-) or follows (as -agra) the other elements of the compound or usually appears between the other elements (as -em-). Following each combining form, the first item of information is the Greek or Latin word, or both a Greek and a Latin word, from which it is derived. Those words that are not printed in Greek characters are Latin. Information necessary to an understanding of the form appears next in parentheses. Then the meaning or meanings of the word are given, followed where appropriate by reference to a synonymous combining form. Finally, an example is given to illustrate the use of the combining form in a compound English derivative.

a-	a- (n is added before words beginning with a vowel) negative prefix. Cf. in-[1]. ametria	alve-	alveus trough, channel, cavity. alveolar
ab-	ab away from. Cf. apo-. abducent	amph-	See amphi-. ampheclexis
abdomin-	abdomen, abdominis. abdominoscopy	amphi-	ἀμφί (i is dropped before words beginning with a vowel) both, doubly. amphicelous
ac-	See ad-. accretion	amyl-	ἄμυλον starch. amylosynthesis
acet-	acetum vinegar. acetometer	an-[1]	See ana-. anagogic
acid-	acidus sour. aciduric	an-[2]	See a-. anomalous
acou-	ἀκούω hear. acouesthesia. (Also spelled acu-)	ana-	ἀνά (final a is dropped before words beginning with a vowel) up, positive. anaphoresis
acr-	ἄκρον extremity, peak. acromegaly	ancyl-	See ankyl-. ancylostomiasis
act-	ago, actus do, drive, act. reaction	andr-	ἀνήρ, ἀνδρός man. gynandroid
actin-	ἀκτίς, ἀκτῖνος ray, radius. Cf. radi-. actinogenesis	angi-	ἀγγεῖον vessel. Cf. vas-. angiemphraxis
acu-	See acou-. osteoacusis	ankyl-	ἀγκύλος crooked, looped. ankylodactylia. (Also spelled ancyl-)
ad-	ad (d changes to c, f, g, p, s, or t before words beginning with those consonants) to. adrenal	ant-	See anti-. antophthalmic
		ante-	ante before. anteflexion
aden-	ἀδήν gland. Cf. gland-. adenoma	anti-	ἀντί (i is dropped before words beginning with a vowel) against, counter. Cf. contra-. antipyogenic
adip-	adeps, adipis fat. Cf. lip- and stear-. adipocellular	antr-	ἄντρον cavern. antrodynia
aer-	ἀήρ air. anaerobiosis	ap-[1]	See apo-. apheter
aesthe-	See esthe-. aesthesioneurosis	ap-[2]	See ad-. append
af-	See ad-. afferent	-aph-	ἅπτω, ἁφ- touch. dysaphia. (See also hapt-)
ag-	See ad-. agglutinant		
-agogue	ἀγωγός leading, inducing. galactagogue	apo-	ἀπό (o is dropped before words beginning with a vowel) away from, detached. Cf. ab-. apophysis
-agra	ἄγρα catching, seizure. podagra		
alb-	albus white. Cf. leuk-. albocinereous	arachn-	ἀράχνη spider. arachnodactyly
		arch-	ἀρχή beginning, origin. archenteron
alg-	ἄλγος pain. neuralgia		
all-	ἄλλος other, different. allergy		

*Compiled by Lloyd W. Daly, A.M., Ph.D., Litt. D., Allen Memorial Professor of Greek, University of Pennsylvania.

598 APPENDIX 6

arter(i)-	ἀρτηρία elevator (?), artery. arteriosclerosis, periarteritis
arthr-	ἄρθρον joint. Cf. articul-. synarthrosis
articul-	articulus joint. Cf. arthr-. disarticulation
as-	See ad-. assimilation
at-	See ad-. attrition
aur-	auris ear. Cf. ot-. aurinasal
aux-	αὔξω increase. enterauxe
ax-	ἄξων or axis axis. axofugal
axon-	ἄξων axis. axonometer
ba-	βαίνω, βα- go, walk, stand. hypnobatia
bacill-	bacillus small staff, rod. Cf. bacter-. actinobacillosis
bacter-	βακτήριον small staff, rod. Cf. bacill-. bacteriophage
ball-	βάλλω, βολ- throw. ballistics. (See also bol-)
bar-	βάρος weight. pedobarometer
bi-¹	βίος life. Cf. vit-. aerobic
bi-²	bi- two (see also di-¹). bilobate
bil-	bilis bile. Cf. chol-. biliary
blast-	βλαστός bud, child, a growing thing in its early stages. Cf. germ-. blastoma, zygotoblast.
blep-	βλέπω look, see. hemiablepsia
blephar-	βλέφαρον (from βλέπω; see blep-) eyelid. Cf. cili-. blepharoncus
bol-	See ball-. embolism
brachi-	βραχίων arm. brachiocephalic
brachy-	βραχύς short. brachycephalic
brady-	βραδύς slow. bradycardia
brom-	βρῶμος stench. podobromidrosis
bronch-	βρόγχος windpipe. bronchoscopy
bry-	βρύω be full of life. embryonic
bucc-	bucca cheek. distobuccal
cac-	κακός bad, abnormal. Cf. mal-. cacodontia, arthrocace. (See also dys-)
calc-¹	calx, calcis stone (cf. lith-), limestone, lime. calcipexy
calc-²	calx, calcis heel. calcaneotibial
calor-	calor heat. Cf. therm-. calorimeter
cancr-	cancer, cancri crab, cancer. Cf. carcin-. cancrology. (Also spelled chancr-)
capit-	caput, capitis head. Cf. cephal-. decapitator
caps-	capsa (from capio; see cept-) container. encapsulation
carbo(n)-	carbo, carbonis coal, charcoal. carbohydrate, carbonuria
carcin-	καρκίνος crab, cancer. Cf. cancr-. carcinoma
cardi-	καρδία heart. lipocardiac
cary-	See kary-. caryokinesis
cat-	See cata-. cathode
cata-	κατά (final a is dropped before words beginning with a vowel) down, negative. catabatic
caud-	cauda tail. caudad
cav-	cavus hollow. Cf. coel-. concave
cec-	caecus blind. Cf. typhl-. cecopexy
cel-¹	See coel-. amphicelous
cel-²	See -cele. celectome
-cele	κήλη tumor, hernia. gastrocele
cell-	cella room, cell. Cf. cyt-. celliferous
cen-	κοινός common. cenesthesia
cent-	centum hundred. Cf. hect-. Indicates fraction in metric system. [This exemplifies the custom in the metric system of identifying fractions of units by stems from the Latin, as centimeter, decimeter, millimeter, and multiples of units by the similar stems from the Greek, as hectometer, decameter, and kilometer.] centimeter, centipede
cente-	κεντέω puncture. Cf. punct-. enterocentesis
centr-	κέντρον or centrum point, center. neurocentral
cephal-	κεφαλή head. Cf. capit-. encephalitis
cept-	capio, -cipientis, -ceptus take, receive. receptor
cer-	κηρός or cera wax. ceroplasty, ceromel
cerat-	See kerat-. aceratosis
cerebr-	cerebrum. cerebrospinal
cervic-	cervix, cervicis neck. Cf. trachel-. cervicitis
chancr-	See cancr-. chancriform
cheil-	χεῖλος lip. Cf. labi-. cheiloschisis
cheir-	χείρ hand. Cf. man-. macrocheiria. (Also spelled chir-)
chir-	See cheir-. chiromegaly
chlor-	χλωρός green. achloropsia
chol-	χολή bile. Cf. bil-. hepatocholangeitis
chondr-	χόνδρος cartilage. chondromalacia
chord-	χορδή string, cord. perichordal
chori-	χόριον protective fetal membrane. endochorion
chro-	χρώς color. polychromatic
chron-	χρόνος time. synchronous
chy-	χέω, χυ- pour. ecchymosis
-cid(e)	caedo, -cisus cut, kill. infanticide, germicidal
cili-	cilium eyelid. Cf. blephar-. superciliary
cine-	See kine-. autocinesis
-cipient	See cept-. incipient
circum-	circum around. Cf. peri-. circumferential
-cis-	caedo, -cisus cut, kill. excision
clas-	κλάω, κλασ- break. cranioclast
clin-	κλίνω bend, incline, make lie down. clinometer
clus-	claudo, -clusus shut. Malocclusion
co-	See con-. cohesion
cocc-	κόκκος seed, pill. gonococcus
coel-	κοῖλος hollow. Cf. cav-. coelenteron. (Also spelled cel-)
col-¹	See colon-. colic
col-²	See con-. collapse

APPENDIX 6 599

colon-	κόλον lower intestine. *colon*ic	di-¹	See dia-. *di*uresis.
colp-	κόλπος hollow, vagina. Cf. sin-. *endocolp*itis	di-²	See dis-. *di*vergent.
com-	See con-. *com*maasculation	dia-	διά (*a* is dropped before words beginning with a vowel) through, apart. Cf. рег-. *dia*gnosis
con-	con- (becomes co- before vowels or *h*; col- before *l*; com- before *b, m,* or *p*; cor- before *r*) with, together. Cf. syn-. *con*traction	didym-	δίδυμος twin. Cf. gemin-. epi*didym*al
		digit-	*digit*us finger, toe. Cf. dactyl-. *digit*igrade
contra-	*contra* against, counter. Cf. anti-. *contra*indication	diplo-	διπλόος double. *diplo*myelia
copr-	κόπρος dung. Cf. sterco-. *copr*oma	dis-	*dis*- (*s* may be dropped before a word beginning with a consonant) apart, away from. *dis*location
cor-¹	κόρη doll, little image, pupil. *iso*cor*ia*		
cor-²	See con-. *cor*rugator	disc-	δίσκος or *disc*us disk. *disco*placenta
corpor-	*corpus, corporis* body. Cf. somat-. intra*corpor*al		
cortic-	*cortex, corticis* bark, rind. *cortic*osterone	dors-	*dors*um back. ventro*dors*al
		drom-	δρόμος course. hemo*drom*ometer
cost-	*cost*a rib. Cf. pleur-. inter*cost*al	-ducent	See duct-. ad*ducent*
crani-	κρανίον or *crani*um skull. peri*crani*um	duct-	*duco, ducentis, ductus* lead, conduct. ovi*duct*
creat-	κρέας, κρεατ- meat, flesh. *creat*orrhea	dur-	*dur*us hard. Cf. scler-. in*dur*ation
-crescent	*cresco, crescentis, cretus* grow. ex*crescent*	dynam(i)-	δύναμις power. *dynam*oneure, neuro*dynam*ic
cret-¹	*cerno, cretus* distinguish, separate off. Cf. crin-. dis*crete*	dys-	δυσ- bad, improper. Cf. mal-. *dys*trophic. (See also cac-)
cret-²	See -crescent. ac*cret*ion	e-	*e* out from. Cf. ec- and ex-. *e*mission
crin-	κρίνω distinguish, separate off. Cf. cret-¹. endo*crin*ology	ec-	ἐκ out of. Cf. e-. *ec*centric
crur-	*crus, cruris* shin, leg. brachio*crur*al	-ech-	ἔχω have, hold, be. syn*ech*otomy
cry-	κρύος cold. *cry*esthesia	ect-	ἐκτός outside. Cf. extra-. *ect*oplasm
crypt-	κρύπτω hide, conceal. *crypt*orchism	ede-	οἰδέω swell. *ede*matous
cult-	*colo, cultus* tend, cultivate. *cult*ure	ef-	See ex-. *ef*florescent
		-elc-	ἕλκος sore, ulcer. enter*elc*osis. (See also helc-)
cune-	*cune*us wedge. Cf. sphen-. *cune*iform	electr-	ἤλεκτρον amber. *electr*otherapy
cut-	*cut*is skin. Cf. derm(at)-. sub*cut*aneous	em-	See en-. *em*bolism, *em*pathy, *em*physis
cyan-	κύανος blue. anthocy*an*in	-em-	αἷμα blood. an*em*ia. (See also hem(at)-)
cycl-	κύκλος circle, cycle. *cycl*ophoria	en-	ἐν (*n* changes to *m* before *b, p,* or *ph*) in, on. Cf. in-². *en*celitis
cyst-	κύστις bladder. Cf. vesic-. nephro*cyst*itis		
cyt-	κύτος cell. Cf. cell-. plasmo*cyt*oma	end-	ἔνδον inside. Cf. intra-. *end*angium
dacry-	δάκρυ tear. *dacry*ocyst	enter-	ἔντερον intestine. dys*enter*y
dactyl-	δάκτυλος finger, toe. Cf. digit-. hexa*dactyl*ism	ep-	See epi-. *ep*axial
		epi-	ἐπί (*i* is dropped before words beginning with a vowel) upon, after, in addition. *epi*glottis
de-	*de* down from. *de*composition		
dec-¹	δέκα ten. Indicates multiple in metric system. Cf. dec-². *dec*agram	erg-	ἔργον work, deed. *en*ergy
		erythr-	ἐρυθρός red. Cf. rub(r)-. *erythr*ochromia
dec-²	*dec*em ten. Indicates fraction in metric system. Cf. dec-¹. *dec*ipara, *dec*imeter	eso-	ἔσω inside. Cf. intra-. *eso*phylactic
		esthe-	αἰσθάνομαι, αἰσθη- perceive, feel. Cf. sens-. an*esthe*sia
dendr-	δένδρον tree. neuro*dendr*ite		
dent-	*dens, dentis* tooth. Cf. odont-. inter*dent*al	eu-	εὐ good, normal. *eu*pepsia
derm(at)-	δέρμα, δέρματος skin. Cf. cut-. endo*derm*, *dermat*itis	ex-	ἐξ or *ex* out of. Cf. e-. *ex*cretion
		exo-	ἔξω outside. Cf. extra-. *exo*pathic
desm-	δεσμός band, ligament. syn*desm*opexy	extra-	*extra* outside of, beyond. Cf. ect- and exo-. *extra*cellular
dextr-	*dexter, dextr*- right-hand. ambi*dextr*ous		
di-¹	*di*- two. *di*morphic. (See also bi-²)	faci-	*faci*es face. Cf. prosop-. brachio*faci*olingual

600 APPENDIX 6

-facient	*facio, facientis, factus, -fectus* make. Cf. poie-. cale*facient*	glyc(y)-	γλυκύς sweet. *glyc*emia, *glycyr*rhizin. (Also spelled gluc-)
-fact-	See facient-. arte*fact*	gnath-	γνάθος jaw. ortho*gnath*ous
fasci-	*fascia* band. *fasci*orrhaphy	gno-	γιγνώσκω, γνω- know, discern. dia*gno*sis
febr-	*febris* fever. Cf. pyr-. *febr*icide		
-fect-	See -facient. de*fect*ive	gon-	See gen-. amphi*gon*y
-ferent	*fero, ferentis, latus* bear, carry. Cf. phor-. ef*ferent*	grad-	*gradior* walk, take steps. retro*grade*
ferr-	*ferrum* iron. *ferr*oprotein	-gram	γράφω, γραφ- + -μα scratch, write, record. cardio*gram*
fibr-	*fibra* fibre. Cf. in-¹. chondro*fibr*oma	gran-	*granum* grain, particle. lipo*gran*uloma
fil-	*filum* thread. *fil*iform	graph-	γράφω scratch, write, record. histo*graphy*
fiss-	*findo, fissus* split. Cf. schis-. *fiss*ion	grav-	*gravis* heavy. multi*grav*ida
flagell-	*flagellum* whip. *flagell*ation	gyn(ec)-	γυνή, γυναικός woman, wife. andro*gyny*, *gynec*ologic
flav-	*flavus* yellow. Cf. xanth-. ribo*flav*in	gyr-	γύρος ring, circle. *gyr*ospasm
-flect-	*flecto, flexus* bend, divert. de*flect*ion	haem(at)-	See hem(at)-. *haem*orrhagia, *haemat*oxylon
-flex-	See -flect-. re*flex*ometer	hapt-	ἅπτω touch. *hapt*ometer
flu-	*fluo, fluxus* flow. Cf. rhe-. *flu*id	hect-	ἑκτ- hundred. Cf. cent-. Indicates multiple in metric system. *hect*ometer
flux-	See flu-. af*flux*ion		
for-	*foris* door, opening. per*for*ated	helc-	ἕλκος sore, ulcer. *helc*osis
-form	*forma* shape. Cf. -oid. ossi*form*	hem(at)-	αἷμα, αἵματος blood. Cf. sanguin-. *hem*angioma, *hemat*ocyturia. (See also -em-)
fract-	*frango, fractus* break. re*fract*ive	hemi-	ἡμι- half. Cf. semi-. *hemi*ageusia
front-	*frons, frontis* forehead, front. naso*front*al	hen-	εἷς, ἑνός one. Cf. un-. *hen*ogenesis
-fug(e)	*fugio* flee, avoid. vermi*fuge*, centri*fug*al	hepat-	ἧπαρ, ἥπατος liver. gastro*hepat*ic
funct-	*fungor, functus* perform, serve, function. mal*funct*ion	hept(a)-	ἑπτά seven. Cf. sept-¹. *hept*atomic, *hepta*valent
fund-	*fundo, fusus* pour. in*fund*ibulum	hered-	*heres, heredis* heir. *hered*oimmunity
fus-	See fund-. dif*fus*ible	hex-¹	ἕξ six. Cf. sex-. *hex*yl-. An *a* is added in some combinations.
galact-	γάλα, γάλακτος milk. Cf. lact-. dys*galact*ia	hex-²	ἔχω, ἑχ- (added to σ becomes ἑξ-) have, hold, be. cachexy
gam-	γάμος marriage, reproductive union. a*gam*ont	hexa-	See hex-¹. *hexa*chromic
gangli-	γάγγλιον swelling, plexus. neuro*gangli*itis	hidr-	ἱδρώς sweat. hyper*hidr*osis
gastr-	γαστήρ, γαστρός stomach. cholangio*gastr*ostomy	hist-	ἱστός web, tissue. *hist*odialysis
gelat-	*gelo, gelatus* freeze, congeal. *gelat*in	hod-	ὁδός road, path. *hod*oneuromere. (See also od- and -ode¹)
gemin-	*geminus* twin, double. Cf. didym-. quadri*gemin*al	hom-	ὁμός common, same. *hom*omorphic
gen-	γίγνομαι, γεν-, γον- become, be produced, originate, or γεννάω produce, originate. cyto*gen*ic	horm-	ὁρμή impetus, impulse. *horm*one
		hydat-	ὕδωρ, ὕδατος water. *hydat*ism
		hydr-	ὕδωρ, ὕδρ- water. Cf. lymph-. achlor*hydr*ia
germ-	*germen, germinis* bud, a growing thing in its early stages. Cf. blast-. *germ*inal, ovi*germ*	hyp-	See hypo-. *hyp*axial
gest-	*gero, gerentis, gestus* bear, carry. con*gest*ion	hyper-	ὑπέρ above, beyond, extreme. Cf. super-. *hyper*trophy
		hypn-	ὕπνος sleep. *hypn*otic
gland-	*glans, glandis* acorn. Cf. aden-. intra*gland*ular	hypo-	ὑπό (*o* is dropped before words beginning with a vowel) under, below. Cf. sub-. *hypo*metabolism
-glia	γλία glue. neuro*glia*		
gloss-	γλῶσσα tongue. Cf. lingu-. tricho*gloss*ia	hyster-	ὑστέρα womb. colpo*hyster*opexy
		iatr-	ἰατρός physician. ped*iatr*ics
glott-	γλῶττα tongue, language. *glott*ic	idi-	ἴδιος peculiar, separate, distinct. *idi*osyncrasy
gluc-	See glyc(y)-. *gluc*ophenetidin	il-	See in-².³. *il*linition (in, on), *il*legible (negative prefix)
glutin-	*gluten, glutinis* glue. ag*glutin*ation	ile-	See ili- [ile- is commonly used to refer to the portion of the

APPENDIX 6   601

	intestines known as the ileum]. ileostomy	lien-	*lien* spleen. Cf. splen-. *lieno*cele
ili-	*ilium (ileum)* lower abdomen, intestines [ili- is commonly used to refer to the flaring part of the hip bone known as the ilium]. *ilio*sacral	lig- lingu-	*ligo* tie, bind. *liga*te *lingua* tongue. Cf. gloss-. sub*lingual*
im-	See in-¹, ². *im*mersion (in, on), *im*perforation. (negative prefix)	lip- lith-	λίπος fat. Cf. adip-. glyco*lip*in λίθος stone. Cf. calc-¹. nephro*lith*otomy
in-¹	ἴς, ἰνός fiber. Cf. fibr-. *ino*steatoma	loc-	*locus* place. Cf. top-. *loco*motion
in-²	*in* (*n* changes to *l*, *m*, or *r* before words beginning with those consonants) in, on. Cf. en-. *in*sertion	log-	λέγω, λογ- speak, give an account. *log*orrhea, embry*ology*
in-³	*in-* (*n* changes to *l*, *m*, or *r* before words beginning with those consonants) negative prefix. Cf. a-. *in*valid	lumb- lute-	*lumbus* loin. dorso*lumb*ar *luteus* yellow. Cf xanth-. *lute*oma
infra-	*infra* beneath. *infra*orbital	ly-	λύω loose, dissolve. Cf. solut-. kerato*ly*sis
insul-	*insula* island. *insul*in	lymph-	*lympha* water. Cf. hydr-. *lymph*adenosis
inter-	*inter* among, between. *inter*carpal	macr-	μακρός long, large. *macro*myeloblast
intra-	*intra* inside. Cf. end- and eso-. *intra*venous	mal-	*malus* bad, abnormal. Cf. cac- and dys-. *mal*function
ir-	See in-¹, ². *ir*radiation (in, on), *ir*reducible (negative prefix)	malac- mamm-	μαλακός soft. osteo*malac*ia *mamma* breast. Cf. mast-. sub*mamm*ary
irid-	ἶρις, ἴριδος rainbow, colored circle. kerato*irid*ocyclitis (Also spelled cary-)	man-	*manus* hand. Cf. cheir-. *man*iphalanx
is- ischi-	ἴσος equal. *is*otope ἰσχίον hip, haunch. *ischi*opubic	mani-	μανία mental aberration. *mani*graphy, klepto*mania*
jact- ject-	*iacio, iactus* throw. *jact*itation *iacio, -iectus* throw. in*ject*ion	mast-	μαστός breast. Cf. mamm-. hyper*mast*ia
jejun-	*ieiunus* hungry, not partaking of food. gastro*jejun*ostomy	medi-	*medius* middle. Cf. mes-. *medi*frontal
jug- junct-	*iugum* yoke. con*jug*ation *iungo, iunctus* yoke, join. con*junct*iva	mega-	μέγας great, large. Also indicates multiple (1,000,000) in metric system. *mega*colon, *mega*dyne. (See also megal-)
kary-	κάρυον nut, kernel, nucleus. Cf. nucle-. mega*kary*ocyte. (Also spelled cary-)	megal-	μέγας, μεγάλου great, large. acro*megal*y
kerat-	κέρας, κέρατος horn. *kerat*olysis. (Also spelled cerat-)	mel- melan-	μέλος limb, member. sym*mel*ia μέλας, μέλανος black. hippo*melan*in
kil-	χίλιοι one thousand. Cf. mill-. Indicates multiple in metric system. *kil*ogram	men- mening-	μήν month. dys*men*orrhea μῆνιγξ, μήνιγγος membrane. encephalo*mening*itis
kine	κινέω move. *kine*matograph. (Also spelled cine-)	ment-	*mens, mentis* mind. Cf. phren-, psych- and thym-. de*ment*ia
labi-	*labium* lip. Cf. cheil-. gingivo*labi*al	mer- mes-	μέρος part. poly*mer*ic μέσος middle. Cf. medi-. *mes*oderm
lact-	*lac, lactis* milk. Cf. galact-. gluco*lact*one	met	See meta-. *met*allergy
lal- lapar-	λαλέω talk, babble. glosso*lal*ia λαπάρα flank. *lapar*otomy	metr-¹	μήτρα womb. endo*metr*itis
laryng-	λάρυγξ, λάρυγγος windpipe. *laryng*endoscope	metr-¹ metr-²	μέτρον measure. stereo*metr*y μήτρα womb. endo*metr*itis
lat-	*fero, latus* bear, carry. See -ferent. trans*lat*ion	micr- mill-	μικρός small. photo*micr*ograph *mille* one thousand. Cf. kil-. Indicates fraction in metric system. *milli*gram, *milli*pede
later-	*latus, lateris* side. ventro*later*al	miss-	See -mittent. intro*miss*ion
lent-	*lens, lentis* lentil. Cf. phac-. *lent*iconus	-mittent	*mitto, mittentis, missus* send. inter*mittent*
lep-	λαμβάνω, ληπ- take, seize. cata*lep*tic		
leuc- leuk-	See leuk-. *leuc*inuria λευκός white. Cf. alb-. *leuk*orrhea. (Also spelled leuc-)		

mne-	μιμνήσκω, μνη- remember	pseudomnesia
mon-	μόνος only, sole. monoplegia	
morph-	μορφή form, shape. polymorphonuclear	
mot-	moveo, motus move. vasomotor	
my-	μῦς, μυός muscle. inoleiomyoma	
-myces	μύκης, μύκητος fungus. myelomyces	
myc(et)-	See -myces. ascomycetes, streptomycin	
myel-	μυελός marrow. poliomyelitis	
myx-	μύξα mucus. myxedema	
narc-	νάρκη numbness. toponarcosis	
nas-	nasus nose. Cf. rhin-. palatonasal	
ne-	νέος new, young. neocyte	
necr-	νεκρός corpse. necrocytosis	
nephr-	νεφρός kidney. Cf. ren-. paranephric	
neur-	νεῦρον nerve. esthesioneure	
nod-	nodus knot. nodosity	
nom-	νόμος (from νέμω deal out, distribute) law, custom. taxonomy	
non-	nona nine. nonacosane	
nos-	νόσος disease. nosology	
nucle-	nucleus (from nux, nucis nut) kernel. Cf. kary-. nucleide	
nutri-	nutrio nourish. malnutrition	
ob-	ob (b changes to c before words beginning with that consonant) against, toward, etc. obtuse	
oc-	See ob-. occlude.	
ocul-	oculus eye. Cf. ophthalm-. oculomotor	
-od-	See -ode¹. periodic	
-ode¹	ὁδός road, path. cathode. (See also hod-)	
-ode²	See -oid. nematode.	
odont-	ὀδούς, ὀδόντος tooth. Cf. dent-. orthodontia	
-odyn-	ὀδύνη pain, distress. gastrodynia	
-oid	εἶδος form. Cf. -form. hyoid	
-ol	See ole-. cholesterol	
ole-	oleum oil. oleoresin	
olig-	ὀλίγος few, small. oligospermia	
omphal-	ὀμφαλός navel. periomphalic	
onc-	ὄγκος bulk, mass. hematoncometry	
onych-	ὄνυξ, ὄνυχος claw, nail. anonychia	
oo-	ᾠόν egg. Cf. ov-. perioothecitis	
op-	ὁράω, ὀπ- see. erythropsia	
ophthalm-	ὀφθαλμός eye. Cf. ocul-. exophthalmic	
or-	os, oris mouth. Cf. stom(at)-. intraoral	
orb-	orbis circle. suborbital	
orchi-	ὄρχις testicle. Cf. test-. orchiopathy	
organ-	ὄργανον implement, instrument. organoleptic	
orth-	ὀρθός straight, right, normal. orthopedics	
oss-	os, ossis bone. Cf. ost(e)-. ossiphone	
ost(e)-	ὀστέον bone. Cf. oss-. enostosis, osteanaphysis	
ot-	οὖς, ὠτός ear. Cf. aur-. parotid	
ov-	ovum egg. Cf. oo-. synovia	
oxy-	ὀξύς sharp. oxycephalic	
pachy(n)-	παχύς thicken. pachyderma, myopachynsis	
pag-	πήγνυμι, παγ- fix, make fast. thoracopagus	
par-¹	pario bear, give birth to. primiparous	
par-²	See para-. parepigastric	
para-	παρά (final a is dropped before words beginning with a vowel) beside, beyond. paramastoid	
part-	pario, partus bear, give birth to. parturition	
path-	πάθος that which one undergoes, sickness. psychopathic	
pec-	πήγνυμι, (πηκ- before τ) fix, make fast. sympectothiene. (See also pex-)	
ped-	παῖς, παιδός child. orthopedic	
pell-	pellis skin, hide. pellagra	
-pellent	vello, pellentis, pulsus drive. repellent	
pen-	πένομαι need, lack. erythrocytopenia	
pend-	pendeo hang down. appendix	
pent(a)-	πέντε five. Cf. quinque-. pentose, pentaploid	
peps-	πέπτω, πεψ- (before σ) digest bradypepsia	
pept-	πέπτω digest. dyspeptic	
per-	per through. Cf. dia-. pernasal	
peri-	περί around. Cf. circum-. periphery	
pet-	peto seek, tend toward. centripetal	
pex-	πήγνυμι, πηγ- (added to σ becomes πηξ-) fix, make fast. hepatopexy	
pha-	φημί, φα- say, speak. dysphasia	
phac-	φακός lentil, lens. Cf. lent-. phacosclerosis. (Also spelled phak-)	
phag-	φαγεῖν eat. lipophagic	
phak-	See phac-. phakitis	
phan-	See phen-. diaphanoscopy	
pharmac-	φάρμακον drug. pharmacognosy	
pharyng-	φάρυγξ, φαρυγγ- throat. glossopharyngeal	
phen-	φαίνω, φαν- show, be seen. phosphene	
pher-	φέρω, φορ- bear, support. periphery	
phil-	φιλέω like, have affinity for. eosinophilia	
phleb-	φλέψ, φλεβός vein. periphlebitis	
phleg-	φλέγω, φλογ- burn, inflame. adenophlegmon	
phlog-	See phleg-. antiphlogistic	
phob-	φόβος fear, dread. claustrophobia	
phon-	φωνή sound. echophony	

APPENDIX 6   603

phor-	See pher-. Cf. -ferent. exophoria	prosop-	πρόσωπον face. Cf. faci-. diprosopus
phos-	See phot-. phosphorus	pseud-	ψευδής false. pseudoparaplegia
phot-	φῶς, φωτός light. photerythrous	psych-	ψυχή soul, mind. Cf. ment-. psychosomatic
phrag-	φράσσω, φραγ- fence, wall off, stop up. Cf. sept-¹. diaphragm	pto-	πίπτω, πτω- fall. nephroptosis
phrax-	φράσσω, φραγ- (added to σ becomes φραξ-) fence, wall off, stop up. emphraxis	pub-	pubes & puber, puberis adult. ischiopubic. (See also puber-)
phren-	φρήν mind, midriff. Cf. ment-. metaphrenia, metaphrenon	puber-	puber adult. puberty
phthi-	φθίνω decay, waste away. ophthalmophthisis	pulmo(n)-	pulmo, pulmonis lung. Cf. pneumo(n)-. pulmolith, cardiopulmonary
phy-	φύω beget, bring forth, produce, be by nature. nosophyte	puls-	pello, pellentis, pulsus drive. propulsion
phyl-	φῦλον tribe, kind. phylogeny	punct-	pungo, punctus prick, pierce. Cf. cente-. punctiform
-phyll	φύλλον leaf. xanthophyll	pur-	pus, puris pus. Cf. py-. suppuration
phylac-	φύλαξ guard. prophylactic	py-	πύον pus. Cf. pur-. nephropyosis
phys(a)-	φυσάω blow, inflate. physocele, physalis	pyel-	πύελος trough, basin, pelvis. nephropyelitis
physe-	φυσάω, φυση- blow, inflate. emphysema	pyl-	πύλη door, orifice. pylephlebitis
pil-	pilus hair. epilation	pyr-	πῦρ fire. Cf. febr-. galactopyra
pituit-	pituita phlegm, rheum. pituitous	quadr-	quadr- four. Cf. tetra-. quadrigeminal
placent-	placenta (from πλακοῦς) cake. extraplacental	quinque	quinque five. Cf. pent(a)-. quinquecuspid
plas-	πλάσσω mold, shape. cineplasty	rachi-	ῥάχις spine. Cf. spin-. encephalorachidian
platy-	πλατύς broad, flat. platyrrhine	radi-	radius ray. Cf. actin-. irradiation
pleg-	πλήσσω, πληγ- strike. diplegia		
plet-	pleo, -pletus fill. depletion	re-	re- back, again. retraction
pleur-	πλευρά rib, side. Cf. cost-. peripleural	ren-	renes kidneys. Cf. nephr-. adrenal
plex-	πλήσσω, πληγ- (added to σ becomes πληξ-) strike. apoplexy	ret-	rete net. retothelium
plic-	plico fold. complication	retro-	retro backwards. retrodeviation
pne-	πνοιά breathing. traumatopnea	rhag-	ῥήγνυμι, ῥαγ- break, burst. hemorrhagic
pneum(at)-	πνεῦμα, πνεύματος breath, air. pneumodynamics, pneumatothorax	rhaph-	ῥαφή suture. gastrorrhaphy
		rhe-	ῥέω flow. Cf. flu-. diarrheal
pneumo(n)-	πνεύμων lung. Cf. pulmo(n)-. pneumocentesis, pneumonotomy	rhex-	ῥήγνυμι, ῥηγ- (added to σ becomes ῥηξ-) break, burst. metrorrhexis
pod-	πούς, ποδός foot. podiatry	rhin-	ῥίς, ῥινός nose. Cf. nas-. basirhinal
poie-	ποιέω make, produce. Cf. -facient. sarcopoietic	rot-	rota wheel. rotator
pol-	πόλος axis of a sphere. peripolar	rub(r)-	ruber, rubri red. Cf. erythr-. bilirubin, rubrospinal
poly-	πολύς much, many. polyspermia	salping-	σάλπιγξ, σάλπιγγος tube, trumpet. salpingitis
pont-	pons, pontis bridge. pontocerebellar	sanguin-	sanguis, sanguinis blood. Cf. hem(at)-. sanguineous
por-¹	πόρος passage. myelopore	sarc-	σάρξ, σαρκός flesh. sarcoma
por-²	πῶρος callus. porocele	schis-	σχίζω, σχιδ- (before τ or added to σ becomes σχισ-) split. Cf. fiss-. schistorachis, rachischisis
posit-	pono, positus put, place. repositor		
post-	post after, behind in time or place. postnatal, postoral	scler-	σκληρός hard. Cf. dur-. sclerosis
pre-	prae before in time or place. prenatal, prevesical	scop-	σκοπέω look at, observe. endoscope
press-	premo, pressus press. pressoreceptive	sect-	seco, sectus cut. Cf. tom-. sectile
pro-	πρό or pro before in time or place. progamous, procheilon, prolapse	semi-	semi- half. Cf. hemi-. semiflexion
proct-	πρωκτός anus. enteroproctia	sens-	sentio, sensus perceive, feel. Cf. esthe-. sensory

APPENDIX 6

sep- σήπω rot, decay. sepsis
sept-¹ saepio, saeptus fence, wall off, stop up. Cf. phrag-. nasoseptal
sept-² septem seven. Cf. hept(a)-. septfan
ser- serum whey, watery substance. serosynovitis
sex- sex six. Cf. hex-¹. sexdigitate
sial- σίαλον saliva. polysialia
sin- sinus hollow, fold. Cf. colp-. sinobronchitis
sit- σῖτος food. parasitic
solut- solvo, solventis, solutus loose, dissolve, set free. Cf. ly-. dissolution
-solvent See solut-. dissolvent
somat- σῶμα, σώματος body. Cf. corpor-. psychosomatic
-some See somat-. dictyosome
spas- σπάω, σπασ- draw, pull. spasm, spastic
spectr- spectrum appearance, what is seen. microspectroscope
sperm(at)- σπέρμα, σπέρματος seed. spermacrasia, spermatozoon
spers- spargo, -spersus scatter. dispersion
sphen- σφήν wedge. Cf. cune-. sphenoid
spher- σφαῖρα ball. hemisphere
sphygm- σφυγμός pulsation. sphygmomanometer
spin- spina spine. Cf. rachi-. cerebrospinal
spirat- spiro, spiratus breathe. inspiratory
splanchn- σπλάγχνα entrails, viscera. neurosplanchnic
splen- σπλήν spleen. Cf. lien-. splenomegaly
spor- σπόρος seed. sporophyte, zygospore
squam- squama scale. desquamation
sta- ἵστημι, στα- make stand, stop. genesistasis
stal- στέλλω, σταλ- send. peristalsis. (See also stol-)
staphyl- σταφυλή bunch of grapes, uvula. staphylococcus, staphylectomy
stear- στέαρ, στέατος fat. Cf. adip-. stearodermia
steat- See stear-. steatopygous
sten- στενός narrow, compressed. stenocardia
ster- στερεός solid. cholesterol
sterc- stercus dung. Cf. copr-. stercoporphyrin
sthen- σθένος strength. asthenia
stol- στέλλω, στολ- send. diastole
stom(at)- στόμα, στόματος mouth, orifice. Cf. or-. anastomosis, stomatogastric
strep(h)- στρέφω, στρεπ- (before τ) twist. Cf. tors-. strephosymbolia, streptomycin. (See also stroph-)

strict- stringo, stringentis, strictus draw tight, compress, cause pain. constriction
-stringent See strict-. astringent
stroph- στρέφω, στροφ- twist. anastrophic. (See also strep(h)-)
struct- struo, structus pile up (against). obstruction
sub- sub (b changes to f or p before words beginning with those consonants) under, below. Cf. hypo-. sublumbar
suf- See sub-. suffusion
sup- See sub-. suppository
super- super above, beyond, extreme. Cf. hyper-. supermotility
sy- See syn-. systole
syl- See syn-. syllepsiology
sym- See syn-. symbiosis, symmetry, sympathetic, symphysis
syn- σύν (n disappears before s, changes to l before l, and changes to m before b, m, p, and ph) with, together. Cf con-. myosynizesis
ta- See ton-. ectasis
tac- τάσσω, ταγ- (τακ- before τ) order, arrange. atactic
tact- tango, tactus touch. contact
tax- τάσσω, ταγ- (added to σ becomes ταξ-) order, arrange. ataxia
tect See teg-. protective
teg- tego, tectus cover. integument
tel- τέλος end. telosynapsis
tele- τῆλε at a distance. teleceptor
tempor- tempus, temporis time, timely or fatal spot, temple. temporomalar
ten(ont)- τένων, τένοντος (from τείνω stretch) tight stretched band. tenodynia, tenonitis, tenontagra
tens- tendo, tensus stretch. Cf. ton-. extensor
test- testis testicle. Cf. orchi-. testitis
tetra- τέτρα- four. Cf. quadr-. tetragenous
the- τίθημι, θη- put, place. synthesis
thec- θήκη repository, case. thecostegnosis
thel- θηλή teat, nipple. thelerethism
therap- θεραπεία treatment. hydrotherapy
therm- θέρμη heat. Cf. calor-. diathermy
thi- θεῖον sulfur. thiogenic
thorac- θώραξ, θώρακος chest. thoracoplasty
thromb- θρόμβος lump, clot. thrombopenia
thym- θυμός spirit. Cf. ment-. dysthymia
thyr- θυρεός shield (shaped like a door θύρα). thyroid

APPENDIX 6   605

tme-	τέμνω, τμη- cut. axono*tme*sis	troph-	τρέφω, τροφ- nurture. a*troph*y
toc-	τόκος childbirth. dys*toc*ia	tuber-	*tuber* swelling, node. *tuber*cle
tom-	τέμνω, τομ- cut. Cf. sect-. ap-pendec*tom*y	typ-	τύπος (from τύπτω strike) type. a*typ*ical
ton-	τείνω, τον- stretch, put under tension. Cf. tens-. peri*tone*um	typh- typhl-	τῦφος fog, stupor. adeno*typh*us τυφλός blind. Cf. cec-. *typhl*ectasis
top-	τόπος place. Cf. loc-. *top*esthesia	un- ur-	*un*us one. Cf. hen-. *un*ioval οὖρον urine. poly*ur*ia
tors-	*torqueo, torsus* twist. Cf. strep-. ex*tors*ion	vacc- vagin-	*vacc*a cow. *vacc*ine *vagin*a sheath. inv*agin*ated
tox-	τοξικόν (from τόξον bow) arrow poison, poison. *tox*emia	vas- vers-	*vas* vessel. Cf. angi-. *vas*cular See vert-. in*vers*ion
trache- trachel-	τραχεία windpipe. *trache*otomy τράχηλος neck. Cf. cervic-. *trachel*opexy	vert- vesic-	*verto, versus* turn. di*vert*iculum *vesic*a bladder. Cf. cyst-. *vesic*o-vaginal
tract-	*traho, tractus* draw, drag. pro*tract*ion	vit- vuls-	*vit*a life. Cf. bi-¹. de*vit*alize *vello, vulsus* pull, twitch. con-*vuls*ion
traumat-	τραῦμα, τραύματος wound. *traumat*ic	xanth-	ξανθός yellow, blond. Cf. flav- and lute-. *xanth*ophyll
tri-	τρεῖς, τρία or *tri-* three. *tri*gonid	-yl zo-	ὕλη substance. cacod*yl* ζωή life, ζῷον animal. micro*zo*aria
trich- trip-	θρίξ, τριχός hair. *trich*oid τρίβω rub. en*trip*sis	zyg-	ζυγόν yoke, union. *zyg*odactyly
trop-	τρέπω, τροπ- turn, react. sito*trop*ism	zym-	ζύμη ferment. en*zym*e

---

(Courtesy of Miller, B.F., and Keane, C.B.: Encyclopedia and Dictionary of Medicine, Nursing, and Allied Health, 2nd ed. Philadelphia, W.B. Saunders Company, 1978.)

RULES FOR FORMING PLURALS

The rules for commonly forming plurals of medical terms are as follows:

1. For words ending in **is**, drop the **is** and add **es**:

    Examples:

Singular	Plural
anastomosis	anastomoses
metastasis	metastases
epiphysis	epiphyses
prosthesis	prostheses

2. For words ending in **um**, drop the **um** and add **a**:

    Examples:

Singular	Plural
bacterium	bacteria
diverticulum	diverticula
ovum	ova

3. For words ending in **us**, drop the **us** and add **i**:

    Examples:

Singular	Plural
calculus	calculi
bronchus	bronchi
nucleus	nuclei

Some exceptions to this rule include viruses and sinuses.

4. For words ending in **a**, retain the a and add **e**:

    Examples:

Singular	Plural
vertebra	vertebrae
bursa	bursae
bulla	bullae

5. For words ending in **ix** and **ex**, drop the **ix** or **ex** and add **ices**:

    Examples:

Singular	Plural
apex	apices
varix	varices

6. For words ending in **on**, drop the **on** and add **a**:

    Examples:

Singular	Plural
ganglion	ganglia
spermatozoon	spermatozoa

(Courtesy of Chabner, D.-E.: Language of Medicine, 2nd ed. Philadelphia, W. B. Saunders Company, 1981.)

SYMBOLS

Symbol	Meaning	Symbol	Meaning
Ⓛ	left	$>$	greater than
Ⓜ	murmur	$\geq$	greater than or equal to
®	right, trademark	$<$	less than
⊙	start of operation	$\leq$	less than or equal to
⊗	end of operation	$\sim$	approximate
□	male	$\simeq$	approximately equal to
○	female	$\pm$	not definite, plus/minus
♂	male	$(+)$	significant
♀	female	$(-)$	insignificant
*	birth	$(\pm)$	possibly significant
†	death	↓	decreased, depression
τ	life (time)	↑	elevation, increased
$\tau\frac{1}{2}$	half-life (time)	⇧	up
$\bar{p}$	after	↑V	increase due to *in vivo* effect
$\bar{a}$	before	↓V	decrease due to *in vivo* effect
$\bar{c}$	with	↑C	increase due to chemical interference during the assay
$\bar{s}$	without	↓C	decrease due to chemical interference during the assay
?	question of, questionable, possible		

→	causes no change transfer to	2d	second
←	is due to	2°	secondary
⊖	normal	2ndry	secondary
$\sqrt{\bar{c}}$	check with	2×	twice
φ	none	×2	twice
V	systolic blood pressure	1×	once
Λ	diastolic blood pressure	°	degree
#	gauge number weight	′	foot
		″	inch
24°	24 hours	$\ddot{\overline{\text{ii}}}$	two
Δt	time interval	/	of per
ΔA	change in absorbance	:	ratio (is to)
ΔpH	change in pH	+	positive present
Δ	prism diopter	−	absent negative
3 = D	delayed double diffusion (test)	$\overline{X}$	average of all X's
606	arsphenamine	α	alpha particle is proportional to
914	neoarsphenamine	≠	does not equal
℞	take	x^2	chi square (test)
6-MP	6-mercaptopurine	σ	1/100 of a second standard deviation
³HT	H_3T, tritiated thymidine		
1°	primary	℈	scruple

℥	ounce	μu	microunit
f℥	fluid ounce	μv	microvolt
μ	micron	μw	microwatt
μμ	micromicron	μγ	milligamma (nanogram)
μc	microcurie	mμ	millimicron
μEq	microequivalent	mμc	millimicrocurie (nanocurie)
μf	microfarad		
μg	microgram	mμg	millimicrogram (nanogram)
μl	microliter	Ω	ohm
μμc	micromicrocurie (picocurie)	ℨ	drachm dram
μμg	micromicrogram (picogram)	f ℨ	fluidrachm fluidram
μM	micromolar	∞	infinity
μr	microroentgen	◠	combined with
μsec	microsecond	X	crossed with, as in hybridization

PREFIXES

M-	mega, 10^6
k-	kilo, 10^3
d-	deci, 10^{-1}
c-	centi, 10^{-2}
m-	milli, 10^{-3}
μ-	micro, 10^{-6}
n-	nano, 10^{-9}